MW01078202

Martin L. Pall

Explaining
"Unexplained Illnesses"
Disease Paradigm for Chronic Fatigue Syndrome, Multiple Chemical Sensitivity, Fibromyalgia, Post-Traumatic Stress Disorder, Gulf War Syndrome, and Others

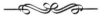
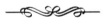
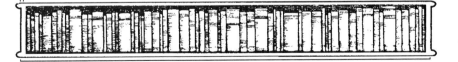

More pre-publication
REVIEWS, COMMENTARIES, EVALUATIONS . . .

"Clinicians often see and recognize clinical pictures long before the science catches up and the pathophysiology has been worked out. Increasingly, clinicians are seeing new patterns of disease such as chronic fatigue syndrome, fibromyalgia, multichemical sensitivity, and post-traumatic stress syndrome. It has been a difficult time for the few clinicians not prepared to accept the psychiatric model. They know their patients are physically ill and have learned many tricks of the trade which have afforded substantial clinical improvements. This book is extremely helpful to these clinicians.

Professor Pall demonstrates how many new syndromes have very much in common clinically even if they can be arrived at in many different ways. These new syndromes can be triggered by infectious stresses, chemical stresses, psychological and emotional traumas but the end clinical picture is often similar. Currently many of these syndromes are classified clinically by how the patients acquire their symptoms but he postulates a common underlying pathophysiology. This model elegantly explains how many different treatment modalities are effective in bringing about the clinical benefits. He identifies a common biochemical pathway which can be damaged in many different ways but results in a wide range of symptoms depending on where the damage is, how severe it is, and how long it has persisted for. His ideas explain what puzzles many clinicians: why is it that once the disease trigger has been identified and removed the disease process continues?

Professor Pall's book has given me huge insight and opens up avenues of possibilities for future interventions. This book is a must-buy for anyone who suffers from any of these problems. It will reassure them that their illness has a physical basis with effective, proven nutritional remedies to guide them toward recovery. Furthermore, it will give them a sound scientific basis with which they can refute the notion that the disease is psychological in origin—something which is also a vital part of the healing process."

Dr. Sarah Myhill, MB, BS
Secretary, British Society of Allergy, Environmental and Nutritional Medicine; Author *Diagnosing and Treating Chronic Fatigue Syndrome*

"Dr. Pall has clearly demonstrated the weight of the molecular evidence regarding these targeted diseases: chemical hypersensitivities, fibromyalgia, chronic fatigue, and post-traumatic stress, and that their causation and progression implicates redox imbalances, or in other words, electronic imbalances. His model is unique in explaining the overlapping nature of these diseases (comorbidity), and explaining why they were previously so difficult to understand, diagnose, and effectively treat. Dr. Pall has integrated a massive amount of molecular/biochemical data in order to present a well-crafted model, which should convince serious-minded scientists and doctors that these conditions are strongly associated with reactive molecular fragments, oxidative species, and that inflammation and immune abnormalities are the consequences. The options for therapy are intriguingly varied, generally with attractive safety profiles. The political/environmental implications of this work are vast, and must be embraced for the health of all across the globe."

Stephen A. Levine, PhD
President and CEO of Allergy Research Group; Co-author, *Antioxidant Adaptation: Its Role in Free Radical Pathology*

Explaining "Unexplained Illnesses"

Disease Paradigm for Chronic Fatigue Syndrome, Multiple Chemical Sensitivity, Fibromyalgia, Post-Traumatic Stress Disorder, Gulf War Syndrome, and Others

HAWORTH RESEARCH SERIES
ON MALAISE, FATIGUE, AND DEBILITATION
Roberto Patarca-Montero, MD, PhD
Editor in Chief

Concise Encyclopedia of Chronic Fatigue Syndrome by Roberto Patarca-Montero

CFIDS, Fibromyalgia, and the Virus-Allergy Link: New Therapy for Chronic Functional Illnesses by R. Bruce Duncan

Adolescence and Myalgic Encephalomyelitis/Chronic Fatigue Syndrome: Journeys with the Dragon by Naida Edgar Brotherston

Phytotherapy of Chronic Fatigue Syndrome: Evidence-Based and Potentially Useful Botanicals in the Treatment of CFS by Roberto Patarca-Montero

Autogenic Training: A Mind-Body Approach to the Treatment of Fibromyalgia and Chronic Pain Syndrome by Micah R. Sadigh

Enteroviral and Toxin Mediated Myalgic Encephalomyelitis/Chronic Fatigue Syndrome and Other Organ Pathologies by John Richardson

Treatment of Chronic Fatigue Syndrome in the Antiviral Revolution Era by Roberto Patarca-Montero

Chronic Fatigue Syndrome, Christianity, and Culture: Between God and an Illness by James M. Rotholz

The Concise Encyclopedia of Fibromyalgia and Myofascial Pain by Roberto Patarca-Montero

Chronic Fatigue Syndrome and the Body's Immune Defense System by Roberto Patarca-Montero

Chronic Fatigue Syndrome, Genes, and Infection: The Eta-1/Op Paradigm by Roberto Patarca-Montero

The Psychopathology of Functional Somatic Syndromes: Neurobiology and Illness Behavior in Chronic Fatigue Syndrome, Fibromyalgia, Gulf War Illness, Irritable Bowel, and Premenstrual Dysphoria by Peter Manu

Handbook of Cancer-Related Fatigue by Roberto Patarca-Montero

Medical Etiology, Assessment, and Treatment of Chronic Fatigue and Malaise: Clinical Differentiation and Intervention by Roberto Patarca-Montero

Explaining "Unexplained Illnesses:" Disease Paradigm for Chronic Fatigue Syndrome, Multiple Chemical Sensitivity, Fibromyalgia, Post-Traumatic Stress Disorder, Gulf War Syndrome, and Others by Martin L. Pall

Explaining "Unexplained Illnesses"

Disease Paradigm for Chronic Fatigue Syndrome, Multiple Chemical Sensitivity, Fibromyalgia, Post-Traumatic Stress Disorder, Gulf War Syndrome, and Others

Martin L. Pall

HPP

Harrington Park Press®
The Trade Division of The Haworth Press, Inc.
New York • London

For more information on this book or to order, visit
http://www.haworthpress.com/store/product.asp?sku=5139

or call 1-800-HAWORTH (800-429-6784) in the United States and Canada
or (607) 722-5857 outside the United States and Canada

or contact orders@HaworthPress.com

Published by

Harrington Park Press®, the trade division of The Haworth Press, Inc., 10 Alice Street, Binghamton, NY 13904-1580.

PUBLISHER'S NOTE
The development, preparation, and publication of this work has been undertaken with great care. However, the Publisher, employees, editors, and agents of The Haworth Press are not responsible for any errors contained herein or for consequences that may ensue from use of materials or information contained in this work. The Haworth Press is committed to the dissemination of ideas and information according to the highest standards of intellectual freedom and the free exchange of ideas. Statements made and opinions expressed in this publication do not necessarily reflect the views of the Publisher, Directors, management, or staff of The Haworth Press, Inc., or an endorsement by them.

This book has been published solely for educational purposes and is not intended to substitute for the medical advice of a treating physician. Medicine is an ever-changing science. As new research and clinical experience broaden our knowledge, changes in treatment may be required. While many potential treatment options are made herein, some or all of the options may not be applicable to a particular individual. Therefore, the author, editor and publisher do not accept responsibility in the event of negative consequences incurred as a result of the information presented in this book. We do not claim that this information is necessarily accurate by the rigid scientific and regulatory standards applied for medical treatment. **No warranty, express or implied, is furnished with respect to the material contained in this book. The reader is urged to consult with his/her personal physician with respect to the treatment of any medical condition.**

Cover design by Kerry E. Mack.

Library of Congress Cataloging-in-Publication Data

Pall, Martin L.
    Explaining 'unexplained illnesses': disease paradigm for chronic fatigue syndrome, multiple chemical sensitivity, fibromyalgia, post-traumatic stress disorder, and Gulf War syndrome, and others/Martin L. Pall.
       p. cm.
    ISBN: 978-0-7890-2388-9 (hard : alk. paper)
    ISBN: 978-0-7890-2389-6 (soft : alk. paper)
    1. Nitric oxide—Pathophysiology. 2. Chronic fatigue syndrome—Etiology. 3. Multiple chemical sensitivity—Etiology. 4. Fibromyalgia—Etiology. 5. Post-traumatic stress disorder—Etiology. 6. Persian Gulf syndrome—Etiology. I. Title.
    [DNLM: 1. Signs and Symptoms. 2. Fatigue Syndrome, Chronic—etiology. 3. Fibromyalgia—etiology. 4. Multiple Chemical Sensitivity—etiology. 5. Persian Gulf Syndrome—etiology. 6. Stress Disorders, Post-Traumatic—etiology. WB 143 P164e 2007]
    RB113.P338 2007
    616'.0478—dc22
                                                                              2006034698

CONTENTS

ABOUT THE AUTHOR

Martin L. Pall, PhD, is Professor of Biochemistry and Basic Medical Sciences at Washington State University in Pullman, where he teaches portions of the medical biochemistry course for first-year medical students. His long-term interests in biological regulatory mechanisms and in free radicals and reactive oxygen/nitrogen species have been key influences in leading him to his conceptual breakthrough in viewing chronic fatigue syndrome (CFS), multiple chemical sensitivity (MCS), fibromyalgia, and related multi-system illnesses. Dr. Pall is a member of the American Society for Biochemistry and Molecular Biology and is on the editorial board of the *Journal of Chronic Fatigue Syndrome* (Haworth). He is on the Scientific Advisory Board of Ariston Pharmaceuticals and the advisory board of the Environmental Law Centre in London, and has advised the South Australian government on multiple chemical sensitivity.

Acknowledgments

I am indebted to many for their help not only with this book but also with the whole process of trying to understand these various diseases. I am indebted to my colleague James Satterlee, who has been involved in this process for over six years and has been supportive throughout. He has specifically been unstinting in his time and commitment to this book, helping with figures, computer problems, and making suggestions about the text. I am indebted to Dr. Marti Wolfe, Ms. AnneElena Foster, and Ms. Jeri Friedman for their suggestions on the text and help with figures and ferreting out flaws that I was unable to see. The remaining flaws are, of course, my own. I am indebted to two dedicated physicians, Dr. Albert G. Corrado and Dr. Grace Ziem, for their unstinting commitment to their patients and to the science. They have both tried to use scientific knowledge of these diseases, as it has developed, to optimize the health of their patients and to use their clinical experience with their patients to help understanding of the science. Dr. Corrado died over five years ago, with much loss to me and to his patients. I am indebted to many colleagues for their interest and support, both here in Pullman and around the world. Among them, I want to particularly acknowledge the support and interest of Dr. James Hurst, who has kept me honest on the chemistry, and Dr. Francisco Saavedra, who has always been willing to talk about these issues. I am indebted to Dr. Paul Cheney for the interest, time, and insight that he has shared on CFS, the "unexplained" place where I first started. I am indebted to Dr. Gordon Baker, Dr. Stephen Levine, and Mr. Jim Seymour for their profound interest and encouragement. I also want to acknowledge my professors and fellow students at Caltech back in the dark ages—it was there that I learned much of what science was about and, most important, how to learn. At Caltech, it was always assumed that we can understand whatever needs to be understood, the key assumption when it came to "unexplained" illnesses.

I am indebted to Washington State University for the sabbatical leave that was spent in large measure researching and writing this book. I believe

Explaining "Unexplained Illnesses"
© 2007 by The Haworth Press, Inc. All rights reserved.
doi:10.1300/5139_a

it is still the case that the most important things in science are done by individuals taking the time to think deeply about the challenges facing us. All efforts to mechanize this process have, in my view, largely failed.

I am especially indebted to Judith, who has kept me sane, or at least semi-sane, through the challenges of the past seven and a half years. I could not possibly have done it without her!

Chapter 1

The NO/ONOO⁻ Cycle and the Cause of Chronic Fatigue Syndrome, Multiple Chemical Sensitivity, Fibromyalgia, and Post-Traumatic Stress Disorder

Man's mind, once stretched by a new idea, never regains its original dimensions.

Oliver Wendell Holmes

A new scientific truth does not triumph by convincing its opponents and making them see the light, but rather because its opponents eventually die, and a new generation grows up that is familiar with it.

Max Planck, translated by Frank Gaynor

TAKE-HOME LESSONS

The chronic, overlapping illnesses chronic fatigue syndrome (CFS), multiple chemical sensitivity (MCS), fibromyalgia (FM), and post-traumatic stress disorder (PTSD) are suggested by several researchers to share a common causal mechanism. The proposed causal mechanism for these illnesses is centered on a vicious cycle, involving elevated levels of two compounds in the body, nitric oxide (NO) and its oxidant product peroxynitrite ($ONOO^-$). Once chronically elevated, these appear to act through known biochemical sequences to stay elevated. These elevation mechanisms constitute a cycle

Explaining "Unexplained Illnesses"
© 2007 by The Haworth Press, Inc. All rights reserved.
doi:10.1300/5139_01

that is responsible for the chronic nature of these illnesses such that regions of the body are flipped over into a pathological state that propagates itself over time through the action of the cycle. This cycle, called the NO/ONOO⁻ cycle (pronounced "no/oh no"), is central to this explanatory model.

Many cases of these multisystem illnesses are initiated by short-term stressors, such as viral or bacterial infection, physical or psychological trauma, or exposure to any of several classes of chemicals. Each of these stressors is known to stimulate responses that raise the levels of nitric oxide. Thus, they all can initiate the NO/ONOO⁻ cycle in a common way. Symptoms are generated by elevated levels of nitric oxide, peroxynitrite, and several other consequences of the NO/ONOO⁻ cycle. Therapy should focus on down-regulating the NO/ONOO⁻ cycle biochemistry rather than on the treatment of symptoms. Observations on animal models of these illnesses provide substantial support for this theory.

The NO/ONOO⁻ cycle mechanism is the only proposed mechanism to explain each of these four illnesses and is, therefore, the only mechanism fulfilling the predictions of researchers that the four share a common causal mechanism. It is proposed, in short, as a major new paradigm of human disease. We will see in subsequent chapters how abundant additional evidence provides further support for this theory of causation.

INTRODUCTION

CFS, MCS, and FM are repeatedly described in the scientific literature as being "unexplained." They are described as unexplained by certain experts, by professional and nonprofessional organizations, and by lay people. Many have even described the symptoms as being unexplained. And yet, many professionals and lay people who have wrestled with the challenges of trying to understand these illnesses have felt that a time would come when we would understand these illnesses as well as we understand such well-accepted diseases as asthma, migraine headache, and multiple sclerosis. I argue that time *has* come.

These illnesses have multiple overlaps, leading several research groups to propose that they may share a common etiologic (causal) mechanism.[1-11] Others have observed similar overlaps with PTSD.[1,12-15] These overlaps suggest a need for a common mechanism to explain not just one but all four of these illnesses.

What I am going to present is a theory of the etiology (cause) of these illnesses that is supported by many different clinical and experimental observations of people suffering from these illnesses, as well as of animal models.

In the evidence presented will be dozens of "coincidences" offered as support for this theory. The question you should ask is the following: Are these just coincidences or do they collectively provide at least suggestive and at most strong support for this theory? What a skeptic needs to argue is that these are all just coincidences, and that their apparent support for this theory can be explained by other means. Any skeptic and I both have a difficult task in front of us. Due to the complexities of these illnesses and the many puzzles that have surrounded them, I need to argue that most or all of these can be well explained by my theory. I also need to suggest further experiments that can confirm or deny important predictions of the theory. What a skeptic needs to show is that the dozens of "coincidences" supporting the theory are just that—coincidences. He or she also needs to show that there is some alternative hypothesis that provides a better fit to the available observations. What you will not find here is a "smoking-gun" type of evidence—something that <u>individually</u> provides strong support for the theory. The complexity of these illnesses almost always provides alternative explanations for any <u>particular</u> piece of evidence. While I do not rule out the possibility of providing such smoking-gun-type evidence through studies in the future, the current argument is based on many hundreds of individual observations and studies, each of which may be individually interpreted in other ways. It is the <u>pattern</u> of evidence that may be convincing, not any individual experiment or observation.

Having said that, I must emphasize that any overall theory that explains in detail the properties of this group of illnesses should be viewed as a major step forward, given the lack of alternative theories providing explanations for this whole group of illnesses. At worst, it gives us a testable framework for further "hypothesis-driven" experimentation, something that has been largely lacking with this group of illnesses. At best, it provides the great beam of light to illuminate our way.

OVERLAPPING MULTISYSTEM ILLNESSES

CFS, FM, and MCS show multiple overlaps with each other. They have many symptoms and other correlates in common. They have high comorbidities. Individuals diagnosed with one have a high probability of meeting the diagnostic criteria for others.[1-11] They also have a common pattern of case initiation: Cases of each are commonly preceded by a short-term stressor, which is followed by a chronic medical condition that typically lasts for years and often for life. The idea that CFS, MCS, FM, and several other types of illnesses share such a common etiology has been proposed by

Miller[1] although the etiologic mechanism was uncertain. Miller asks in the title of her paper "Are we on the threshold of a new theory of disease?" Buchwald and Garrity[2] (p. 2052) concluded a study of CFS, MCS, and FM patients by suggesting that: "Despite their different diagnostic labels, existing data, though limited, suggests that these illnesses may be similar if not identical conditions. . . ." Donnay and Ziem[4] advanced a similar point of view, suggesting that CFS, FM, and MCS "may simply reflect different aspects of a common underlying medical condition" (p. 78).

The common features of CFS, MCS, and FM also links them to PTSD, which I have suggested, following the lead of four other investigators,[1,12-14] may also share a common etiologic mechanism.[15] Gulf War syndrome and probably some other postconflict syndromes have elements of all four of these.[16-20] For the purpose of this book, I will refer to these four illnesses as well as the Gulf War syndrome as <u>multisystem illnesses</u>. The implication here is that they share a common etiologic mechanism. In any case, we need a term to identify all of them. This does not rule out the possibility that other types of illnesses and well-accepted diseases may also share this common mechanism, and I will discuss several other suitable candidates in Chapter 14.

PRECEDING STRESSORS

Cases of each of the four multisystem illnesses are preceded by short-term stressors, which vary from one illness to another. These short-term stressors apparently induce cases of these illnesses. One important question is how can these stressors induce these chronic illnesses. In CFS the initiating stressor is commonly either a viral or bacterial infection.[21-28] The diversity of infectious agents implicated in the initiation of cases of CFS[21-28] demonstrates that we cannot ascribe apparent induction of CFS to a single type of infectious agent. In FM both infection, again involving multiple agents,[29-34] and physical trauma[34-40] are reported to be involved. The types of physical trauma involved typically include a bad fall, an automobile accident, or a major surgery.[34-40] Head and neck trauma seem to be most commonly involved.[39,40] MCS initiation commonly involves chemical exposure, either a single high-level exposure or multiple lower-level exposures.[41-45] The chemicals involved in initiation of MCS fall mainly into four classes, organophosphorus and carbamate pesticides and two other classes of pesticides, and volatile organic solvents. Many of the solvents are hydrophobic, but others such as formaldehyde are not.[41-45] The symptomatic patterns of MCS cases initiated by organophosphorus pesticides and organic solvents are reported to be quite similar to each other.[44] PTSD initiation commonly follows severe psychological stress. The case definition of PTSD given in DSM-IV[46] demands such stress ("trauma") as a required diagnostic feature.

These various stressors are clearly very diverse, with no obvious common features that might explain how they can produce a similar biological response in humans, such that they may each be able to induce this group of illnesses. An <u>important coincidence</u> is that there is substantial evidence that each of these stressors can increase the levels of nitric oxide, an important compound in the body. This common <u>nitric oxide</u> response provides a partial explanation for the similar responses to these stressors. I have reviewed the evidence supporting this common response,[21,47-52] and it is instructive to discuss the diverse mechanisms that lead each to increased nitric oxide levels.

Infection is known to stimulate the synthesis and secretion of certain small protein messengers known as <u>inflammatory cytokines</u>, several of which induce* an enzyme known as the <u>inducible nitric oxide synthase</u>[†] (iNOS), which then synthesizes increased levels of nitric oxide.[21] The mechanisms of this response have been extensively studied, and it is clear that infection through this mechanism can lead to substantial increases in nitric oxide and its oxidant product, <u>peroxynitrite</u>.[‡] Both of these are central to the vicious cycle mechanism—the NO/ONOO⁻ cycle discussed in this book. The reaction involved here is that nitric oxide reacts with another compound in the body, known as <u>superoxide</u>, to form peroxynitrite (Figure 1.1).

Physical trauma involving the head (traumatic head or brain injury) is also known to increase nitric oxide levels, acting to stimulate the activity of

Peroxynitrite synthesis

$$NO^{\bullet} \; + \; OO^{\bullet -} \longrightarrow ONOO^-$$

Nitric oxide   Superoxide   Peroxynitrite

FIGURE 1.1. Peroxynitrite synthesis. The very rapid reaction of a molecule nitric oxide with superoxide yields one molecular of peroxynitrite.

---

*Induce means to synthesize greatly increased amounts—in this case, induction of iNOS causes increased amounts of this enzyme to be synthesized, leading to increased levels of its product, nitric oxide. Induction typically acts by increasing the amount of RNA encoding the protein (messenger RNA), which in turn directs increasing synthesis of the protein.

†Pronounced SIN-thays.

‡Pronounced purr-OX-ee-NYE-trite.

a neural transmitter system in the brain known as the NMDA* system,[54-61] and it is known that increased NMDA activity leads to increases in nitric oxide and peroxynitrite.[50] NMDA receptors are also known to occur in the spinal column and in the neck, so it is reasonable to suppose that neck trauma may produce a similar response. Physical trauma in other parts of the body is also reported to produce increases in nitric oxide,[62] but the mechanism is not known.

Of the two classes of chemicals that appear most often to induce MCS, the organophosphorus and carbamate pesticides act to raise acetylcholine levels, which stimulate, in turn, another set of neurotransmitter receptors in the nervous system known as the muscarinic receptors.[49-51] It is known that stimulation of three of the five muscarinic receptors leads to increases in nitric oxide levels.[63-65] This muscarinic stimulation also leads to increases in NMDA stimulation, thus producing increases in nitric oxide through that mechanism as well.[50] The action of volatile organic solvents has been a more difficult issue to resolve but these appear to act mainly by stimulating a receptor known as the vanilloid receptor,[52] the receptor for the "hot" compound (capsaicin) in hot red peppers. It is known that stimulation of the vanilloid receptor increases nitric oxide levels[66-71] and can also lead to increased NMDA stimulation, leading to additional increases in nitric oxide.[72-80] Some of the important properties of the three neurotransmitter systems discussed here, the NMDA and muscarinic and vanilloid receptor systems, will be reviewed in Chapter 2.

Severe psychological stress in PTSD also appears to act by excessive stimulation of NMDA receptors in the brain, and is thought to have a substantial role in initiation of PTSD.[81-83] In animal models, it has been reported that NMDA antagonists can block the PTSD-like response.[84-89] In one study, it was shown that inhibition of the synthesis of nitric oxide in an animal model also blocked the physiological response (gastric mucosal damage) being studied.[90] These studies show that severe psychological stress can produce increased nitric oxide levels acting through increased NMDA activity.

There is another type of observation that suggests that these different stressors act in a similar fashion: there is considerable "cross-talk" among them, where a stressor primarily implicated in initiating one of these illnesses is found to have a role in initiating another (Table 1.1). An example is where psychological stress is a risk factor for FM, CFS, or MCS or where organophosphorus pesticide exposure is a risk factor for CFS or FM. This

---

*Many acronyms including NMDA are pronounced by reading the letters.

TABLE 1.1. Some examples of "cross-talk" of stressors.

Stressor implicated	Illness response	The more usual stressor	References
Organophosphorus exposure	CFS	Infection	91, 92
Psychological stress	CFS and FM	Infection or physical trauma	93, 94
Childhood sexual abuse	CFS	Infection	95
Psychiatric trauma	CFS	Infection	96
Early life stress	MCS-animal model	Pesticide or organic solvent exposure	97
Early life stress	MCS	Pesticide or organic solvent exposure	98
Traumatic head injury	PTSD	Severe psychological stress	99, 100
Sexual and physical abuse	FM	Infection or physical trauma	101
Solvent exposure	CFS	Infection	102, 103

evidence of cross-talk among these stressors provides further evidence suggesting that each of these is acting through a similar response. Because the only known common response is the increase in nitric oxide, this supports a critical role of nitric oxide in the mechanisms of these illnesses. Before leaving this issue of cross-talk, I wanted to mention the studies of Abou-Donia and coworkers on the synergistic role of psychological stress and chemical exposure in inducing an MCS-like response in an animal model.[104,105] Such synergism among different stressors is suspected from many observations in humans but is much more readily demonstrated in animal model studies.

We have, then, an important coincidence where each of these diverse stressors, viral or bacterial infection, physical trauma, organophosphorus/carbamate pesticide exposure, volatile organic solvent exposure, and severe psychological stress can lead to a common biochemical response—increased levels of nitric oxide and presumably its oxidant product, peroxynitrite, as well. How might this short-term elevation lead to a chronic illness? It was proposed earlier that elevated levels of peroxynitrite and also nitric oxide can lead to certain increased levels of both nitric oxide itself and also of superoxide (the other precursor of peroxynitrite), thus leading to a chronic elevation of nitric oxide and peroxynitrite.[21,47-52] The mechanisms thought to be involved in this vicious cycle, almost all involving well-described biochemical and physiological mechanisms, are discussed in the following text.

In addition to the six stressors that are well documented to initiate multisystem illnesses, there are six additional stressors that are candidate initiators* for these illnesses. These candidates are less well documented in their initiation of these illnesses. I will discuss evidence elsewhere in this book that these six candidate initiators are known to produce responses that can increase, in turn, nitric oxide levels, and most of them have been shown to produce increases in nitric oxide in animal models. We have, then, a common apparent response to all 12 initiators of multisystem illnesses increasing nitric oxide levels. The question facing the reader is whether this is because nitric oxide has a key role in such initiation or whether this pattern is just coincidental.

NOMENCLATURE: THE NO/ONOO⁻ CYCLE

The vicious cycle initiated by nitric oxide and peroxynitrite is diagrammed in Figure 1.2. It is the central concept in this etiologic theory and

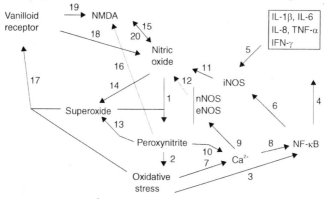

FIGURE 1.2. The NO/ONOO⁻ cycle. The elevated nitric oxide/peroxynitrite vicious cycle (NO/ONOO⁻ cycle) predominantly involves those two compounds but involves many other elements. These include superoxide, intracellular calcium, the transcription factor NF-κB, inflamatory cytokines (upper right corner), oxidative stress, vanilloid receptor activity, and NMDA receptor activity. Mitochondrial (energy metabolism) dysfunction is also involved in certain of the arrows. Each arrow represents the stimulation of one element by another, and the sequences of arrows constitute positive feedback loops that maintain the cycle.

*These six stressors, discussed later in the book, are carbon monoxide exposure, toxoplasmosis infection, ciguatoxin poisoning, organochlorine pesticide exposure, pyrethroid pesticide exposure, and thimerosal exposure.

we need a name for it. I have decided to name the cycle the NO/ONOO¯ cycle,* using the structures of nitric oxide (NO) and peroxynitrite (ONOO). We will see in subsequent chapters that the NO/ONOO¯ cycle appears to vary somewhat in different tissues, both because certain aspects of the Figure 1.2 diagram are more active in some tissues than in others and because still additional mechanisms appear to be involved in some tissues. It seems to consistently involve nitric oxide and peroxynitrite at its center, however, supporting this nomenclature.

Five Principles of Proposed Mechanism

The NO/ONOO¯ cycle as an explanatory model can be summarized in five different principles:

1. Short-term stressors that initiate cases of multisystem illnesses act by stimulating nitric oxide synthase (NOS) activity and consequently produce increased levels of nitric oxide and its oxidant product peroxynitrite.
2. Initiation is converted into a chronic illness through the action of vicious cycle mechanisms through which chronic elevation of nitric oxide and peroxynitrite is produced and maintained.
3. Symptoms and signs of these illnesses are generated by elevated levels of nitric oxide and/or other important consequences of the proposed mechanism, that is elevated levels of peroxynitrite or inflammatory cytokines, oxidative stress, and elevated NMDA and vanilloid receptor activity.
4. Because the compounds involved, nitric oxide, superoxide and peroxynitrite have quite limited diffusion distances in biological tissues and because most of the mechanisms involved in maintaining the NO/ONOO¯ cycle act at the level of individual cells, the fundamental mechanisms are local. The consequence of this is that one tissue may be impacted by this underlying biochemistry while an adjacent tissue may be largely unaffected. The tissue distribution may be propagated indefinitely over time by these local vicious cycle mechanisms. This can lead to many differences in symptoms, depending on the tissue distribution variation, from one case to another. This is such an important principle that I have devoted an entire chapter to it (Chapter 4).
5. Therapy should focus on down-regulating elements of the NO/ONOO¯ cycle rather than just on providing symptomatic relief.

---

*Pronounced, of course, no, oh no! I am greatly indebted to AnneElena Foster for suggesting this name.

These principles make it clear that one needs to distinguish between <u>initial causes</u> of these illnesses and <u>ongoing causes</u>. The first is responsible for the initiation of each illness and the second is responsible for the properties of the chronic phase of the illness. This distinction between initial causes and ongoing causes has sometimes been obscured in some of the scientific literature on CFS and FM.

I will discuss many of the <u>shared symptoms and signs</u> of these illnesses (principle 3) and their proposed causal mechanisms in Chapter 3. The symptoms and signs thought to be <u>specific to one of these multisystem illnesses</u> will be discussed in the chapter dedicated to that illness.

A Brief Note on Nomenclature

The basic theory of these multisystem illnesses developed in this book can be described using any of three alternative and almost synonymous terms: <u>etiologic theory</u>, <u>overall mechanism</u>, and <u>explanatory model</u>. Each of these conveys similar information, but each emphasizes a distinct perspective. Etiologic theory emphasizes etiology or causal role. Overall mechanism emphasizes the specific biochemical mechanisms most centrally involved and how they may interrelate with each other. Explanatory model emphasizes how this view may explain the many properties of these illnesses. You will see each of these terms used in this book to emphasize one or another of these aspects.

Proposed Vicious Cycle Mechanisms

I have described these mechanisms in a series of four papers[21,47,50,52] and the summary here includes each of these four contributions. Vicious cycles are often made up of what are known as positive feedback loops, which are distinguished from the more common negative feedback loops often described in living organisms. Positive and negative here do not describe whether these are good or bad but simply describe the effect of the overall design of the control circuitry. Let me give you a simple example. In a refrigerator, a thermostat is set to turn on the compressor that cools the refrigerator when it gets above a set temperature. This is a negative feedback loop. It acts to keep the refrigerator at or near the set temperature, therefore stabilizing it.

If, instead, the thermostat was connected to an electric heater inside the machine, whenever it got above the temperature set point, it would turn on the heater and would heat up the "refrigerator" and keep the thermostat engaged. The consequence is that once the heater turned on, it would stay on and keep the chamber heated. So if the thermostat was set at 35°C, it would not be engaged until you had a very hot day that went above that temperature. Once it did, it would probably stay above that temperature due to the influence of the electric heater being turned on. This is a positive feedback loop. It tends to be inherently unstable—if it is below the temperature at which the thermostat will be engaged, it may stay there, but once it gets above that temperature, it will probably <u>flip over into another state</u> and then stay there because of the influence of the heater on the temperature.

POSITIVE FEEDBACK LOOPS IN THE NO/ONOO⁻ CYCLE

We have a combination of instability with the ability to flip from one state to another while the individual states may have substantial stability. It is this inherent <u>combination of instability and stability</u> that makes vicious cycle mechanisms attractive models for chronic multisystem illnesses. Once the initial stressor flips over the physiology into a pathological state, it tends to stay in the pathological state, therefore maintaining the illness indefinitely. It turns out that there are multiple known mechanisms that may act as positive feedback loops in response to peroxynitrite or nitric oxide and these loops are diagrammed in Figure 1.2.

I realize, of course, that Figure 1.2 is complex and perhaps intimidating to the reader. I hope to lead you through it one step at a time. However, it is important before doing so to consider why you may need to understand it. The mechanisms behind Figure 1.2 are important in four different ways:

- They provide plausible, known mechanisms for the generation of a vicious cycle centered on elevated levels of nitric oxide and peroxynitrite.
- They make important predictions about which biochemical and physiological changes should be observed in these illnesses, predictions that can be tested via both existing and future observations.
- Because the symptoms and signs of these illnesses are predicted to be produced by the elements of the NO/ONOO⁻ cycle, those elements provide the basis to explain the mechanisms producing these symptoms and signs.
- They may help us to understand the challenges facing us in terms of effective therapy for these illnesses. The complexities of these mechanisms suggest that multiple therapeutic approaches may be more effective than single approaches. According to this etiologic theory, the <u>whole issue of therapy for multisystem illnesses should be focused on Figure 1.2.</u>

I have called the proposed mechanism the NO/ONOO⁻ cycle mechanism, based on the structures of nitric oxide and peroxynitrite, but as you will see, it involves a number of other important parameters.

One of the questions that you need to keep in mind when looking at Figure 1.2 is whether the proposed mechanisms diagrammed in that figure are what is known as physiologically relevant—do they actually occur in these multisystem illnesses and therefore help explain their etiology? We will be coming back to that question repeatedly.

The individual arrows in Figure 1.2 represent proposed stimulatory mechanisms by which increased activity of one parameter may be expected to stimulate a second parameter. They are numbered so we can focus on one arrow at a time. As we work through those numbers roughly in order, you should keep referring back to the figure. Arrow1 leading from nitric oxide and superoxide to peroxynitrite represents the rapid reaction between the first two compounds to yield the third (peroxynitrite), as we discussed above. Excessive peroxynitrite, due to its activity as a potent oxidant, will lead to oxidative stress (arrow 2), a state where there is an imbalance between free radicals and other oxidants (too much of these) and antioxidants (too little of these). Oxidants, including those derived from peroxynitrite,[106-110] are known to stimulate a transcription factor known as NF-κB (pronounced and sometimes written NF-kappa B). NF-κB is a protein that binds to certain genes and stimulates their activity, thus increasing the production of the proteins encoded by these genes. Among the genes stimulated by NF-κB are five inflammatory cytokine genes, for the cytokines IL-1β, IL-6, IL-8, TNF-α, and IFNγ*, as well as the gene for the inducible nitric oxide synthase (iNOS) (arrows 4 and 6).[109-115] These five cytokines are small protein molecules. Each of them acts as a chemical messenger involved in inflammation of tissues, and they each cause cells to increase their iNOS† activity (arrow 5). It follows that increased NF-κB activity will be expected to lead to increased iNOS activity by directly stimulating the activity of the iNOS gene itself (arrow 6) and indirectly through the action of these five inflammatory cytokines (arrows 4 and 5).[21] So we have our first potential positive feedback loop, with too much nitric oxide leading to too much peroxynitrite, oxidative stress, NF-κB activity, inflammatory cytokine activity, and iNOS activity, potentially leading to too much nitric oxide.

---

*IL stands for interleukin. TNF stands for tumor necrosis factor. IFN stands for interferon. The three Greek letters are beta, alpha, and gamma and are pronounced as such.

†Pronounced EYE-naws.

Before leaving this topic, it may be worthwhile to discuss a few of the details of the regulation of NF-κB. Certain stressors can act to increase NF-κB activity, including bacterial and viral infections and also oxidative stress. NF-κB activity is determined by another protein called Iκ-B, which is degraded in response to stressors, leading the released NF-κB to move into the nucleus of the cell where it can activate certain target genes. These target genes include the inflammatory cytokine genes and the iNOS gene. Interestingly, the mechanism by which oxidants lead to increase NF-κB activity is still being investigated[116-119] and is not yet sufficiently understood.

Oxidants may also be expected to influence another important parameter, that of intracellular (cytoplasmic) calcium levels (designated Ca^{2+}). Ca^{2+} levels are thought to be stimulated by oxidative stress in general (arrow 7) and by peroxynitrite in particular (arrow 10). Under most conditions, intracellular calcium is kept very low, well below the levels of calcium that surround the cells of the body, and these levels are kept low by calcium pump mechanisms that pumps calcium that may have leaked into cells out again to keep these levels low. There are thought to be several mechanisms by which oxidants in general and peroxynitrite in particular may be expected to lead to a rise in Ca^{2+}.[120-128] The one that is best documented is that peroxynitrite is known to inactivate pump mechanisms that pump Ca^{2+} out of the cytoplasm of the cell.[123-128] The expected rise in intracellular Ca^{2+} is expected to have two important consequences: Ca^{2+} is known to stimulate the transcription factor NF-κB (arrow 8)[129,130] and also will stimulate the activity of two other nitric oxide synthase enzymes, designated nNOS and eNOS. Both nNOS and eNOS are discussed in more detail in Chapter 2, and the important feature that these two enzymes share is that they are both calcium-dependent, so their activity in the cell is stimulated by intracellular calcium. It follows that increased calcium may be expected to increase nitric oxide synthesis (arrow 12) by stimulating both nNOS and eNOS activity, as well as less directly, by stimulating NF-κB activity (arrows 4, 5, 6, and 11). So we have additional positive feedback loops producing increases in nitric oxide levels. One point worth noting here is that intracellular calcium level is determined primarily by the balance of activities that lead to calcium leakage into the cytoplasm of the cell versus activities that lead to calcium being pumped out of the cytoplasm. Intracellular calcium is little affected by the amount of calcium in the diet, so dietary calcium is not a major concern here.

There are several mechanisms that may be expected to increase the levels of superoxide, the other precursor of peroxynitrite (arrows 13 and 14). Arrow 14 represents three different proposed mechanisms. It is known that most of the superoxide in the cell is generated in the mitochondrion, the

portion (organelle) of the cell that generates usable energy in the form of
ATP (discussed further in Chapter 2). It is known that the mitochondrial
superoxide dismutase, the enzyme in mitochondria that gets rid of superoxide, is inactivated by peroxynitrite and this was proposed as a possible
positive feedback loop by a prominent research group.[131,132] In this way, too
much peroxynitrite may be expected to raise the levels of superoxide by
lowering its breakdown, which could then react with nitric oxide to form
too much peroxynitrite (arrows 13 and 1). These are not the only mechanisms that may lead to increased superoxide. Peroxynitrite inactivates components in what is called the electron transport chain in the mitochondrion
and nitric oxide is known to inhibit an enzyme called cytochrome oxidase
in that same chain. Both of these effects appear to produce increased generation of superoxide (arrows 13 and 14),[21] potentially providing for further
positive feedback activity.

Peroxynitrite has several actions that deplete energy in the form of ATP,
including its effects on the mitochondrial electron transport chain discussed
in the preceding paragraph—these are all discussed in more detail in Chapter 2. Such energy depletion is known to generate increased superoxide in
tissues that do not have enough blood flow (ischemia) through a distinct
mechanism outside of the mitochondrion—the generation of increased activity of an enzyme known as xanthine oxidase,[133,134] and this mechanism
may plausibly be expected to occur in these multisystem illnesses because
of energy depletion produced by peroxynitrite and nitric oxide (again, arrows 13 and 14). It is known that, when the enzyme xanthine oxidase works,
it generates superoxide as a product. It is reported that excessive NMDA
stimulation leads to increased xanthine oxidase activity,[135] linking it to another mechanism suggested here. Furthermore, the enzyme xanthine dehydrogenase can be reversibly converted to xanthine oxidase by the oxidation
of certain cysteine residues in the protein,[136,137] a process stimulated by oxidative stress that has been linked to excessive NMDA activity.[135,137] These
observations strongly suggests that increased superoxide production via increased xanthine oxidase activity is a plausible part of the NO/ONOO⁻ cycle.

We have seen so far that multiple plausible mechanisms may be expected
to act as positive feedback loops, increasing levels of both nitric oxide and
superoxide, thus potentially generating chronic elevation of their levels and
those of peroxynitrite. The mechanisms we have discussed so far are general
ones, potentially relevant to many different cell types and tissues. Before
leaving them, it is important to point out that they involve what is basically
inflammatory biochemistry. Not only does one have increased nitric oxide,
peroxynitrite, and oxidative stress when tissues are inflamed, but inflammation also involves increased levels of inflammatory cytokines as well as

increased NF-κB activity. It should not be surprising, therefore, that even though the multisystem illnesses are not classified as inflammatory conditions, they each have <u>important aspects of inflammatory biochemistry</u>.

The remaining cycle mechanisms are more specific, mainly influencing nervous tissues in the central nervous system and the peripheral nervous system. They involve two neurotransmission systems discussed earlier, the NMDA receptor system and the vanilloid receptor. The vanilloid receptor, which was also discussed earlier due to its apparent role in MCS, has been reported in a series of studies to show substantially increased activity under inflammation.[139-144] Part of this increase is reported to be produced by oxidants, including superoxide,[145,146] leading to arrow 17. When the vanilloid receptor is stimulated, it is known to produce increases in both nitric oxide (arrow 18) and also NMDA activity (arrow 19). The NMDA receptor itself is known to generate increases in nitric oxide and also of peroxynitrite (arrows 15 and 1).[50] Both the vanilloid receptor and the NMDA receptor act, when stimulated, to allow calcium to enter the cells by opening channels in the plasma membrane surrounding the cell, channels through which calcium ions flow very readily. This, in turn, stimulates the two forms of nitric oxide synthases, nNOS and eNOS, which, as discussed earlier, are calcium-dependent enzymes. It follows from this that arrows 15 and 19 should go to the Ca^{2+} in Figure 1.2, but this figure was too complicated already and so this was omitted.

The regulation of the NMDA receptor was discussed in detail in one of my papers on MCS.[50] In the hippocampus and several other regions of the brain, nitric oxide stimulates neurons to release L-glutamate, the neurotransmitter that stimulates NMDA receptors, thus producing more nitric oxide (double-headed arrows 15, 20). In addition the NMDA receptor becomes increasingly more sensitive to stimulation when the cell in which it is present is depleted of energy (ATP). Due to the effects of peroxynitrite in inhibiting energy metabolism, which were discussed earlier, this is expected to also lead to increases in NMDA activity (arrow 16).

Before leaving this discussion, it is important to point out that, in addition to the various positive feedback loops constituting this complex proposed vicious cycle mechanism, there are also some negative feedback loops that may be viewed as lowering these responses. For example, while NF-κB activity is known to be stimulated by oxidants and these are reported to include peroxynitrite, its activity is known to be lowered by nitric oxide—an opposite effect. In addition, while NF-κB activity is known to induce the inducible nitric oxide synthase, both directly and indirectly as we have discussed, which may be expected to raise oxidative stress through the effects of peroxynitrite, it also has some antioxidant effects. It is reported to induce increased synthesis of glutathione, the most important antioxidant synthesized in the body. These negative feedback loop type responses may be important in avoiding the responses that lead to these multisystem illnesses, preventing some but not other cases of these illnesses.

This, then, completes the outline of the cycle mechanisms implicit in Figure 1.2. Of the 20 arrows in the figure, representing 22 different mechanisms (two extra because arrow 13 represents three distinct mechanisms, not just one), and of those 22, 19 are all very well documented. Three are reported but not yet well documented (the superoxide generation in response to nitric oxide and peroxynitrite and vanilloid receptor stimulation by oxidants). While these three may be questioned based on limited empirical evidence, the mechanisms presumably involved in their action are well documented. So most of Figure 1.2 is based on very solid biochemistry and physiology, but some aspects of it can be questioned. From the figure, one can suggest a number of possible observations that would provide confirmation for the proposed mechanisms for the chronic phase of multisystem illnesses: increased levels of nitric oxide, iNOS activity, peroxynitrite, oxidative stress, NF-κB activity, vanilloid activity, and NMDA activity. Further support for the physiological relevance of these proposed mechanisms may also be sought through possible roles of nitric oxide, peroxynitrite, etc., in the generation of symptoms and other correlates of these illnesses.

PLAUSIBILITY:
EVIDENCE FOR REAL POSITIVE FEEDBACK LOOPS INVOLVING NITRIC OXIDE

One question about this proposed NO/ONOO⁻ cycle mechanism, involving positive feedback loops, concerns whether it occurs in real living organisms and real living tissues. The fact that one can make an outline, such as we have seen in Figure 1.2 that is predicted to comprise a complex vicious cycle does not necessarily mean that such a cycle really occurs. Most of the diagrammed cycle is based on well-documented mechanisms, but again we should still question whether the entire proposed cycle reflects what actually goes on in living tissues. There may be countervailing influences that may prevent such a cycle from occurring. It is important, therefore, to determine whether such a cycle really acts in animals or people. Clear evidence for such positive feedback loop mechanisms has been published in a number of studies. In such studies, nitric oxide levels have been artificially raised and have been shown to produce increased nitric oxide synthesis. This has been shown in studies with the drugs as nitroglycerine or nitroprusside, which are known to act by breaking down chemically to release nitric oxide. These drugs have been shown <u>to produce a rise in the enzymatic synthesis of nitric oxide</u> via increased nitric oxide synthase activity.[147-158] So we see evidence in these studies that increased nitric oxide can lead to increased nitric oxide synthesis. Consistent with the mechanisms in Figure 1.2, all three nitric oxide synthases have been shown to be involved in such increased synthesis.[147-158] Other evidence for such vicious cycle mechanisms in vivo comes from studies where iNOS activity has been stimulated and where this leads to increased activity of nNOS or eNOS as well. I am only aware of one study where peroxynitrite was used to determine whether it might generate a vicious cycle response, and in that study peroxynitrite induced inflammatory colitis, a chronic inflammatory response including elevated levels of nitric oxide and presumably peroxynitrite itself.[159] It was shown that the nitric oxide synthesis increase was necessary to produce the inflammatory reaction,[160] providing further evidence consistent with a vicious cycle initiated by peroxynitrite.

All of these observations tend to confirm the existence of a vicious cycle mechanism involving excessive nitric oxide and thus the existence of part of the NO/ONOO⁻ cycle. The question that must be raised <u>is whether it is physiologically relevant to the multisystem illnesses</u>.

ANIMAL MODELS

It is often possible to conduct studies demonstrating causality using animal models of human disease, demonstrations that would be either impossible or much more difficult in humans. Consequently, there have been many key studies using animal models that have been important in our understanding of human disease. Having said that, it is important to point out that there is always considerable debate about how well any given animal model reflects the human condition. There are quite a number of animal models that may provide insights into each of the four multisystem illnesses. However, none of these have been studied with the goal of testing predictions of the NO/ONOO⁻ cycle. So we have to settle for observations made for other reasons that may shed some light on this etiologic theory.

The research group of Chao and coworkers has published a series of papers on a mouse model of CFS,[161-164] where apparent fatigue is induced by injection of a bacterial extract. There are no live bacteria involved so there is no apparent infectious agent involved in this CFS-like response. It is known that this bacterial extract can increase the synthesis of nitric oxide[165] and that it induces increased and prolonged synthesis of inflammatory cytokine levels in this model.[161,162,164] So some of the elements the NO/ONOO⁻ cycle have been studied and shown to occur in this model. Chao and coworkers also reported that the brains of these apparently fatigued mice have dysfunctional mitochondria and therefore are expected to have defective energy metabolism, possibly explaining the fatigue response.[163] It is known, as I have discussed, that peroxynitrite attacks a number of the components of the mitochondrion, therefore producing mitochondrial dysfunction, providing a possible explanation for such mitochondrial dysfunction in this animal model.

It should be clear from this discussion that this animal model is not consistent with a chronic infection mechanism for CFS, given that no live infectious agent is involved. However, there are three properties of this animal model that are consistent with predictions of our proposed mechanism: It is induced by an agent that induces increased nitric oxide synthesis, it involves increased and prolonged inflammatory cytokine synthesis, and it involves mitochondrial dysfunction. Still, there are many different experiments that have not been done in that model. Can one block or lower the apparent fatigue response by using nitric oxide synthase inhibitors, by lowering NF-κB activity, or by using compounds that function as superoxide dismutase mimics to lower superoxide levels? Does the NMDA receptor or the vanilloid receptor have a role? These are questions that could be asked of this animal model but have not been asked.

An animal (rat) model of PTSD has been the focus of considerable study. It has been shown with this model that treatment with an NMDA antagonist, thus lowering NMDA receptor activity, can block both the behavioral and physiological changes induced by the severe psychological stress (reviewed in Reference 48). This provides strong evidence that NMDA stimulation has a key role in PTSD. In a single study, it was reported that using a nitric oxide synthase inhibitor blocked the development of a characteristic physiological response in this model.[90] Thus, there is experimental evidence for a key role for nitric oxide as well.

A number of animal models of MCS are reported to have an NMDA receptor role (reviewed in Reference 50). In one model, a mouse model, it was shown that not only was the sensitization response blocked by using a nitric oxide synthase inhibitor, but that it was blocked by using a mouse missing the nNOS form of nitric oxide synthase and that the response was stimulated by feeding the mouse arginine to stimulate nitric oxide synthase activity. Three different types of studies provide convincing evidence for a key role of nitric oxide in this mouse model of MCS.

With one exception described in Chapter 8, there are no animal models described in the Medline database as animal models for fibromyalgia (FM).

However, there are extensively studied animal models afflicted with excessive pain, the cardinal symptom of FM. These may be viewed as animal models of fibromyalgia and may also be relevant to the other multisystem illnesses, given how common excessive pain is in CFS, MCS, and PTSD. These animal models are commonly described as having hyperalgesia, excessive pain response to stimuli that normally produced only modest pain, or as having allodynia, pain responses to stimuli that normally would produce no detectable pain. I will refer to both of these as hyperalgesia because allodynia is commonly found with hyperalgesia.

Animal models of hyperalgesia have been found to involve all of the parameters described in Figure 1.2. Not only are all of these parameters involved, they each are reported to have substantial causal roles in producing the excessive pain response.[166-187] So there is evidence that pain in hyperalgesia is produced by excessive levels of nitric oxide,[166-170] NF-κB activity,[170-172] intracellular (cytoplasmic) calcium levels,[167,169,174-177] inflammatory cytokine activity,[168,172,181-183] NMDA activity,[166,167,174,177,178] vanilloid receptor activity.[167,169,179,180] superoxide,[184,185] and peroxynitrite.[184,186,187] The pattern of evidence is a bit more complex here, because there are changes both in the tissues showing increased pain sensitivity and in the central nervous system regions involved in the processing of pain information, both involving elements of our proposed vicious cycle mechanism. I will discuss these aspects in some detail in Chapter 3. The relevance of hyperalgesia mechanisms to FM is still more complex, as I will discuss in Chapter 8.

These results implicating the elements of the NO/ONOO⁻ cycle mechanism are quite striking. It is difficult to see how all of these could have important causal roles in producing excessive pain in hyperalgesia, unless they are all linked together by the sorts of interactions diagrammed in Figure 1.2. These mechanisms diagrammed were based entirely on the basic biochemistry and physiology involved and on the various types of evidence linking them to these multisystem illnesses. I was unaware of this extensive evidence from hyperalgesia studies until I started researching this chapter, and here we find evidence from hyperalgesia studies alone providing substantial support for the types of interactions proposed in Figure 1.2. This provides independent verification for both the plausibility and physiological relevance of these proposed mechanisms in real living systems. The physiological relevance of these proposed mechanisms to multisystem illnesses is suggested, from these studies, by the importance of excessive pain in each of the multisystem illnesses.

One can summarize the animal model studies discussed here as follows: An animal model of CFS is consistent with the NO/ONOO⁻ cycle and inconsistent with a chronic infection model, but has not been studied for possible causal roles for nitric oxide, peroxynitrite, NMDA activity, and so on. We have animal models of both PTSD and MCS that provide substantial support for our NO/ONOO⁻ cycle mechanism, specifically providing evidence for important causal roles for excessive NMDA activity and excessive nitric oxide levels. Finally, and most strikingly, hyperalgesia animal models as possible models for FM and the excessive pain common in the other illnesses provide evidence for causal roles of all of the important parameters in our etiologic theory of these illnesses—nitric oxide, superoxide, peroxynitrite, intracellular calcium levels, NF-κB activity, inflammatory cytokines, NMDA activity, and vanilloid receptor activity.

WHAT ABOUT ILLNESSES WITH NO APPARENT PRECEDING STRESSOR?

The majority of cases of these illnesses are preceded by one or more readily apparent stressors, and in the Gulf War syndrome, the military personnel were exposed to over a dozen plausible stressors. However, there are cases where no such stressor is apparent. How can one explain this? One possible explanation is that there was a stressor that was not apparent. One such stressor is carbon monoxide exposure, as proposed by Albert Donnay.[188,189] Carbon monoxide being both odorless and colorless is a possible stressor that may not be readily detected. Interestingly, there is a literature, which I reviewed earlier, reporting that carbon monoxide exposure can induce symptoms similar to those of these multisystem illnesses[48] and that in some individuals these symptoms are chronic despite having no concurrent carbon monoxide exposure.[48] Can this be due to initiation of the NO/ONOO⁻ cycle? It is known that carbon monoxide exposure can induce increased nitric oxide synthesis in tissues and can also induce oxidative stress that may be reasonably explained by peroxynitrite elevation.[50] So this view may well be compatible with the proposed mechanisms discussed here and may provide an explanation of some of these illnesses without apparent preceding stressors. I doubt that this is the explanation for all of these, and perhaps there are other possible but not apparent stressors that may have a role, including other odorless chemicals. Perhaps some are initiated by chronic infections rather than acute infections, such as has been proposed for some Lyme disease cases. Some may have a high genetic predisposition toward developing these illnesses such that obvious stressors are not needed to initiate the cycle. It is clear that we have much to learn about these cases with no apparent preceding stressor, but I see no incompatibility between the existence of these cases and the NO/ONOO⁻ cycle mechanisms.

WHY DO SOME BECOME ILL BUT NOT OTHERS?

Clearly the occurrence of stressors that precede and presumably initiate cases of these multisystem illnesses is much more common than are these illnesses. Why do some of these stressor events lead to these illnesses but others do not? Clearly, most infections do not lead to cases of CFS, and when groups of individuals have similar exposure to chemicals, such as in sick building syndrome situations, some become ill with MCS while others do not. Among the factors that may be involved are the following:

1. Genetics is one important factor, and a genetic role in susceptibility has been reported in all four of these multisystem illnesses: CFS,[190-195] FM,[195-203] MCS,[204-206] and PTSD.[207-210] Thus, clearly individuals vary in innate susceptibility.

2. Hormonal factors are likely to be important. Glucocorticoids such as cortisol lower iNOS induction and may have a role, therefore, in these illnesses.[21] These illnesses are more common after puberty than before, so the sex hormones may well have a role. Specifically, estrogen may have an important role, given its many reported interactions with nitric oxide synthesis mechanisms. However, some of these estrogen effects are predicted to increase nitric oxide synthesis—but others are predicted to decrease nitric oxide synthesis. I would like to suggest that estrogen effects may provide an explanation for why all four of these multisystem illnesses are more common in women than in men, but the evidence at this point is unconvincing, one way or the other. There may be other hormonal factors to consider as well.

3. The strength of the stressors involved may be a key factor. Clearly, all of these stressors come in different strengths, producing variation in the body's biochemical response to them. Of the infectious agents reported to be involved in CFS, herpes virus infections seem to be quite common, and it is reported that herpes viruses are quite active in inducing a high inflammatory cytokine response,[211-213] providing a possible explanation for their apparent role here. The cross talk of vari types of stressors may have a role here, given their common influence on nitric oxide levels. I have discussed the possible role of tissue hypoxia induced by excessive exercise in the possible initiation of CFS.[47] Other factors may have a role, such as excessive sunlight exposure, which increases nitric oxide levels.[214]

4. I have discussed the possible role of several nutritional factors previously.[21] There are literally dozens of antioxidants in the diet, many of which lower NF-κB activity or may lessen the effects of peroxynitrite

and its breakdown products. Magnesium has a key role in lowering NMDA receptor activity (discussed in Chapter 2) as well as possibly having a role in limiting nitric oxide synthesis in some tissues.[21] It is known that magnesium levels in the diet of the United States and some other Western countries have declined substantially over the last century; it is reported that marginal magnesium deficiencies are quite common and may have an important role producing increased susceptibility to these illnesses. Could changes in magnesium nutrition be responsible for some of the perception that these illnesses may have become more prevalent over the years? The amino acid arginine is the precursor for nitric oxide synthesis, and the level of arginine pools in the body is known to substantially influence nitric oxide synthesis. In contrast, the amino acid lysine competes with arginine for transport into cells, so the ratio of arginine to lysine may be important in determining susceptibility. The amino acid cysteine is known to often be the rate limiting precursor in the synthesis of glutathione, the most important antioxidant synthesized in the body, and so its levels may be important here. There may be other significant nutritional factors as well.

5. The cells of the immune system are quite active in producing nitric oxide and may consequently have a special role. It has been proposed that changes in the development of the immune system including its Th1/Th2 balance may have a role in predisposing towards asthma and a similar predisposition may also be a possibility in these multisystem illnesses.

ARE THERE BIOLOGICAL PRECEDENTS FOR VICIOUS CYCLE MECHANISMS?

Obviously, when one proposes what is, in essence, a new paradigm, there are no currently accepted precedents for it. Still, in science one always looks for precedents not only to increase the plausibility of the approach but also to determine where a new view may fit into the structure of science. We have here a vicious cycle theory to explain the etiology of these multisystem illnesses. This explanatory model may be viewed as having two general aspects. Firstly, it has the property of having a series of interactive controlling mechanisms that can flip over into another state, with both the old and new states having substantial stability. Secondly, the relevance to medicine depends on how the state influences the health of the individual. Let us talk about a precedent for each of these.

Back in the dark ages, when I was in graduate school, I became aware of an interesting study of the lactose or *lac* control system[215] of the common bacterium *Escherichia coli* (*E. coli*). The *lac* system controls the synthesis of two important proteins that determine the ability of this bacterium to grow on the sugar lactose, the *lac* permease, which concentrates lactose into the cell, and the enzyme β-galactosidase, which metabolizes lactose, allowing it to be used as an energy source. If you grow these bacteria in media not containing lactose or similar compounds, they make almost none of these two proteins, but if you grow them in medium containing high levels of lactose or another inducer known as TMG, they make a lot of both of them. If you put them into medium containing only low levels of TMG, they will stay in whatever state they were when they were put into that medium. If they are uninduced, having almost none of these proteins, they stay indefinitely in the uninduced state. However, if they were previously induced, the high levels of the *lac* permease allow them to concentrate the TMG into the cell and therefore stay induced.[215] In this way, a simple bacterium can be in either of two states, which in a medium containing low TMG can be maintained indefinitely. One of the components involved here is the *lac* permease, a protein with no obvious regulatory function but one that has an important regulatory influence under these conditions. So we have, in essence, a "vicious" cycle mechanism but one that is benign with regard to the function of the organism. Surely, if a simple bacterium can have alternative quasi-stable states as well as a mechanism to flip from one state to another, something as complex as a human being should be able to do likewise. Are there examples of such quasi-stable states that are important in human health?

The best such example relevant to human health is the example of rheumatic heart disease, an autoimmune disease.[216-218] Rheumatic heart disease is initiated by certain streptococcal (bacterial) infections in which the bacteria carry an antigen that is similar to an antigen present in the human heart. Antibodies induced by the bacterium react with and are maintained by the human heart antigen, initiating a long-term antibody response that attacks the heart tissue and produces the damage of rheumatic heart disease. In this way a short-term stressor, the infection by a bacterium carrying a specific antigen, initiates a vicious cycle involving the immune system that produces human disease. This is a precedent for a vicious cycle in human disease, albeit quite a distinctive one from the NO/ONOO⁻ cycle. It may share features with the NO/ONOO⁻ cycle in that it may be difficult to reverse once it has flipped over into a pathological state. Other autoimmune diseases may share this property of being initiated by a short-term stressor, such as reactive arthritis.

There is another human illness model that may involve a vicious cycle mechanism, albeit one that is not well understood. This is drug addiction, where short-term exposure to a drug produces long-term changes in the nervous system, leading to addiction. Miller[1] has drawn parallels between addiction and MCS, suggesting an intriguing connection between addiction and the multisystem illnesses.

SOME KEY CONCEPTS

Sydney Brenner, the 2002 Nobel Laureate and one of the most insightful observers of biomedical science, stated[219] "but there is now a crisis developing in biology, in that completely unstructured information does not enhance understanding." He added that "We need a framework to put all of this knowledge and data into, that is going to be the problem in biology." Laurence Pilgeram, when discussing this same issue, stated[220] "this immense mass of uncollated and non-integrated data does not permit understanding biological mechanisms or function. The crux of the problem seems to be that we have developed a current generation of scientists with a mind set on automation who use this generation of data as a substitute for thinking. . . ." What clearly is needed is the development of cogent and coherent theories that can be used to organize and test the relevance of all of this unstructured data. Given the claimed "unexplained" nature of the multisystem illnesses, there is no area of medical science that may be more in need of such theory. This is what I have attempted to do. What each reader needs to decide is whether my analysis has merit.

At this point, we have a series of short-term stressors, viral and bacterial infection, physical trauma, severe psychological stress, organophosphorus and carbamate pesticide exposure, and volatile organic solvent exposure, and several others, each of which is reported to precede and apparently induce the multisystem illnesses and each of which is also reported to increase nitric oxide levels. So one question that must be asked is whether this relationship to nitric oxide of this very diverse set stressors is just coincidental.

I introduced five principles describing the proposed etiologic mechanism for these illnesses. The first is that short-term stressors initiate these illnesses by increasing nitric oxide and its oxidant product peroxynitrite. The second is that increases in these compounds initiate the NO/ONOO⁻ cycle centered on elevated levels of these two compounds but involving a series of other factors including increased oxidant stress, intracellular calcium, NF-κB activity, inflammatory cytokines, nitric oxide synthesis via three synthases, superoxide, NMDA activity, and vanilloid receptor activity. The NO/ONOO⁻ cycle, converts a short-term stressor into a chronic illness, maintaining itself indefinitely. This is an attractive explanatory model for these illnesses, given the need to explain how such a short-term stressor can produce chronic illness in the absence of any clear, permanent damage to the body.

At this point, we have not discussed any evidence linking this proposed vicious cycle to real people suffering from these illnesses, but we have discussed several other types of support:

- The mechanisms involved in the individual steps of the NO/ONOO⁻ cycle are all supported by substantial evidence with most of them being very well established.
- A number of studies have shown that artificially raising nitric oxide levels, often using a drug that breaks down to release nitric oxide, can lead to an increased synthesis of nitric oxide via an increased activity of one or more nitric oxide synthases, thus confirming a key prediction of the NO/ONOO⁻ cycle mechanism.
- Animal models of CFS, MCS, and PTSD are consistent with predictions of this etiologic theory. While the CFS model has not been tested for a causal role for the important parameters of the cycle, studies of models of MCS and PTSD report a causal role of both NMDA receptor activity and nitric oxide in the biological response characteristic of the model. These results are important because they confirm important predictions of the theory in these animal models, including an important role for nitric oxide itself.
- Animal model data on hyperalgesia, a possible animal model for FM, provide the most convincing evidence supporting the NO/ONOO⁻ cycle. In hyperalgesia, reports link <u>each of the individual components</u> of the NO/ONOO⁻ cycle, nitric oxide, superoxide, peroxynitrite, intracellular calcium, and so on, with causing the excessive pain response. It is difficult to see how this could occur except through the action of a vicious cycle mechanism similar or identical to that proposed in this chapter.

We will see how well these concepts hold up in subsequent chapters.

Chapter 2

Important Components
and Their Properties

TAKE-HOME LESSONS

Several of the elements of the NO/ONOO⁻ cycle are explored in some detail, including the properties of nitric oxide (NO), which is synthesized by three distinct enzymes known as nitric oxide synthases. All three nitric oxide synthases, iNOS, nNOS, and eNOS, have roles in elevating nitric oxide in the NO/ONOO⁻ cycle. Nitric oxide has important normal (physiological) functions, but functions here mostly in a pathophysiological role, acting to a great extent through its product peroxynitrite. Superoxide, another important cycle element, reacts with nitric oxide to form peroxynitrite. Superoxide is generated in five distinct ways. It is produced by the electron transport chain in the part of the cell involved in energy metabolism (the mitochondrion) and also when the nitric oxide synthases are uncoupled from a cofactor. Peroxynitrite is a potent oxidant, and it or its products initiate oxidative chain reactions and cause damage to both proteins and DNA. When its levels are sufficiently elevated, it can cause programmed cell death (apoptosis), an important mechanism in neurodegenerative diseases. Peroxynitrite attacks several of the important proteins in mitochondria, acting along with superoxide and nitric oxide to lower energy metabolism. Such energy metabolism dysfunction lowers the availability of ATP, the energy currency in cells, and is an important part of NO/ONOO− cycle biochemistry. Increased activity of two neurotransmission "receptors," the NMDA receptors and the vanilloid receptors are part of the NO/ONOO⁻ cycle. The activation of either of these receptors allows calcium to flow into the cells, activating the nNOS and eNOS nitric oxide synthases and increasing nitric oxide levels. There are several well-accepted diseases that often

Explaining "Unexplained Illnesses"
© 2007 by The Haworth Press, Inc. All rights reserved.
doi:10.1300/5139_02

occur along with chronic fatigue syndrome (CFS), multiple chemical sensitivity (MCS), fibromyalgia (FM), and post-traumatic stress disorder (PTSD) including asthma, migraine headache, tinnitus, and autoimmune diseases such as lupus and rheumatoid arthritis. These are all said to be "comorbid conditions" with the multisystem illnesses, because people with these four illnesses have high probabilities of also being diagnosed with these diseases. Each of these comorbid diseases shares elevation of multiple elements of the NO/ONOO⁻ cycle as part of their disease mechanism. I argue, therefore, that we can explain these comorbidities as being due to the elevated levels of NO/ONOO⁻ cycle elements in CFS, MCS, FM, and PTSD as well as in these comorbid diseases. To my knowledge, these comorbidities have never been previously explained, but they are easily explained by the NO/ONOO⁻ cycle mechanism.

INTRODUCTION

Several components that make up the NO/ONOO⁻ cycle mechanism are central to this book. They explain how symptoms and other properties of these multisystem illnesses may be generated, how they interact with other illnesses including well-accepted diseases, and, most importantly, how they may be treated. Some of the components have already been adequately discussed, including the role of intracellular calcium, NF-κB, and the inflammatory cytokines. Other components requiring further discussion include nitric oxide, superoxide, and peroxynitrite, mitochondrial function and three neurotransmitter systems, the NMDA, and vanilloid and muscarinic systems. I discuss in this chapter much of the fundamental science, giving you the basics to understand the important properties of each of these. I also provide further evidence for the relevance of each component to the NO/ONOO⁻ cycle explanatory model. In Chapter 3, I discuss mechanisms by which the elements of this vicious cycle mechanism can produce the many shared symptoms of these multisystem illnesses.

NITRIC OXIDE

Nitric oxide is a compound found in many different organisms, made up of one atom of oxygen (O) and one atom of nitrogen (N). It is a free radical, having an unpaired electron in its structure, and is often represented as NO$^{\bullet}$ or $^{\bullet}$NO where the dot represents the unpaired electron. Many free radicals are highly reactive, having half-lives in our bodies on the order of 1 μs to

1 ms, whereas nitric oxide is relatively stable, having a half-life on the order of 1 s. Nitric oxide has important <u>physiological</u> roles in the body, performing important functions in the blood circulatory system, the nervous system, and the immune system. However, it also plays what are called <u>pathophysiological</u> roles, that is roles that are damaging to the body, such that nitric oxide has important causal roles in disease. It is neither always a good guy nor always a bad guy. The pathophysiological roles show up when there is excessive nitric oxide—when the levels are too high. Our main interest here is in the pathophysiology of nitric oxide, but it is important to remember that it is found in the body for good reasons and that it performs important normal functions in the human body. Some of these normal functions, such as its role controlling the vasculature (blood vessels), learning and memory in the brain, and controlling the immune system may also help explain some of the symptoms of the multisystem illnesses that involve these functions.

There are three different enzymes in the body that make nitric oxide, called nitric oxide synthases,[1-3] designated nNOS, iNOS, and eNOS.* These stand for neural NOS, inducible NOS, and endothelial NOS. nNOS is found in many neurons in the brain, the spinal cord, and the peripheral nervous system, but it is also found in many other types of cells. eNOS is found in the endothelial cells that line the blood vessels, but it is also found in many other cells in the body. iNOS is inducible[†] and found only in very low amounts unless it is induced, typically under inflammatory conditions. The inflammatory cytokines, you will recall, are active in inducing iNOS. The iNOS gene is activated by the transcription factor NF-κB. iNOS is induced to particularly high levels in the cells of the immune system and in the glial cells in the brain, but it is also induced in many other cell types. iNOS induction is similar to the induction of other proteins such that, following induction, the iNOS gene is stimulated to make much more RNA, which then directs the synthesis of much more iNOS protein. Most of the regulation of iNOS is via regulation of the level of RNA.

In contrast, the nNOS and eNOS proteins are typically present in more or less constant amounts in a particular type of cell, while varying from one cell type to another. The activity of these enzymes, their ability to produce nitric oxide, is, however, regulated. These are both calcium-dependent enzymes,

---

*Pronounced NYE-trick OX-eyed SIN-thays, en-NAWS, eye-NAWS, and ee-NAWS. nNOS is sometimes called NOS1, iNOS, NOS2, and eNOS, NOS3.

[†]Inducible means it is made in only low amounts except when some signal, such as the presence of inflammatory cytokines, causes it to be made in much higher amounts.

which means that they produce essentially no nitric oxide unless the calcium ion Ca^{2+} is present. The cytoplasm of cells, where these enzymes are found, typically have very low levels of calcium present, as was discussed in Chapter 1. This is because calcium influx into the cytoplasm is limited and regulated, and there are mechanisms to pump calcium out of the cell and also to store it elsewhere in the cell so that it does not have access to the nNOS and eNOS enzymes. These cellular mechanisms are responsible for determining the level of cytoplasmic calcium. The amount of calcium consumed in the diet has little effect. Due to these mechanisms, the actual activity of nNOS and eNOS in producing nitric oxide is low under most circumstances. However, anything that increases the levels of cytoplasmic calcium will greatly increase their activity in producing nitric oxide. The pattern of regulation of these three enzymes is summarized in Exhibit 2.1. The NO/ONOO$^-$ cycle involves both types of regulation, iNOS induction and stimulation of nNOS and eNOS activity by calcium. Accordingly, all three of these enzymes may have a role in producing excessive nitric oxide in multisystem illnesses.

All enzymes have one or more compounds that they act on (substrates) and one or more compounds that they produce (products). The nitric oxide synthases act on the amino acid L-arginine, an amino acid that is found in foods and, to a limited extent, is made in the body. From each molecule of arginine they use up, they produce one molecule of nitric oxide and one molecule of the amino acid citrulline. Nitric oxide in the body has a half-life of circa 1 s, as discussed earlier, and is typically measured in blood samples not directly but through its breakdown products, nitrite and nitrate. Citrulline is much more stable. It can be measured directly, as we have done in serum samples from CFS patients and controls. At the common concentrations of arginine in the cell, the nitric oxide synthases are only partially saturated. Consequently, their activity in producing nitric oxide is increased with

EXHIBIT 2.1. The Pattern of Regulation of Three Enzymes

Nitric oxide synthase	Primary mode of regulation
iNOS	Synthesis of mRNA, which regulates, in turn synthesis of the protein (induction)
nNOS	Cytoplasmic Ca^{2+} concentration
eNOS	Cytoplasmic Ca^{2+} concentration

increased arginine in the diet and decreased if the arginine pools in the body are depleted. Typically in multisystem illnesses, the arginine pools appear to be relatively low, presumably because much of the arginine has been used up making nitric oxide.

The mechanism of the nitric oxide synthases is very complex, involving several different cofactors, one of which is tetrahydrobiopterin. It has recently been shown that when nitric oxide synthases have limited tetrahydrobiopterin and limited arginine, they produce superoxide in place of nitric oxide. Because superoxide is another component of the $NO/ONOO^-$ cycle mechanism, rather than improving these illnesses because of the lowered nitric oxide production, it is possible that arginine limitation and tetrahydrobiopterin depletion may exacerbate them. Tetrahydrobiopterin availability may be a key factor here, because it is oxidized by peroxynitrite.*

The physiological importance of nitric oxide was discovered relatively recently but has also been the focus of many different research studies over the last 19 years. The journal *Science* declared it the molecule of the year in 1992. The Nobel Prize for physiology and medicine in 1998 was given to Furchgott, Ignaro, and Murad for the discovery and early biological studies of nitric oxide, its role in controlling the blood vessels in the body, and the basic biochemistry and physiology involved in its action. This area of research has been extensively studied and is well understood.

Actions of Nitric Oxide in the Body

Nitric oxide acts through two well-documented pathways in the body and, in addition, has some other effects that are less well understood. The first pathway to be elucidated was the cyclic GMP[†] pathway.[3,4] Nitric oxide binds to an enzyme known as the soluble guanylyl cyclase, which it activates, stimulating this enzyme to produce its product, cyclic GMP, often designated cGMP.[‡] The cyclic GMP, in turn, stimulates another enzyme, discussed subsequently, which catalyzes changes in many different proteins in cells, producing changed responses. The enzyme guanylyl cyclase is

---

*This issue is discussed in Chapter 12, because it may be an important focus for future research of multisystem illnesses. It is also a possible focus for therapy.

†Pronounced cyclic gee em pee. In most cases in this book, acronyms written as capital letters are simply pronounced by reading out the names of the letters.

‡Cyclic GMP levels are raised by the drug Viagra, which acts to inhibit the enzyme that breaks down cyclic GMP. Many people seem to think that Viagra raises nitric oxide levels, but that is incorrect.

called the <u>receptor</u> for nitric oxide, in that it binds nitric oxide, with such binding producing specific biological changes. There are many other receptors in cells, some of which we will discuss later in this chapter. Most of the <u>normal physiological changes</u> produced by nitric oxide are produced through its ability to increase cyclic GMP levels. The enzyme that is regulated by cyclic GMP is called the G-kinase. It acts by modifying (phosphorylating) proteins in the cell. Cyclic GMP acts, then, to modify many proteins in the cell, producing biological responses.*

The second well-documented pathway for nitric oxide is due to its reaction with the compound superoxide to form the potent oxidant peroxynitrite.[5-7] Both superoxide and peroxynitrite, you may recall, are key players in the NO/ONOO⁻ cycle mechanism. The reaction between superoxide and nitric oxide is said to be "diffusion limited," which means it is almost unlimited. Almost any time a molecule of nitric oxide bumps into a molecule of superoxide, they react to form a molecule of peroxynitrite. Peroxynitrite, being such a potent oxidant, can produce much damage to living cells. The production of peroxynitrite is thought to be central to one of two major pathways in the generation of oxidative stress in the body. Much of the pathophysiology of nitric oxide is caused through the production of peroxynitrite, but some is also produced by excessive production of cyclic GMP.

There is evidence for the presence of other mechanisms of action of nitric oxide but these are not well understood. One of these other proposed mechanisms involves the production of chemical structures known as *S*-nitrosothiols[8] on proteins in cells. Many proteins have groups on them known as thiols or SH groups, and nitrosothiols can be produced from them. However, nitric oxide cannot react directly with these thiols because the reaction requires an oxidation reaction as well as the presence of nitric oxide. The factors that may influence this reaction in cells to form these nitrosothiols are uncertain. Furthermore, both superoxide[9] and peroxynitrite[10] are reported to react with nitrosothiols, destroying these structures. Because nitric oxide, superoxide and peroxynitrite are all predicted to be elevated, it is unclear whether we would expect such *S*-nitrosothiols to be elevated in these multisystem illnesses. I will discuss this again in the chapter on FM because it may be relevant to some observations made about that illness.

---

*The G-kinase is responsible for producing the vasodilation (dilation of the blood vessels), which was the first demonstrated biological response to nitric oxide in mammals.

SUPEROXIDE

Superoxide is another relatively unreactive free radical[11] that is formed in four different ways in human and other animal cells. Three of these are likely to be relevant to our NO/ONOO$^-$ cycle mechanism. Superoxide is found in two interconvertible forms in cells. The predominant form is designated OO$^{\bullet-}$, with the dot indicating again an unpaired electron and the minus sign indicating a negative charge. About 1/1000th of it in the human body is found as the acid form HOO$^\bullet$. Because most superoxide is negatively charged, a form that does not move through biological membranes readily, most of it is retained within the part of the cell in which it was formed. It does not, in general, move very far from its origin.

Superoxide resembles nitric oxide in that it does fulfill some functions in cells, serving as an intracellular signaling molecule. It is when there are excessive levels of superoxide that it has pathophysiological effects.

Superoxide is sufficiently damaging to cells such that they take great pains to lower its level. There are enzymes that degrade superoxide, superoxide dismutases (SODs), found in essentially all organisms that live in the presence of oxygen from the air.[11] In humans and other animals, there are three SODs, one found in the mitochondrion,* the part of the cell involved in energy (ATP) metabolism, one found in the cytoplasm of the cell and a third that is secreted outside of cells. Each SOD is encoded by its own gene and each has a distinct structure.

Five distinct mechanisms of superoxide production are summarized in Exhibit 2.2. Each of these may have a role in the NO/ONOO$^-$ cycle mechanism.

It has long been thought that the main source of superoxide in cells under normal conditions is what is called the electron transport chain in the mitochondrion, an important sequence involved in energy metabolism. The importance of the electron transport chain in the generation of superoxide was recently confirmed in studies of transgenic mice. It was shown that mice that do not have a gene for the mitochondrial superoxide dismutase (gene knockout mice) die shortly after birth, even if they overproduce the other superoxide dismutases.[12] In contrast, mice that lack the other superoxide dismutases can survive, although they do suffer from oxidative stress. It may be inferred that the mitochondrial superoxide dismutase is an essential enzyme. This shows that much superoxide is produced inside of the mitochondrion and that much of this never gets out. It must, therefore, be destroyed by the mitochondrial SOD or it will cause lethal damage. One of

---

*Pronounced mye-toe-KOND-ree-on, the plural of which is mitochondria.

EXHIBIT 2.2. Mechanisms of Superoxide Production

Mechanism	Possible relation to NO/ONOO⁻ cycle
Superoxide generation by electron transport chain in mitochondria	Increased by both peroxynitrite and nitric oxide; increased levels produced by peroxynitrite-mediated inactivation of the mitochondrial SOD
Superoxide generation by uncoupled nitric oxide synthases	Expected to be increased by peroxynitrite oxidation of tetrahydrobiopterin cofactor
Superoxide generation by NADPH oxidase activity in cells of immune system	May be increased by inflammatory biochemistry
Superoxide generation by xanthine oxidase activity	Increased by lowered oxidative energy metabolism and also by oxidative conversion of xanthine dehydrogenase to xanthine oxidase
Superoxide generation by cytochrome P450s	Probably none

the component mechanisms of the NO/ONOO⁻ cycle is the destruction of the mitochondrial SOD by peroxynitrite, leading to higher superoxide and more peroxynitrite production, leading to further damage to the mitochondrion. Other parts of the NO/ONOO⁻ cycle involve reported actions of both nitric oxide and peroxynitrite increasing the production of superoxide by the electron transport chain. The mitochondrial damage produced by excessive mitochondrial superoxide appears to be important in generating fatigue in these fatiguing illnesses, as I discuss in Chapter 3. Its role in generating excessive peroxynitrite may have many potential consequences.

There are other major sources of superoxide in the body. Phagocytes, cells that ingest and kill bacteria and fungi, produce what is called a respiratory burst that uses a large amount of oxygen to generate superoxide, which is used, in turn, to generate a number of different oxidants to kill the ingested microorganisms. The enzyme involved in producing this respiratory burst is called NADPH oxidase. This can be a substantial source of superoxide and other oxidants in infected tissues. Enzymes called cytochrome P450s are another source of superoxide, often producing superoxide as a product of the enzyme reaction.

There are two additional sources of superoxide. Hypoxia (low oxygen stress) increases conversion of the enzyme xanthine dehydrogenase to xanthine oxidase because of the effect of hypoxia on intracellular calcium levels and energy metabolism. Xanthine oxidase generates superoxide when it oxidizes compounds such as hypoxanthine. Xanthine oxidase activity may also be increased when cells are depleted of reduced glutathione, and such depletion occurs whenever cells are under oxidative stress. Both of these increases in xanthine oxidase activity are expected to occur under the influence of NO/ONOO⁻ cycle biochemistry, and thus the xanthine oxidase generation of superoxide is part of the cycle.

One additional mechanism of superoxide is cause by uncoupling of nitric oxide synthases, caused, in part, by lowered availability of the cofactor tetrahydrobiopterin. Because tetrahydrobiopterin is oxidized by peroxynitrite, this may be an important part of the cycle, as well (Exhibit 2.2).

Which of the mechanisms of superoxide generation are most likely to have a substantive role in producing increased superoxide levels in the NO/ONOO⁻ cycle? My judgment is that superoxide from the electron transport chain of the mitochondrion and from partial uncoupling of nitric oxide synthases are likely to be the most important. However, xanthine oxidase activity may also play a substantive role.

PEROXYNITRITE

Peroxynitrite is formed by the very rapid reaction of nitric oxide with superoxide.[5-7] The acid form of the molecule, comprising about 1/4 of the total at the normal acidity of the cells of the body (pH), is unstable and is the primary oxidant. Most of the effects of peroxynitrite are produced not by the peroxynitrite itself but rather from its breakdown products. The chemistry of peroxynitrite is complex and has only become clear during the past decade or so. The acid form of peroxynitrite can break down to form two reactive free radicals, hydroxyl radical ($HO^{\bullet}$) and NO_2 radical ($^{\bullet}NO_2$), each of which can react to cause damage to biologically important molecules. However, in the body, before this happens, most of the peroxynitrite reacts with abundantly available carbon dioxide, to form a molecule: O_2COONO^- that breaks down to form $^{\bullet}CO_3$ (carbonate radical) and $^{\bullet}NO_2$ (NO_2 radical). Most of the damage produced by peroxynitrite in living organisms is thought to be mediated through the action of carbonate radical and NO_2 radical, rather than by peroxynitrite itself. There are a number of compounds, possible drugs or "agents," often called peroxynitrite scavengers, which may protect the body from the effects of peroxynitrite. While a few of these

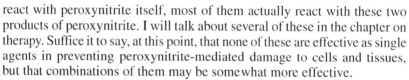

react with peroxynitrite itself, most of them actually react with these two products of peroxynitrite. I will talk about several of these in the chapter on therapy. Suffice it to say, at this point, that none of these are effective as single agents in preventing peroxynitrite-mediated damage to cells and tissues, but that combinations of them may be somewhat more effective.

What types of damage do peroxynitrite and its products produce in the human body? There are several types of such damage including the following:

1. Inactivation of certain specific proteins known as iron-sulfur proteins, including several types of proteins of this class that are important in mitochondria.
2. Modifications of proteins by such changes as nitration and oxidation to form such products as protein carbonyls and 3-nitrotyrosines.
3. Several types of damage to DNA including nicking of DNA chains.
4. Peroxynitrite initiates oxidative chain reactions, including oxidation of lipids in biological membranes, a process known as lipid peroxidation.
5. The oxidant products of peroxynitrite stimulate the activity of the transcription factor NF-κB, discussed in Chapter 1, as well as of another transcription factor known as AP-1, because both of these transcription factors are stimulated by a variety of oxidants.

Each of these types of damage is important in explaining the biological consequences of excessive peroxynitrite. Four out of five may be targets of therapy designed to minimize such consequences. Oxidant damage will generate oxidative stress with many consequences to the organism. Three of these, 1, 3, and 4, are all thought to be important in the impact of peroxynitrite on energy metabolism and consequent depletion of ATP, the energy currency of the cell.

EFFECTS OF PEROXYNITRITE, SUPEROXIDE, AND NITRIC OXIDE ON ENERGY METABOLISM AND MITOCHONDRIA

All three of these compounds, peroxynitrite, superoxide, and nitric oxide, have well-documented effects on energy metabolism that may be expected to lower the level of ATP, the energy currency of the cell. Of these three, I would expect the peroxynitrite effects to be the most important in these multisystem illnesses, but all three may have substantial roles. Because of the central role of energy metabolism in almost everything living organisms must do, it is important to examine how these compounds in the body may be expected to impact energy metabolism.

Peroxynitrite is expected to lower energy (ATP) levels in cells by three distinct pathways, as discussed earlier. It attacks several different important proteins in mitochondria, most of which are iron-sulfur proteins.[13,14] These proteins occur in both the electron transport chain in the mitochondrion and in what is known as the citric acid cycle. I will describe in Chapter 5 the evidence that two enzymes in the citric acid cycle known to be attacked by peroxynitrite have low activity in CFS. Peroxynitrite attack on iron-sulfur proteins leads to irreversible damage—the only way this activity can be restored is to resynthesize the damaged proteins from scratch.

A pathway leading to lowered ATP levels involves the attack of peroxynitrite products on DNA, producing nicks along the backbone of the DNA molecule. These nicks, in turn, stimulate an enzyme known as the poly (ADP-ribose) polymerase,[15,16] which uses the compound NAD as a substrate. The main function of NAD is through its reduced form, NADH, which feeds into the electron transport chain in the mitochondrion and is essential for normal energy metabolism. It follows that excessive peroxynitrite will lead to excessive poly(ADP-ribose) polymerase activity, lowering NAD/NADH pools and greatly impacting the production of ATP. This pathway has been studied in detail[15,16] and has been shown to be important in ATP-depletion under a number of inflammatory conditions. This is another physiologically important way that peroxynitrite can lead to lowered energy levels and ATP-depletion.

A third mechanism of action of peroxynitrite involves its stimulation of the oxidation of fatty acids found in the membranes of the cell—a process known as lipid peroxidation. This will cause many different changes in cell function. When it occurs in the inner membrane of the mitochondrion, it impacts energy metabolism. Because such inner membrane lipid peroxidation is also produced by superoxide and because so much superoxide is produced adjacent to the inner membrane, it is probably the case that superoxide may be a more important cause of inner membrane lipid peroxidation than is peroxynitrite. In any case, a recent clinical trial suggests that membrane regeneration after inner membrane lipid peroxidation may be a fruitful target for therapy in these illnesses.[17]

Nitric oxide can lower ATP pools via two different mechanisms. It can inhibit the last enzyme in the electron transport chain of the mitochondrion, an enzyme known as cytochrome oxidase.[18-20] Both nitric oxide and superoxide can inhibit one of the iron-sulfur proteins in the citric acid cycle that is inactivated by peroxynitrite, the enzyme aconitase.[21-23] Both of these two functions are important for energy metabolism including the generation of

ATP. I will discuss evidence, in Chapter 5, suggesting that the aconitase enzyme has low activity in CFS patients.

I will be returning to these mechanisms in four different contexts in Chapter 3. Elsewhere in this book, we will discuss several types of evidence regarding energy metabolism dysfunction in multisystem illnesses including:

1. The evidence for energy metabolism dysfunction in these illnesses
2. The evidence for specific dysfunction of targets of these mechanisms
3. The role of energy metabolism dysfunction in generating the symptoms and signs in these multisystem illnesses
4. The effectiveness of therapy focused on improving energy metabolism in patients suffering from these illnesses

PEROXYNITRITE AND APOPTOSIS

One important response that many cell types have when exposed to high levels of peroxynitrite is apoptosis,* programmed cell death. Apoptosis is a process whereby cells go through a specific sequence of events, leading to their death. It is an orderly process, unlike necrosis (unprogrammed cell death), and it leads to a noninflammatory process whereby the body can efficiently clean up the remains of the dead cells. Apoptosis is normally involved in a number of important processes, in early development of the anatomy of the body, in the development of the immune system so as to avoid autoimmune responses, in getting rid of potentially precancerous cells etc. It is also involved in a number of pathophysiological processes, the most important being in the death of cells in the brain during neurodegenerative diseases. This neurodegeneration process in such diseases as Alzheimer's disease, Parkinson's disease, amyotrophic lateral sclerosis, and in Huntington's disease involves peroxynitrite, excessive NMDA activity, excessive nitric oxide excessive superoxide, and other elements of the NO/ONOO⁻ cycle. Peroxynitrite is known to be able to induce apoptosis in a large number of cell types and, consequently, may be expected to increase apoptotic cell death in these multisystem illnesses.[24,25] There are seven reports of increased apoptosis occurring in these illnesses,[26-32] although it is uncertain whether such increased apoptosis has an important role in generating the symptoms of these illnesses. There are also two reports of the failure to detect increased apoptosis in CFS patients,[33,34] but both of these used the often criticized Oxford criteria for CFS diagnosis and may be flawed because of the use of these criteria.

---

*Pronounced either ay-pop-TOE-sis or a-pop-TOE-sis.

We now shift the discussion to three neurotransmitter systems that are mainly active in the nervous system, each of which is proposed to have specific roles in these multisystem illnesses.

NMDA RECEPTORS

The NMDA receptors in the nervous system (reviewed in References 35-37) are found in diverse nerve cells (neurons) in the brain, spinal cord, and the peripheral nervous system, and are also found in some non-neuronal cells. They are stimulated by the amino acid glutamate and also by the closely related amino acid aspartate. Glutamate (actually L-glutamate) is the most important excitatory neurotransmitter in the brain, being released by many different types of neurons and stimulating other neurons at contacts between these cells called synapses. Excitatory neurotransmitters act to stimulate the next neuron (known as the postsynaptic neuron) to fire an electrical impulse. In contrast, there are inhibitory neurotransmitters that tend to inhibit firing. The most important inhibitory neurotransmitter in the brain is GABA, a compound synthesized from glutamate. You might well imagine that the ratio between glutamate and GABA is crucial in regulating brain properties, and it is this ratio, not just the absolute amounts, that is involved in some issues of toxicity. The glutamate/GABA ratio also a possible target of therapy. GABA is synthesized from glutamate in a vitamin B_6-dependent process, and so a B_6 deficiency will produce a high glutamate/GABA ratio. People and animals who are very deficient in vitamin B_6 suffer from seizures due to an imbalance in this ratio, a very serious response.

The NMDA receptors are not the only class of receptors stimulated by glutamate in the nervous system. There are three other classes, called AMPA receptors, kainate receptors, and metabotropic receptors. When it was found that there seemed to be different types of receptors for glutamate, neurobiologists searched for compounds that might be able to specifically stimulate one class but not the others, so that the role of each class could be studied. It was found that the compound *N*-methyl-D-aspartate (abbreviated NMDA) could stimulate the NMDA receptors but not the other receptors, thus leading people to name this receptor the NMDA receptor. However, it should be noted that *N*-methyl-D-aspartate is *not* used in the body to stimulate this receptor—glutamate and aspartate are the physiological stimulators. The AMPA and kainate receptors also have specific compounds that stimulate them, and these compounds have also led to the names used for these receptors. These receptors tend to be concentrated in the outer membrane of the neuronal cell at the synapse, so that when one neuron (the presynaptic cell) releases glutamate (or aspartate) at the synapse, the postsynaptic cell can be stimulated by it, often firing an electrical pulse as a consequence. Such stimulation is essential for the functioning of the nervous system, but when there is too much glutamate release or the receptors are hypersensitive to stimulation, it can lead to excessive stimulation and what is called excitotoxicity—too much excitation leading to damage of the nervous system.

Excitotoxicity most often involves excessive stimulation of the NMDA receptors, but the AMPA and kainate receptors also are involved in some situations. Excessive NMDA stimulation is known to have important roles in a number of neurodegenerative disorders, including Parkinson's disease, Alzheimer's disease, amyotrophic lateral sclerosis (ALS or Lou Gehrig's disease), and AIDS-related dementia. Excessive NMDA activity is also an important element in Huntington's disease, a fatal genetic neurodegenerative disease. Brain damage found in a number of the most important diseases of the brain involves excessive NMDA activity. A drug recently approved for the treatment of Alzheimer's disease, memantine, is a known inhibitor (antagonist) of the NMDA receptors, providing additional evidence for an important role of excessive NMDA activity in this disease. In studies of the properties of receptors, compounds that stimulate their characteristic response are called agonists and compounds that inhibit these responses are called antagonists. In this context, glutamate and aspartate are NMDA agonists and memantine is an NMDA antagonist.

The mechanisms by which NMDA stimulation leads to excitotoxicity are diagrammed in Figure 2.1. It can be seen that, when the NMDA receptors are activated, they allow calcium ions to flow into the cell, leading to increased nitric oxide synthesis. It is known that the increased nitric oxide also leads to increases in peroxynitrite synthesis.

There are several features of the NMDA receptors that make their description more complex. There are actually four, not one, structurally distinctive NMDA receptors. They are stimulated by the amino acid glycine and also by compounds known as polyamines, as well as by glutamate and aspartate. It is not clear that these additional features are important to our understanding of multisystem illnesses, but future evidence may implicate one or more of them.

Role of Excessive NMDA Activity in Multisystem Illnesses

There is evidence for a role of excessive NMDA activity in all four of these multisystem illnesses, although the evidence is stronger in some than in others. I will provide documentation for NMDA roles in the chapters on these individual illnesses. In three of them, FM, MCS, and PTSD, excessive

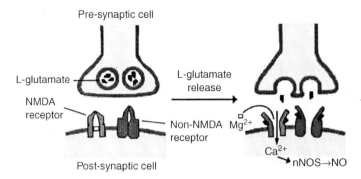

FIGURE 2.1. Activation of the NMDA receptor. NMDA receptors in the post-synaptic cell are typically stimulated by glutamate release by the presynaptic cell, opening a channel that allows calcium ions (Ca^{2+}) to flow into the cell. This, in turn activates the nNOS and eNOS nitric oxide synthases, increasing the production of nitric oxide and also its oxidant product peroxynitrite. In this figure, a second glutamate receptor (AMPA or kainate), on the right side of the post-synaptic cell, is also involved that indirectly acts to increase the sensitivity of the NMDA receptor to stimulation.

NMDA activity is likely to have a role in initiation of many cases of these illnesses. In all four, as we will discuss in subsequent chapters, there is also evidence for a role in the chronic phase of the illnesses. In FM, CFS, and MCS, there are studies reporting improved symptoms in the chronic phase in response to NMDA antagonists. The weakest evidence for excessive NMDA activity is in CFS, where the only evidence I am aware of is from clinical observations of physicians, reporting that NMDA antagonists or other drugs that indirectly lower NMDA activity are useful in therapy. One other potentially important observation is that magnesium has been reported to be a useful therapeutic agent in CFS, FM, and MCS (discussed in Chapter 15), and magnesium ions are known to lower NMDA activity, with the ions blocking the ion channel that might otherwise be opened on the stimulation of the NMDA receptors (Figure 2.1).[35,36]

What are the mechanisms involved in excitotoxicity in response to excessive NMDA activity? As was discussed in Chapter 1, stimulation of this receptor leads to the influx of calcium ions into the cell, leading to stimulation of the two calcium-dependent nitric oxide synthases, nNOS and eNOS. Because nNOS is usually found in much higher amounts in neurons than is eNOS, most of the increase in nitric oxide on NMDA stimulation is thought to be due to nNOS (Figure 2.1). It is known that NMDA stimulation leads to excessive peroxynitrite production as well.[39] While peroxynitrite synthesis is not the only consequence of NMDA overstimulation involved in excito-toxicity, it appears to be the most important such response.[37]

Some of the potential interactions among NMDA receptors, nitric oxide, peroxynitrite, and glutamate stimulation, are diagrammed in Figure 2.2. In addition to the sequence from the preceding paragraph, NMDA→nitric oxide→peroxynitrite, there are several potential interactions. One is that ni-tric oxide is known to act as what is known as a retrograde messenger in the brain, diffusing from the postsynaptic cell to the presynaptic cell and then acting to stimulate the release of glutamate neurotransmitter. This sequence is thought to act in a highly selective fashion in learning and memory, selec-tively strengthening the activity of certain synapses and thus laying down the changes required for memory. What are the consequences if this happens much more broadly in MCS and possibly in the other multisystem illnesses?

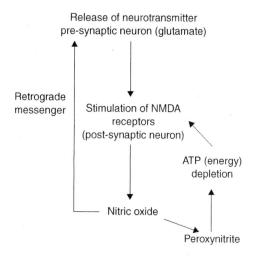

FIGURE 2.2. Neural sensitization cycle. This cycle, at least part of which is involved in what is known as long-term potentiation, the mechanism of learning and memory, may have an important role in MCS and possibly some other multisystem illnesses. When overstimulated by chemicals, the stimulation of NMDA receptors can lead to excessive nitric oxide and peroxynitrite production. The nitric oxide can act as a "retrograde messenger" diffusing to the presynaptic cell and stimulating the release of glutamate neurotransmitter, thus leading to increased NMDA stimulation. Peroxynitrite, due to its ability to attack important components in mitochondria, can lower energy metabolism which stimulates NMDA activity via two distinct mechanisms.

One can already see the potential for a vicious cycle (Figure 2.2), which is part of the broader NO/NO/ONOO⁻ cycle outlined in Chapter 1.

There is also a potential role for peroxynitrite, also outlined in Figure 2.2. Peroxynitrite leads to lowered mitochondrial function and lowered production of ATP, the energy currency of the cell. Any time that ATP is depleted in cells containing NMDA receptors, these receptors become hypersensitive to stimulation.[39] The mechanism here is that the electrical potential across the outer (plasma) membrane of the cell where these receptors are located becomes depleted because of the role of ATP in maintaining that potential. Depletion of the membrane potential causes the magnesium ions to dissociate much more easily from the NMDA receptors, leading to these receptors to be very readily stimulated by glutamate and aspartate. This, in turn, can become part of the vicious cycle diagrammed in Figure 2.2 as well as part of the larger NO/ONOO⁻ cycle discussed in Chapter 1.

NMDA studies also give us the opportunity to test other aspects of the NO/ONOO⁻ cycle. Because NMDA stimulation is known to increase levels of nitric oxide and peroxynitrite, one can raise the question about whether these relatively direct responses lead to the other types of changes predicted by the NO/ONOO⁻ cycle. Does NMDA stimulation lead to increases in iNOS activity, NF-κB activity, superoxide production, or increases in inflammatory cytokine induction, as predicted from the mechanisms of that cycle? There is, in fact, evidence for each of these. NMDA stimulation causes increases in iNOS activity,[40-43] NF-κB activity,[43,44] superoxide levels,[44-47] and synthesis of inflammatory cytokines.[43] With regard to the elevation of superoxide levels, three specific mechanisms proposed as part of the NO/ONOO⁻ cycle and discussed earlier in this chapter are reported— increased generation of superoxide by the electron transport chain in the mitochondrion,[47-49] the peroxynitrite inactivation of the mitochondrial superoxide dismutase,[48,49] and the increase in xanthine oxidase activity[50,51]— have all been reported to be caused by excessive NMDA stimulation. These studies provide important support for the existence and role in living organisms of many of the important mechanisms proposed to be part of our NO/ONOO⁻ cycle. As was the case with some of the evidence discussed in Chapter 1, this provides important evidence for the plausibility of the overall proposed mechanism. What we need to produce is evidence for the physiological relevance of this proposed mechanism in these multisystem illnesses. I have discussed here some such evidence, and considerably more such evidence will be presented later in the book. Not surprisingly, much of this book will either directly or indirectly be concerned with the physiological relevance of the NO/ONOO⁻ cycle mechanisms to these illnesses.

THE VANILLOID RECEPTOR

The potential role of the vanilloid receptor in these multisystem illnesses was first brought to my attention by Dr. Julius Anderson at a couple of meetings at which we both spoke. We have coauthored a paper on this subject, relating its properties specifically to an apparent important role in MCS.[52] The vanilloid receptor was first described because of its role as the receptor for capsaicin, the "heat" in hot chilli peppers and similar capsicum peppers.[54-57] It appears to be stimulated by a large number of diverse chemicals[52,53] and is also stimulated by acid (low pH) and by heat.[54-56] Thus, it is not surprising from the heat stimulation that vanilloid stimulation by capsaicin and other compounds perceived as hot produces the perception of heat. The stimulation by heat, pH, and diverse chemicals seems to have been used in the body such that vanilloid functions in different regions of the body appear to be quite distinct from each other.

The vanilloid receptor has some important similarities to the NMDA receptor. When it is stimulated, it opens up channels in the plasma membrane of the cell, allowing calcium ions to flow into the cell,[53,55] and this influx of calcium produces an increase in nitric oxide synthesis.[52,54] Increased peroxynitrite synthesis is expected to also follow, but this, to my knowledge, has never been studied.

Part of the NO/ONOO⁻ cycle involves vanilloid stimulation leading to increased NMDA stimulation. Vanilloid stimulation of NMDA activity has been shown to occur via one pathway and may be expected to occur by a second pathway. It has been shown that many vanilloid-receptor-containing neurons release glutamate as their neurotransmitter,[52] leading in turn to stimulation of NMDA receptors in the postsynaptic neuron. One may expect that, in addition to this established mechanism, increased nitric oxide and peroxynitrite synthesis via vanilloid stimulation may lead to increased NMDA activity, as outlined in Figure 2.2. This sequential stimulation of vanilloid receptors and NMDA receptors appears to be involved in a number of responses. For example, cough responses are known to be produced by capsaicin acting as a vanilloid agonist, while they are blocked by NMDA antagonists, such as the drug dextromethorphan.

How might vanilloid receptor stimulation have a role in these multisystem illnesses? It is expected that excessive vanilloid stimulation will be able to stimulate the NO/ONOO⁻ cycle as was outlined in Chapter 1. Dr. Anderson and I have argued that this is what happens when organic solvents trigger sensitivity responses in MCS.[52] In addition, it is expected that there will be excessive vanilloid activity as a consequence of its involvement in the NO/ONOO⁻ cycle. There is evidence for such excessive vanilloid activity that has been published in both FM and MCS, and these will be discussed in subsequent chapters.

MUSCARINIC RECEPTORS

The muscarinic receptors are receptors in neurons, muscle, and some other tissues that are stimulated by the neurotransmitter acetylcholine.[57] They are not the only class of receptor stimulated by acetylcholine; there is another class called the nicotinic receptors. Because most of the pathophysiological consequences of excessive acetylcholine are due to the action of the muscarinic receptors, that will be the focus of our discussion. The muscarinic receptors are not part of the NO/ONOO⁻ cycle mechanism discussed in Chapter 1, so why are we discussing them here? Basically because they appear to have important roles in the initiation of MCS and some CFS cases by pesticides, and it makes sense, therefore, to discuss them here because they have some properties that relate to the NMDA and vanilloid receptors. There is another reason to discuss them—even though they were not included in our overall vicious cycle mechanism, there is an argument that they should have been—an argument supported by some observations on both CFS and MCS.

There are five types of muscarinic receptors, designated M1, M2, . . . , M5. The M1, M3, and M5 receptors are similar to each other. Each of these, when stimulated, produces increased levels of cytoplasmic calcium in the cell. Coincidentally, all of these have odd numbers, so they can be referred to together as the M-odd receptors. The mechanism by which the M-odd receptors produce increases in intracellular calcium is different from the mechanisms by which the NMDA receptors and vanilloid receptors produce the same final response. M-odd receptors trigger synthesis of the chemical messenger, designated IP3, which leads to release of intracellular calcium from certain calcium stores that are sequestered away in the cell. So rather than allowing calcium from outside the cell to flow in, as do the NMDA and vanilloid receptors, they release otherwise sequestered calcium that is already in the cell but was not previously accessible to the cytoplasm of the cell. The increased calcium in the cytoplasm will, of course, increase the synthesis of nitric oxide by nNOS and eNOS, the two calcium-dependent nitric oxide synthases, thus increasing nitric oxide levels.

What role do these receptors have in MCS? Cases of MCS are typically triggered by exposure to either certain pesticides or organic solvents.[39,58,59] The pesticides that are often involved are either organophosphorus or carbamate pesticides, both of which exert their toxicity in insects and in vertebrates by acting as inhibitors of the enzyme acetylcholinesterase, the enzyme that breaks down acetylcholine. By inhibiting the breakdown of acetylcholine, they produce excessive accumulation of acetylcholine, and most of the toxicity produced is through excessive muscarinic stimulation. Excessive muscarinic stimulation not only directly increases production of nitric oxide, but also increases stimulation of the NMDA receptors,[39] which produces, in turn, increases in nitric oxide and peroxynitrite. You can see, from this, how these pesticides will be expected to feed into our NO/ONOO⁻ cycle mechanism. For the first time, we have a detailed explanation for how the organophosphorus and carbamate pesticides, repeatedly implicated in MCS, may act to initiate sensitivity responses.

COMORBID DISEASES

These multisystem illnesses are known to be comorbid with a number of well-accepted diseases, with known properties. Multisystem illnesses are often found in individuals who are also afflicted with these other diseases. Presumably one can explain this comorbidity if the well-accepted disease and the multisystem illness share common causal elements. We predict, therefore, that the elements of the NO/ONOO⁻ cycle will also be found in these comorbid diseases—an important and testable prediction. What are these potentially important comorbid diseases?

Patarca-Montero[60] reports the following well-accepted diseases are comorbid with fibromyalgia: allergies, migraine headache, hepatitis C infection, inflammatory bowel disease, rhinitis, and systemic lupus erythematosis (an autoimmune disease), as well as other evidence for other possible autoimmune diseases. Bell[61] describes a number of apparent comorbid diseases in CFS, including allergy, asthma, headaches including apparent migraines and tinnitus. Ashford and Miller[58] list a large number of apparent responses to chemical exposure that closely resemble well-accepted diseases including conjunctivitis, rhinitis, sinusitis, inner ear dysfunction including vertigo and tinnitus, gastroenteritis, inflammatory bowel disease, migraine headache, seizures, asthma, and autoimmune responses including systemic lupus erythematosis and rheumatoid arthritis. Yunus[62] lists such well-recognized diseases as migraine headaches, systemic lupus erythematosis, and rheumatoid arthritis being comorbid with CFS and FM. Neumann and Buskila[63] report that FM is often comorbid with rheumatoid arthritis, systemic lupus erythematosis, and chronic viral infections, suggesting a common pathogenesis, and Nicolodi and Sicuteri[64] emphasize the high prevalence of migraine among FM sufferers.

All of these comorbid diseases are inflammatory diseases, and therefore they all share with the NO/ONOO⁻ cycle such inflammatory markers as increased nitric oxide and inflammatory cytokines. Many of them are known to share other aspects of the proposed cycle, including elevated levels of peroxynitrite. For example, asthma involves nitric oxide, peroxynitrite, inflammatory cytokine and NF-κB elevation, and vanilloid and NMDA hyperactivity. Autoimmune diseases, including rheumatoid arthritis and lupus, are reported to have elevated iNOS activity and peroxynitrite as well as NF-κB and cytokine elevation at the sites of the autoimmune-related inflammation. Tinnitus involves essentially all of the elements of the vicious cycle as do migraine headaches. I will discuss these issues in more detail in Chapter 7 and Chapter 14. In general, the role of inflammatory biochemistry and physiology in these comorbid diseases provides a direct explanation for their reported comorbidity with multisystem illnesses. Any alternative etiologic theory needs to provide an alternative explanation for these comorbidity patterns.

IMPORTANT EXPLANATIONS

Chapters 1 and 2 were designed to focus on mechanism rather than explanation. Despite that focus, they provide us with important explanations of these often claimed "unexplained illnesses." Some of these explanations go to the heart of the most puzzling aspects of these illnesses:

1. The diverse stressors that apparently initiate these illnesses all can act through a common biochemical response—increasing nitric oxide levels.
2. The pattern of short-term stressor followed by chronic illness is explained through the stressors initiating a vicious cycle—the NO/ONOO⁻ cycle. The fact that the cycle is based on well-documented biochemistry and physiology and also that the elements of the cycle show up in hyperalgesia and in response to NMDA stimulation gives the cycle considerable credence.
3. A number of animal models are initiated by short-term stressors similar to those initiating the human condition and are characterized by elevation of elements of the NO/ONOO⁻ cycle in the chronic phase of illness. It can be seen from this that animal models fit well with and are explained by the properties of the cycle.
4. Positive reported therapeutic responses to magnesium supplements, carnitine supplements, NMDA antagonists, and a mixture designed to

stimulate regeneration of the inner mitochondrial membrane are all explained by the NO/ONOO$^-$ cycle. I will discuss in other chapters further examples of reported therapeutic responses that are also explained by this explanatory model. The complexity of the cycle explains, in addition, the challenge of effective therapy—it suggests that multiple elements of the cycle and multiple positive feedback loop mechanisms may have to be down-regulated in order to obtain much more normal function.

5. The reported increase in apoptotic cell death in these multisystem illnesses may be explained as being due to peroxynitrite induced apoptosis.

6. The reported role of excessive NMDA activity in both initiation and in the chronic phase of these illnesses is explained by the role of NMDA stimulation in producing nitric oxide and peroxynitrite and the proposed role of increased NMDA activity as part of the cycle.

7. Comorbidity between these multisystem illnesses and well-accepted diseases is explained by the well-known involvement of elements of the cycle in these diseases.

Additional important explanations are discussed in subsequent chapters.

Chapter 3

Generation of Symptoms and Signs of Multisystem Illnesses

In the absence of a paradigm or some candidate for a paradigm, all facts that could possibly pertain to the development of a given science are likely to be seen as equally relevant.

Thomas S. Kuhn

TAKE-HOME LESSONS

Seventeen distinct symptoms and signs are shared by at least two, and in most cases all four, of the multisystem illnesses. They include a diversity of symptoms and signs, categorized as biochemical, physiological, immunological, psychiatric, and others that are difficult to classify. Of these 17 symptoms, 16 can be explained as being produced by one or more of the elements of the NO/ONOO⁻ cycle. These explanations are not yet established as mechanisms in these illnesses. However, they provide plausible mechanisms linking the NO/ONOO⁻ cycle with this diversity of symptoms and signs, showing that they should no longer be considered unexplained.

It is difficult to see how the complexities of these multisystem illnesses could be explained as being due to anything other than aberrations in their underlying biochemistry. The fit between the NO/ONOO⁻ cycle biochemistry and the diverse symptoms and signs of illness provides a compelling argument for its central role.

GOAL

One of the most important evidence that these multisystem illnesses may share a common etiologic mechanism is that they share so many symptoms

Explaining "Unexplained Illnesses"
© 2007 by The Haworth Press, Inc. All rights reserved.
doi:10.1300/5139_03

and signs. It seems likely, therefore, that each symptom or sign is generated by a particular mechanism in each of these four multisystem illnesses. The goal of this chapter is to document the existence of many of these common features and then propose plausible explanations for each of them. Specifically, I will be looking for explanations that are predicted to be a response to one or more components of the NO/ONOO⁻ cycle mechanism.

Part of the rationale for the discussion in this chapter is the widespread claim that the symptoms of these multisystem illnesses are "unexplained" or "medically unexplained." This claim has been largely made by those advocating a psychogenic "mechanism" for these illnesses, arguing that they are what are known as somatization disorders.* A requirement for a diagnosis of somatization disorder is that the symptoms are largely unexplained by any known physiological mechanism. This claim of unexplained symptoms has been repeatedly made about these multisystem illnesses, often while ignoring the explanations that are already in the scientific literature. The claim that these symptoms are unexplained is often linked to a related claim, that these symptoms are so diverse that no possible physiological mechanism can generate them, again arguing in the view of those making these claims for a psychogenic etiology. This chapter argues strongly against both of these claims.

It is my hope that by the end of this chapter, you will be convinced that there exist plausible mechanisms linking each of these shared symptoms with the NO/ONOO⁻ cycle mechanism. Clearly, some of these explanations will be more speculative than others. Some will be more detailed than others. Each of these proposed mechanisms is presented <u>as a plausible explanation, not as a clearly established mechanism in multisystem illnesses</u>.

Most of the symptoms and signs are ones where one sees aberrations in some fraction but not all of the individuals afflicted by the multisystem illnesses. There is a stunning variation in symptoms seen from one individual to another, a variation that needs to be explained. I will discuss my explanation for these variations in Chapter 4. In any case, it needs to be kept in mind that these symptoms and signs of these multisystem illnesses are all more common relative to normal controls, but they rarely occur, if ever, in all patients with these illnesses.

---

*Somatization disorders are defined by psychiatrists as having certain diagnostic features and are assumed to be generated by some psychogenic mechanism. It is assumed that there are changes in body properties found in people suffering from somatization disorders that are produced by some type of psychological mechanism.

COMMON SYMPTOMS AND SIGNS
OF MULTISYSTEM ILLNESSES

There are a large number of common symptoms and signs in these illnesses. Most of these have been reported in all four of these illnesses, but others are only reported in two or three. Generally, it is unclear to me, when these have only been reported in two or three, whether this is because they have not been studied adequately in the others. Several of these symptoms in multiple chemical sensitivity (MCS) are reported to become exacerbated in response to chemical exposure, linking them to the general mechanism of chemical sensitivity.

The following are symptoms or signs that are in common among these multisystem illnesses:

1. Energy metabolism/mitochondrial dysfunction has been reported in chronic fatigue syndrome (CFS) (seven references cited in Reference 1)[1-4] and in fibromyalgia (FM).[5-14] It has also been reported in the brains of an animal model of CFS.[15] It has not been studied, to my knowledge, in MCS or in post-traumatic stress disorder (PTSD).

2. Increased levels of markers for oxidative stress have been reported in CFS,[16-23] MCS,[24] FM,[25-28] and in animal models of PTSD. The only study done in PTSD in humans showed mixed results with some markers significantly elevated but not others,[29] whereas animal models of PTSD showed increased oxidative stress.[30-32] An animal model of CFS was reported to show oxidative stress and to respond to antioxidant therapy.[33]

3. Changes in brain PET scans have been reported in CFS,[34-37] MCS,[38,39] FM,[40,41] and PTSD.[42-45]

4. Changes in brain SPECT scans have been reported in CFS,[46-49] MCS,[50-52] FM,[53] and PTSD.[54-58]

5. Immune system dysfunction including, especially low natural killer (NK) cell function, has been reported in CFS,[59-63] MCS,[64,65] FM,[66,67] and PTSD.[68-71]

6. Elevated levels of inflammatory cytokines have been reported in CFS,[63,72-74] FM,[67,75,76] and PTSD[77-80] but have never been studied in MCS, to my knowledge. However, chemicals known to be involved in chemical sensitivity responses in MCS have been reported to produce elevations of such cytokines.[81,82]

7. Hypothalamic-pituitary-adrenal (HPA) axis dysfunction has been reported in CFS,[61,82-86] MCS,[64,65,91,92] FM,[67,87-90] and PTSD,[93-98] as well as in an animal model for MCS.[99]

8. Anxiety is considered a classic symptom of PTSD and has also been reported in CFS,[61,100,101,105] MCS,[64,65,104,105] and FM.[67,102,103]

9. Depression has been reported in CFS,[61,100,105] MCS,[64,65,105] FM,[67,102,103] and PTSD.[106,107]

10. Rage has been reported to be fairly common in PTSD[110] and to occur occasionally in CFS[108] and to occur in response to chemical exposure in some cases of MCS.[109]

11. Cognitive dysfunction/learning and memory dysfunction has been reported in CFS,[61,100,101,111-115] MCS,[64,65] FM,[67,102,103,116] and PTSD.[107,117-119]

12. Multiorgan pain, especially headache pain, joint pain, and muscle pain, are reported in CFS,[61,100,101,115] MCS,[64,65] FM,[67,102,103,115] and PTSD.[107,117,120,121]

13. Fatigue is reported in CFS,[61,100,101] MCS,[64,65] FM,[67,102,103,116] and PTSD.[107,117,122,123]

14. Sleep dysfunction, including unrefreshing sleep, is reported in CFS,[61,100,101,115] MCS,[64,65] FM,[67,102,103] and PTSD.[107,117,122,123]

15. Circulatory dysfunction, particularly orthostatic intolerance, has been reported in CFS,[124,125] MCS,[126] FM,[67] and PTSD.[127,128]

So, we have at least 15 different overlapping symptoms and signs, some of which are clearly classified as biochemical (mitochondrial dysfunction and oxidative stress), some as immunological (low NK cell function), some as psychiatric (anxiety, depression and rage), one circulatory (orthostatic intolerance), and some as possibly neurological [cognitive dysfunction, brain positron emission tomography (PET) scan, and single-photon emission computed tomography (SPECT) scan changes], while others may be still more difficult to classify. I think you will see that these classifications appear to break down further as we discuss possible mechanisms.

PROPOSED MECHANISMS
FOR OVERLAPPING SYMPTOMS AND SIGNS

My goal here is to take the various elements in our NO/ONOO⁻ cycle mechanism—nitric oxide, superoxide, peroxynitrite, oxidative stress, cytoplasmic calcium, inflammatory cytokines, vanilloid receptor activity, and NMDA receptor activity—and show how one or more of them may be responsible for each of these symptoms. The prediction of this etiologic theory is that one or more of them should provide an explanation for the symptoms and signs reported. Some of these proposed mechanisms, but not others, have been discussed earlier in one of my papers.[115]

Three of these, namely item numbers 1, 2, and 6 of the preceding list, can be seen to come straight out of our discussions in Chapter 1 and Chapter 2. Energy metabolism/mitochondrial dysfunction (#1) is seen as being a consequence of the known effects of peroxynitrite and, to a lesser extent, superoxide and nitric oxide on mitochondrial/energy metabolism that were discussed in Chapter 2. Oxidative stress (#2) is seen as being a consequence of the effects of elevated levels of peroxynitrite, a potent oxidant, and its free radical breakdown products, as discussed in Chapter 2. Elevated levels of inflammatory cytokines (#6) are part of the NO/ONOO⁻ cycle mechanism and are seen as being caused by increased activity of NF-κB, which is, in turn, produced by other components of the NO/ONOO⁻ cycle. These proposed mechanisms are all direct consequences of elements from the proposed etiology. Let me say, before going on, that the challenge facing advocates of any alternative etiologic theory, whether primarily physiological or psychogenic, is to show that either the data documenting these symptoms and other signs are wrong or that they can provide better explanations for their existence than I have done.

The brain PET scan abnormalities (#3) and SPECT scan abnormalities (#4) bring other mechanisms to the fore. These are often interpreted in terms of blood flow (perfusion) and may, therefore, reflect changes in blood flow in different regions in the brain. Certainly, blood flow is influenced by the metabolic activity of different organs and is specifically influenced by nitric oxide (increased flow), peroxynitrite, and the oxidant products isoprostanes (decreased flow). However, each of these also reflect additional mechanisms that may be equally or more important. PET scans use a compound fluorodeoxyglucose as what is known a probe in order to look at changed brain properties. Fluorodeoxyglucose is concentrated in tissues at rates that depend on their metabolic rates because of its similarities to glucose, the main support for energy metabolism in the brain.[129-131] So, PET scans reflect the energy metabolism of the tissues involved. They may reflect the energy metabolism dysfunction that is caused by peroxynitrite, superoxide, and nitric oxide. The PET scan/energy metabolism connection was shown by Pietrini and coworkers (p. 161),[129] who state that fluorodeoxyglucose PET scan studies allow one to "measure in vivo regional cerebral glucose metabolism." Similarly, Holthoff et al.[130] interpreted such studies of changes in brains of depressive patients in terms of glucose metabolism, just as Silverman et al.[131] did for Alzheimer's patients and others with cognitive dysfunction. So, we can explain the PET scan abnormalities reported in the brains of persons with all four of these illnesses as being due, at least in part, to energy metabolism dysfunction in regions of the brain.

SPECT scans reflect a different aspect of the proposed biochemistry. The probe that is used in SPECT scan studies accumulates in tissues depending on whether or not it is reduced by the compound reduced glutathione.[132,133] Reduced glutathione is the most important antioxidants that is synthesized in the body, and it is depleted whenever tissues are under oxidative stress. It follows that oxidative stress produced by elevated levels of peroxynitrite and its breakdown products will deplete reduced glutathione in tissues and lead to lowered accumulation of the probe used in SPECT scan studies. I would argue, therefore, that SPECT scan studies of the brains of people afflicted by these illnesses are showing the pattern of oxidative stress in their brains, stress that may be generated by excessive peroxynitrite.

The interactions of the elements of the NO/ONOO$^-$ cycle with the immune system are expected to be a bit more complex. The immune system is known to be especially susceptible to oxidative stress, responding to both oxidants and antioxidants. For example, Meydani et al.[134] state that "cells of the immune system are particularly sensitive to changes in oxidant-antioxidant balance" (p. 1462S). Oxidants will be expected to lower its activity. However, both the inflammatory cytokines and nitric oxide itself tend to increase certain aspects of immune activity, and so one might expect complex effects with some immune system functions being stimulated and others being inhibited. What about low NK cell function, the best-documented change in immune function reported in these multisystem illnesses? It is reported to be lowered by oxidants and is specifically lowered by superoxide,[135-137] one of our NO/ONOO$^-$ cycle components. Consequently, the lowered NK cell function may be due to the action of superoxide and/or other oxidants in these multisystem illnesses. A role for such oxidants in this process is supported by a study reporting improved NK cell function in MCS patients after treatment with high doses of the antioxidant vitamin C.[138] One of the puzzles I am faced with is that, although superoxide and other oxidants are known to lower NK cell function, nitric oxide is known to raise NK cell function, leaving it difficult to predict where the balance is likely to be in these multisystem illnesses in response to the NO/ONOO$^-$ cycle mechanism. Interestingly, Ogawa and coworkers[139] reported that isolated NK cells from CFS patients were less stimulated by nitric oxide than were control NK cells, showing that some mechanism (superoxide and other oxidants?) caused the CFS cells to be less responsive to nitric oxide. These observations suggest that the effects of superoxide and other oxidants in lowering NK cell function are likely to dominate any effects of nitric oxide in stimulating NK cell function in these multisystem illnesses.

We have now gone through six of our symptoms and signs. The explanation for #7, <u>HPA axis dysfunction</u>, is the least satisfactory, in my judgment. I discussed this issue in my first paper on CFS,[1] asking whether the HPA axis dysfunction might be due to chronic elevation of nitric oxide levels. I came to the conclusion that the evidence was confusing at best, because both increased activity and decreased activity had been reported in response to nitric oxide. A similarly confusing state was described in a review on this subject.[140] Neither of these allowed one to assess whether <u>chronic nitric oxide elevation</u> (presumably most relevant to multisystem illnesses) produces effects distinct from those of short-term nitric oxide increases. So, no even tentative mechanism can be supported involving nitric oxide.

Perhaps a different perspective is needed here. The components of the NO/ONOO⁻ cycle, nitric oxide, peroxynitrite, oxidative stress, inflammatory cytokines, and NF-κB activity, are all parts of inflammatory biochemistry, so we expect important similarities between these multisystem illnesses and chronic inflammatory diseases. Several of these chronic inflammatory diseases have been studied and have been reported to have HPA axis dysfunction as well, including rheumatoid arthritis, lupus, migraine, atopic dermatitis, asthma, multiple sclerosis, sepsis, psoriasis, and inflammatory bowel disease.[90,96,141-145] It appears, therefore, that some aspect of chronic inflammatory biochemistry may lead to HPA axis dysfunction, even though we cannot point to what specific aspect may be involved. This is an indication that there is a mechanism that can lead to HPA axis dysfunction in response to chronic inflammatory biochemistry, but I am unable to provide a specific mechanism.

There is one other aspect of HPA axis dysfunction that I will return to in Chapter 5. The pattern of HPA axis dysfunction reported in CFS differs substantially from that reported in these other multisystem illnesses. That shows there must be at least two distinct mechanisms potentially involved here. This distinction may be important for explaining in what critical way CFS may differ from the other multisystem illnesses.

The two psychiatric symptoms, <u>anxiety</u> (#8) and <u>depression</u> (#9) appear to be explained by some studies of animal models. Anxiety has been reported in animal models to be produced by injecting the compound *N*-methyl-D-aspartate (the compound that specifically stimulates the NMDA receptors) into the amygdala region of the brain, as well as by drugs that stimulate NMDA activity. Anxiety is lowered by NMDA antagonists, drugs that lower NMDA responses.[146-149] The amygdala is the region of the brain that is centrally involved in response to severe psychological stress, and so such an anxiety response should not be surprising. The anxiety-inducing effect of NMDA stimulation appears to be produced through the calcium increases produced on NMDA stimulation.[149] One question I will ask in the following paragraph is whether nitric oxide has a role in this process. One of the drugs inducing increased anxiety and NMDA activity in animal models also produces anxiety in humans,[146] suggesting a similar mechanism applies in humans as well. What this observation suggests is that, if the amygdala of a person afflicted by a multisystem illness is impacted by the NO/ONOO⁻ cycle mechanism, one would predict that anxiety responses will be produced by the elevated NMDA activity.

One of the interesting things here is that, in a number of studies, lowering nitric oxide or the cGMP pathway from nitric oxide is reported to tend to increase anxiety-like behavior,[150-153] suggesting that nitric oxide helps protect from anxiety. In other studies, it is reported that increasing the nitric oxide/cGMP cascade induces anxiety responses,[154,155] and so, here, nitric oxide appears to increase anxiety. This appears, at first glance, to be a very confusing situation, but it is possible to suggest a consistent explanation for these observations. It appears that, when nitric oxide levels are either above normal or below normal, they may induce anxiety responses. In any case, the interpretation of the NMDA studies appears to be straightforward, in that excessive NMDA stimulation in the amygdala can produce anxiety-like responses, providing a mechanism consistent with the NO/ONOO⁻ cycle.

Depression (#9) in animal models and in humans is produced by excessive levels of nitric oxide[156-161] and by inflammatory cytokines that induce the iNOS gene and thus produce increases in nitric oxide.[162-164] Depression is reported to be caused by excessive nitric oxide in humans, with nitrate (marker of nitric oxide) levels being elevated.[156,157] An antidepressive drug has been shown to act as a nitric oxide synthase inhibitor.[160] Excessive glutamate, acting in part through its stimulation of NMDA receptors, is also reported to be involved in depression.[159] It is not completely clear what parts of the brain are responsible for these responses. All of these observations implicate excessive nitric oxide, and mechanisms that produce it, in causing psychological depression.

Studies of anxiety and depression mechanisms and how these responses may be generated in some cases of multisystem illnesses are of great interest because they suggest that anxiety and depressive responses are a consequence of the biochemistry of these illnesses rather than being the cause of these illnesses.

Rage, a third psychiatric symptom, has been found in animal models to be generated by excessive NMDA stimulation of certain regions of the midbrain, especially the periacqueductal gray region of the midbrain.[165-168]

We have a second psychiatric symptom occurring in some cases of multisystem illnesses, which is produced by excessive NMDA stimulation but involving a different region of the brain than does the anxiety response. This emphasizes the inference, which we will discuss more extensively in Chapter 4, that, depending on the tissues impacted by the biochemistry and physiology of the NO/ONOO⁻ cycle in different cases of these illnesses, there will be very different symptoms and signs produced.

Cognitive, learning, and memory dysfunction in these illnesses may be another area where the known biochemistry and physiology of brain function may provide important insights on possible mechanisms. The brain is a very high-energy organ, with approximately 10 times the basal metabolic rate of the body as a whole, and is known to be especially sensitive to energy deprivation from hypoxia and other stressors. Therefore, the energy metabolism dysfunction in regions of the brain, suggested by the PET scan studies discussed earlier, will be expected to have substantial impact on brain function. In addition, both NMDA receptors and nitric oxide have very important roles in learning and memory.[169-179] All regulatory systems function well only if the regulatory signals involve change appropriately between low and high levels. It follows that inappropriate elevations of both NMDA receptor activity and nitric oxide levels may be expected to disrupt the normal process of learning and memory and to lead to cognitive dysfunction. These two different plausible mechanisms for cognitive/learning and memory dysfunction are actually expected to interact with each other in a profound way. As was discussed in Chapter 2, NMDA receptors become hypersensitive to stimulation when the cells in which they occur are deprived of energy in the form of ATP. Thus, the energy metabolism dysfunction will exacerbate the excessive NMDA activity and consequent excessive nitric oxide levels. Indeed, it is exactly these sorts of interactions from the NO/ONOO⁻ cycle mechanism that makes this mechanism so pernicious. In conclusion then, it is reasonable to infer that the cognitive/learning and memory dysfunction reported in these multisystem illnesses may be generated to a substantial extent by a combination of energy metabolism dysfunction in regions of the brain and inappropriate elevation of both NMDA activity and nitric oxide synthesis. Both of these latter two disrupt the normally balanced process of learning and memory.

Multiorgan pain should be considered in light of the discussion in Chapter 1 on the mechanism of excessive pain in hyperalgesia, which involves each of the elements in our NO/ONOO⁻ cycle mechanism. That evidence, as you will recall, provides substantial support that the NO/ONOO⁻ cycle mechanism exists and that it is relevant to the generation of excessive pain. Because vicious cycles act in a cyclical fashion, it is often difficult to determine what the final actor is (or actors are) in producing the final response—in this case, pain. It is known, for example, that excessive nitroglycerine, a drug that acts by releasing nitric oxide, can produce headache and other organ pain, but that does not tell you whether nitric oxide acts relatively directly or whether it might act via peroxynitrite, via NF-κB, etc. There is some evidence that nitric oxide can act relatively directly because, in some cases, pain responses are mediated through the action of cyclic GMP,[180] and cyclic GMP synthesis is directly stimulated by nitric oxide. In general, one can say that elements of our NO/ONOO⁻ cycle can be involved in the generation of pain and that, in some cases, nitric oxide is the most directly acting element in the cycle.

However, establishing that each of the important elements of our vicious cycle has a role here provides only an initial understanding. There are mechanisms described as <u>primary hyperalgesia</u> at the site of the damaged tissue and also as <u>secondary hyperalgesia</u>, in which the neural circuits of the spinal cord have a key role.[181] Primary hyperalgesia involves vanilloid receptor stimulation, nitric oxide/peroxynitrite elevation, and a variety of inflammatory responses. Secondary hyperalgesia also involves nitric oxide, NMDA receptors, and, again, inflammatory responses.[181] The data processing in the spinal cord involved in the generation of secondary hyperalgesia is considered to be quite similar to the central sensitization mechanisms thought to be involved in MCS (Chapter 7). Secondary hyperalgesia is characterized by a more widespread pain than that produced by the initial tissue damage that leads to the primary hyperalgesia response. What we have here are two areas of the nervous system communicating with each other to produce hyperalgesia from changes in both the damaged peripheral tissue and from the spinal cord processing. The vanilloid receptors in nociceptors (pain receptors) in the initial impacted tissue, including what are known as C-fibers, send nerve processes to the spinal cord, where they release glutamate neurotransmitter, which stimulates, in turn, the NMDA receptors. The spinal cord, in turn, sends processes to the peripheral tissues, which, via neurogenic inflammation and other mechanisms, stimulate the inflammatory and pain responses in the peripheral tissue (secondary hyperalgesia). There are two important take-home lessons here. First, we have two regions of the nervous system that reciprocally stimulate each other, and so the response is not limited to one region. These types of neuronal interactions raise the possibility that other mechanisms in these illnesses may simultaneously involve more than one region of the nervous system. The second take-home lesson is that we have two regions of the nervous system that have elements of our NO/ONOO⁻ cycle, which have a role in the generation of excessive pain.

While all of these multisystem illnesses are often characterized by excessive pain, FM is characterized by particularly widespread excessive pain. There are a number of research laboratories that have proposed that "pain centers" in the brain are impacted and have a key role in producing the widespread excessive pain in FM. Consequently, FM may involve additional regions of the nervous system in pain responses. I discuss this issue in Chapter 8.

Fatigue is one of the more intriguing symptoms of these multisystem illnesses. Most of the consideration of fatigue in these illnesses has focused on what neurological or psychological mechanisms may be involved in the perception of fatigue. However, it may be argued that fatigue is generated in response to a more fundamental biochemical parameter—that of energy metabolism. Diseases characterized by energy metabolism dysfunction all produce fatigue: various types of anemia,[182-185] where inadequate oxygen is distributed to the tissues; hypoglycemia,[186-188] where inadequate blood sugar is available for energy metabolism; and diseases of mitochondrial dysfunction caused by mutations in the mitochondrial DNA or nuclear DNA that influence mitochondrial function.[189-192] Anemia is so closely linked to fatigue that it has often been called "tired blood,"[182] and treatments that alleviate anemia in various diseases are known to alleviate fatigue.[183-185] All of these links suggest that fatigue may be caused by energy metabolism dysfunction, but they do not prove it. The most important studies supporting a causal link are the those of clinical trials aimed at improving mitochondrial function, with each reporting lessening of fatigue as a consequence of such treatment.[193-198] Two of these studies specifically involved fatigue in CFS or CFS-like illness,[195,197] and these provide substantial support for the relevance of mitochondrial dysfunction to fatigue in these multisystem illnesses. In addition to the apparent role of energy metabolism dysfunction in generalized fatigue, there is an extensive scientific literature reporting that muscle fatigue is both correlated with and caused by lowered ATP levels[199-202]; so, we have direct evidence that muscle fatigue is caused by lowered energy metabolism. Interestingly, it has been proposed by a research group at Stanford University that sleep acts to improve energy levels in the brain.[203] I would argue, therefore, that fatigue may be caused by energy metabolism dysfunction, which is produced in these illnesses by excessive levels of peroxynitrite, superoxide, and nitric oxide, as was discussed in Chapter 2. Nicolson's group[196,197] has also observed this close linkage between energy metabolism dysfunction and fatigue. While the neurological mechanisms leading to the perception of fatigue may well be important, the fundamental cause of lowered energy metabolism may be viewed as more important. One other point that needs to be made is that fatigue is commonly reported as a symptom of a wide variety of inflammatory diseases, not surprising given the roles of nitric oxide, peroxynitrite, and superoxide in inflammation and their actions lowering mitochondrial function.

Before leaving this issue of fatigue in these illnesses, I want to say that this interpretation of the cause of fatigue in these illnesses has great intuitive appeal to those who suffer from them. You feel like you don't have enough energy because . . . you don't have enough energy!

Sleep disturbance is a common symptom of these multisystem illnesses. Sleep is known to be disturbed by several components of the NO/ONOO$^-$ cycle, including inflammatory cytokines, NF-κB, and nitric oxide itself.[204-206] There is no question that several components of the cycle can lead to substantial sleep disturbances. Interestingly, the report that sleep acts to restore energy metabolism in the brain,[203] discussed earlier, may provide a possible explanation for the normal role of sleep in dispelling fatigue, hence closing the circle for the interactive mechanisms of energy metabolism dysfunction, fatigue, and sleep.

Orthostatic intolerance is a phenomenon in which the vasculature and blood pressure are not regulated properly. In normal individuals, when a person stands up from a seated or lying down position, the blood pressure adjusts to maintain adequate blood flow to the brain. In persons with orthostatic intolerance, this control is inadequate, sometimes leading to fainting. There have been two proposed mechanisms for this in multisystem illnesses. One is based on the action of nitric oxide as a vasodilator such that excessive nitric oxide may be expected to lead to excessive vasodilation and therefore inability to get sufficient constriction under these conditions in the lower parts of the body, leading to excessive pooling of the blood in the lower parts of the body. I proposed this mechanism in one of my papers,[115] and it was later proposed by De Meirleir's group,[207] who were apparently unaware of the earlier proposal. This proposal was based on the notion of excessive nitric oxide and so is obviously consistent with our overall proposed mechanism. The role of nitric oxide in such vasodilation has been shown to be important in POTS,[208] the mechanism involved in many cases of orthostatic intolerance. The second proposed mechanism is the failure of the sympathetic nervous system to properly control the vasculature. Interestingly, this is also consistent with a NO/ONOO$^-$ cycle mechanism because it is known that excessive nitric oxide can produce sympathetic dysfunction.[209-211] For example, Krukoff[209] stated that "A growing body of evidence supports the hypothesis that NO acts to decrease sympathetic output to the periphery . . ." (p. 474). We have two alternative explanations, both consistent with the NO/ONOO$^-$ cycle and both involving excessive levels of nitric oxide. A list of the symptoms and signs of multisystem illnesses explained by the elevated nitric oxide/peroxynitrite mechanism is provided in Exhibit 3.1, along with the proposed explanations.

In summary, then, I have presented explanations for 14 of the 15 symptoms and signs of these multisystem illnesses. In one, HPA axis dysfunction, we have evidence that an explanation consistent with the proposed overall mechanism exists but we do not know what that explanation is. Two other explanations for correlates of these illnesses are provided in Exhibit 3.1 and are discussed in the following text. I will also discuss more specific explanations for the individual illnesses in the appropriate chapters of this book. It can be seen from this that these symptoms (and signs) can no longer be considered to be unexplained. If someone wishes to argue that there are better explanations than these available, he or she is free to make that argument. It may also be possible argue that one or more of my explanations are flawed. But it is no longer acceptable to claim that these symptoms are unexplained.

COMPARISON WITH INFLUENZA

Most of the symptoms we have been discussing are often described as being flulike, being generated for periods of a few days to perhaps two or three weeks in response to influenza infection and in response to infection with many other infectious agents. Such infectious agents as HIV, anthrax, Q-fever, and many others have been described as initially generating flulike symptoms during the initial infectious process. These symptoms in influenza are produced by the body's response to infection and specifically by the elevated levels of inflammatory cytokines produced following infection. This leads to excessive levels of nitric oxide, superoxide, and peroxynitrite.[212] These responses are all parts of the NO/ONOO⁻ cycle mechanism, as you have seen. It follows that sufficient elevation of their levels may be expected to produce the same or quite similar symptoms as would our cycle. When I first realized this, I said to myself, "great, all I need to do is go into the scientific literature find out how the individual symptoms of influenza are generated and propose the same mechanisms for multisystem illnesses." The only problem is, as far as I have been able to determine, no one is concerned about how most of the individual symptoms of influenza are generated.*

---

*There is one exception to this, namely, fever in influenza has been extensively studied. Fever is the flulike symptom that does <u>not</u> regularly occur in the multisystem illnesses, and so it is not relevant here.

EXHIBIT 3.1. Explanations for Symptoms and Signs

Symptom/sign	Explanation based on elevated nitric oxide/peroxynitrite theory
Energy metabolism/ mitochondrial dysfunction	Inactivation of several proteins in the mitochondrion by peroxynitrite; inhibition of some mitochondrial enzymes by nitric oxide and superoxide
Oxidative stress	Peroxynitrite, superoxide and other oxidants
PET scan changes	Energy metabolism dysfunction leading to change transport of probe; changes in perfusion by nitric oxide, peroxynitrite, and isoprostanes
SPECT scan changes	Depletion of reduced glutathione by oxidative stress; perfusion changes as under PET scan changes
Low NK cell function	Superoxide and other oxidants acting to lower NK cell function
Elevated cytokines	NF-κB stimulating of the activity of inflammatory cytokine genes
Anxiety	Excessive NMDA activity in the amygdala
Depression	Elevated nitric oxide leading to depression; cytokines and NMDA increases acting in part or in whole via nitric oxide.
Rage	Excessive NMDA activity in the periaqueductal gray region of the midbrain
Cognitive/learning and memory dysfunction	Lowered energy metabolism in the brain, which is very susceptible to such changes; excessive NMDA activity and nitric oxide levels and their effects of learning and memory
Multiorgan pain	All components of cycle have a role, acting in part through nitric oxide and cyclic GMP elevation
Fatigue	Energy metabolism dysfunction
Sleep disturbance	Sleep impacted by inflammatory cytokines, NF-κB activity, and nitric oxide

Orthostatic intolerance	Two mechanisms: Nitric oxide-mediated vasodilation leading to blood pooling in the lower body and nitric oxide-mediated sympathetic nervous system dysfunction
Irritable bowel syndrome	Sensitivity and other changes produced by excessive vanilloid and NMDA activity, and increased nitric oxide
Intestinal permeabilization leading to food allergies	Permeabilization produced by excessive nitric oxide, inflammatory cytokines, NF-κB activity, and peroxynitrite; peroxynitrite acts in part by stimulating poly(ADP-ribose) polymerase activity

Yes, we know they are generated by the inflammatory cytokine response, but <u>exactly how</u> cytokines lead to symptoms is not known. Our ignorance about influenza is not quite complete as there are papers implicating nitric oxide,[207,208] superoxide,[209] and NMDA activity[210] in some of the most damaging aspects of lethal forms of influenza. But the point still stands—the mechanism behind the standard symptoms of influenza, those most similar to the symptoms of multisystem illnesses, are undetermined.

The comparison between multisystem illnesses and influenza may be illustrative in three different ways. First, no one worries terribly much about how most flu symptoms are generated, because no one is trying to argue that flu is a somatization disorder—because flu is known to be an infectious disease, we are spared all of the psychological speculation and focus on "unexplained symptoms." Second, it undercuts the argument that this great diversity of symptoms cannot be explained as being due to a physiological mechanism—if it can happen in flu and many other infectious diseases, it can also happen in multisystem illnesses. Third, it provides some support for the inference that what is aberrant in multisystem illnesses is the body's reaction to the stressors that initiate them. This increases the plausibility of a mechanism whereby a vicious cycle mechanism makes these symptoms chronic.

There is, however, an inference that may be derived from this comparison that I believe to be wrong. In CFS, the majority of cases appear to be initiated by an infection. This has led many to suggest that CFS is a chronic infection and that the symptoms are generated by the continued action of an infectious agent. There may be a few cases like this, perhaps some involving the Lyme disease bacterium. However, the failure to produce convincing evidence for such a chronic infection being the primary cause of CFS after over 30 years of study suggests that this is not the primary mechanism.*

GASTROINTESTINAL TRACT ABERRATIONS IN MULTISYSTEM ILLNESSES

Aberrations of the gastrointestinal (GI) tract are commonly reported in persons with multisystem illnesses. It has been suggested that improving such GI tract function may be a key approach to therapy.[217,219] This suggestion makes sense given the key role of the GI tract in the absorption of any compounds taken orally for therapy as well as in absorption of important nutrients. It also makes sense given the potential role of GI tract inflammation in exacerbating the symptoms of these illnesses. Of these GI tract dysfunctions, I will focus on three interrelated ones—irritable bowel syndrome (IBS), intestinal hyperpermeability, and food allergies.

IBS has been reported to be a common comorbid[†] condition in multisystem illnesses. It is reported to be common in patients with CFS,[219,220] FM,[220-223] MCS,[64,65] and PTSD.[224-226] Some of these studies have suggested that IBS may share a common etiologic mechanism with some of these multisystem illnesses.[220,227] I will return to this issue of possible common etiology shortly.

There is a second area of GI tract aberration that is reported to occur in these illnesses, involving both increased intestinal permeability, sometimes called "leaky gut syndrome" and consequent development of food allergies. The intestinal epithelia are composed of continuous sheets of cells that serve to drastically limit access of food proteins to the rest of the body. Inflammation in the intestine can lead to large increases in the permeability of the intestine,[228-230] resulting in increased absorption of incompletely digested food proteins, allowing for an immune response[231-233] causing them to become important allergens. Consumption of these food proteins can then increase the intestinal inflammation, causing exacerbation and continuation of this problem. This sequence of events is thought to occur in CFS.[217,218,234] Food intolerances/allergies also occur in other multisystem illnesses including MCS.[235-237] The reaction of food antigens with antibodies is reported to produce a number of inflammatory responses, including

---

*This does not rule out roles for opportunistic infections exacerbating the symptoms of CFS.

†Comorbid conditions, as you may recall from Chapter 1, are conditions that often occur together in the same patients.

iNOS induction and consequent increased nitric oxide synthesis, increased NF-κB activity, and inflammatory cytokine induction,[238-242] potentially up-regulating NO/ONOO⁻ cycle biochemistry.

One question that needs to be raised is whether the mechanisms causing IBS and intestinal permeabilization to be chronic may be similar or identical to the NO/ONOO⁻ cycle. There are two general properties about the GI tract that make such a possible mechanism plausible. There is a major center of the nervous system activity whose function is to control the GI tract, known as the enteric nervous system.[243] This major nervous control center, sometimes called "the brain of the gut," has several features that may cause the enteric nervous system to be a focus of the NO/ONOO⁻ cycle mechanisms. It is known that the enteric nervous system uses nitric oxide,[244,245] NMDA receptors,[246] and vanilloid receptors[247] for major roles in its functioning. Consequently, it has properties consistent with those needed for NO/ONOO⁻ cycle biochemistry. Furthermore, the GI tract also has over 50 percent of the body's immune system cells, and given the importance of immune system cells in producing nitric oxide, superoxide, and other oxidants, this may lend itself to possible NO/ONOO⁻ cycle activity in the GI tract as well. The influence on the GI tract of combinations of immune and neurological influences was discussed in an earlier review.[248]

Are any of the components in the NO/ONOO⁻ cycle known to be involved in either IBS or in intestinal permeabilization? In both cases, the answer is yes. IBS is reported to be produced by pain and irritation apparently mediated, at least in part, by elevated levels of vanilloid activity.[247,249-252] Nitric oxide is suggested to have a role as well,[253-255] and the combination of these roles, provides a possible explanation for the elevated IBS activity in multisystem illnesses. Furthermore, IBS has hyperalgesia symptoms, showing excessive pain response to mechanical stress.[256] The excessive pain sensitivity in animal models of IBS has been shown to involve excessive NMDA activity[257,258] as well as excessive vanilloid activity.[249,259] It should be noted that the etiology of IBS has been uncertain. These observations suggest that a NO/ONOO⁻ cycle mechanism focused on the GI tract and enteric nervous system may explain this previously unexplained medical condition. The peripheral and also central pain-processing changes reported in IBS[260] are similar to changes reported in FM, as we will discuss in Chapter 8.

Intestinal permeabilization is reported to involve nitric oxide,[261-271] peroxynitrite,[266-271] inflammatory cytokines,[262,263] and excessive NF-κB activity.[264] Therefore, many of the parameters of our NO/ONOO⁻ cycle mechanism have important causal roles in intestinal permeabilization. The most directly acting of these is likely to be peroxynitrite, given the role of poly-ADP-ribosylation in the permeabilization process[267-269] and the known role of peroxynitrite in stimulating poly-ADP-ribosylation, as discussed in Chapter 2. While the mechanisms that maintain chronic hyperpermeability of the intestine are likely to involve other features not part of the basic NO/ONOO⁻ cycle, such as bacterial infection, stimulation by food antigens- and other mechanisms of oxidative stress generation, aspects of the NO/ONOO⁻ cycle may be important and perhaps of central importance.

SUMMARY: WHERE ARE WE?

I believe that this chapter is by far the most wide-ranging attempt to explain the diverse symptoms and signs of these multisystem illnesses that has been published to date. Of the 17 (including the two GI tract responses as symptoms), we have plausible mechanisms to explain 16 and one (HPA axis dysfunction) where no plausible specific mechanism is apparent based on the literature but where we have evidence that such a mechanism exists. Clearly, any proposed etiologic mechanism for these illnesses must be judged, in part, by its ability to provide such explanations for their diverse symptoms. It is difficult to compare these explanations with those of other etiologic theories when we have no comparable alternative set of explanations or any comparable etiologic theory for these four illnesses. It seems to me it would be extraordinary that, if the NO/ONOO⁻ cycle theory were wrong, it would still be possible to provide so many plausible mechanisms to explain many of these previously unexplained symptoms and signs. Each such plausible mechanism is linked to one or more components of the NO/ONOO⁻ cycle.

This chapter presents cogent evidence and arguments that the diverse symptoms of these illnesses are no longer unexplained. It is offered in addition to my published studies of MCS, discussed in Chapter 7, that have provided detailed explanations for many of the most puzzling features characteristic of that illness. It is my contention that these symptoms can no longer be considered "unexplained" or "medically unexplained." Those advocating a psychogenic or any other etiology for these illnesses can no longer make those arguments without ignoring their responsibilities as scientists to pay attention to published evidence.

At this point in the book, after three chapters, we have explored six most important types of evidence providing support for the NO/ONOO⁻ cycle theory of these illnesses:

1. As many as 12 short-term stressors initiate these illnesses with all apparently able to increase nitric oxide levels. Is this coincidental?
2. The various animal models of these illnesses all provide evidence supporting the NO/ONOO⁻ cycle theory, providing evidence for an important role for nitric oxide and in most cases NMDA activity. In some cases, there is additional evidence for oxidative stress and peroxynitrite. In the case of hyperalgesia models, there is evidence supporting a role for all of the elements in our proposed vicious cycle mechanism. Is this pattern of evidence coincidental?
3. We have evidence from studies of drugs known to act by releasing nitric oxide that they can induce increases in nitric oxide synthesis, suggestive of a vicious cycle mechanism.
4. We also have evidence that excessive NMDA receptor stimulation leads to changes predicted by the NO/ONOO⁻ cycle mechanism, including increased NF-κB activity, increased iNOS activity, increased inflammatory cytokine levels, and increased superoxide levels, the last via three predicted mechanisms. These observations provide important confirmation for the existence of many of the predicted features of the NO/ONOO⁻ cycle.
5. The various well-accepted diseases that are comorbid with these multisystem illnesses are all inflammatory in nature, providing an immediate explanation for their comorbidity based common causal elements with NO/ONOO⁻ cycle biochemistry. Is this coincidental?
6. Finally, we have 16 diverse symptoms and signs of these overlapping multisystem illnesses, which can all be explained based on the proposed elevated nitric oxide/peroxynitrite etiology. Is this coincidental?

We have a detailed proposed mechanism for all four multisystem illnesses, which is extensively supported based on these six important considerations. We will see how well it holds up as we proceed further into the book.

A SET OF PRINCIPLES

When one looks at a new scientific paradigm, it is useful to use sets of basic principles to assess its merits. One set* that may be applied to the NO/ONOO⁻ cycle is the following:

It is <u>integrative</u>: It integrates into a common scheme a wide variety of previously unexplained diseases/illnesses.

---

*I am indebted to Dr. Marti Wolfe for suggesting this set of principles.

It is <u>comprehensive</u>: It encompasses a wide variety of observations about these illnesses/diseases including their patterns of case initiation, the nitric oxide increases produced by their initiating stressors, their chronic nature, and many of their shared symptoms and signs of the chronic phase of these diseases. It is supported by many of the properties of animal models of these illnesses.

It is <u>parsimonious</u>: It explains by a relatively simple conceptual framework many previously unexplained observations.

It is <u>fundamental</u>: Because it is based primarily at the biochemical level, it explains much of the complexity of these illnesses/diseases through the impact of a common biochemistry on a variety of organismal functions.

Chapter 4

The Local versus Systemic Nature of the NO/ONOO⁻ Cycle Mechanism and Its Implications for Nomenclature and Treatment

TAKE-HOME LESSONS

Much of the mechanism of the NO/ONOO⁻ cycle is local, impacting one tissue but not necessarily an adjacent tissue. Different people suffering from these illnesses may have distinct tissues impacted by NO/ONOO⁻ cycle biochemistry, leading to almost infinite variation of symptoms and signs produced by this variation in tissue distribution. This is proposed to be responsible for the extraordinary variation in symptoms and signs reported in comparisons of one patient with another. This variation creates fundamental problems with regard to any separation of this spectrum of illnesses into distinct classes with regard to nomenclature and with regard to the basic concept of differential diagnosis of these illnesses.

LOCAL NATURE OF THE NO/ONOO⁻ CYCLE

This chapter is focused on two issues that initially may not appear to be important. The first is that the primary mechanism of the NO/ONOO⁻ cycle is a local one, where one tissue may be impacted by this biochemistry but other tissues nearby may be largely unaffected. It follows from this that one individual suffering from one of these illnesses may have a particular tissue distribution of the underlying biochemistry, while another may have a very

Explaining "Unexplained Illnesses"
© 2007 by The Haworth Press, Inc. All rights reserved.
doi:10.1300/5139_04

different tissue distribution. The variation of tissue distribution will, in turn, produce variation in symptoms. So, the second issue raised in this chapter is that the tremendous variation in symptoms from one case to another may be largely produced by variation in tissue distribution of the biochemistry. The symptomatic variation produces, as you will see, several very important medical consequences.

Why do I say that the primary predicted mechanism is local? Basically because the in vivo half-lives of nitric oxide, peroxynitrite, and superoxide are short, allowing them to diffuse only relatively short distances away from where they were produced. In addition, most of the positive feedback loops that produce the NO/ONOO⁻ cycle, as we discussed in Chapter 1 and Chapter 2, act at the cellular level, so they act on individual cells and do not necessarily spread from one tissue to another. A prediction from this is that one tissue may be impacted with little or no impact on an adjacent tissue. The other prediction is that, because of the vicious cycle mechanisms, a particular tissue distribution in an individual may be propagated over time indefinitely so that the differences in symptoms from one individual to another may be relatively stable.

The half-life of nitric oxide in tissues is about 1 s, allowing it to diffuse in tissues only about 1 mm or less.[1-3] Peroxynitrite and superoxide are much more limited in their likely diffusion, mainly staying in or in the region of the cell in which they are generated,[1] with superoxide being the most limited of all. We know this for superoxide because mice lacking the enzyme in the mitochondrion that destroys superoxide, the mitochondrial superoxide dismutase, cannot survive despite the fact that they have another similar enzyme outside of the mitochondrion;[4,5] so most of the damage created by superoxide synthesized in the mitochondrion occurs within the cellular compartment in which it is synthesized. So, each of these compounds has limited ability to diffuse away, and *when coupled with NO/ONOO⁻ cycle mechanisms that act within individual cells, there is a potential to propagate a particular tissue distribution in a particular individual essentially indefinitely.*

Okay, you may ask, why should I care about that? One reason you should care is that it explains the puzzling diversity of symptoms that one sees from one individual to another. This variation of symptoms in chronic fatigue syndrome (CFS), fibromyalgia (FM), and multiple chemical sensitivity (MCS) was observed by Taylor and coworkers,[6] who state that "These illnesses exhibit enormous fluctuation in symptom severity between and within individuals" (p. 1). When Sorg[7] reviewed the symptoms often found in cases of MCS, she reported over 40 different symptoms, most of which occur only in some cases and many of which only occur only in a minority of cases. These do not fall into just a few specific symptomatic patterns, raising the issue of why there is such a puzzling variation in symptoms, both qualitative and quantitative in these illnesses. In the 1994 paper developing a case definition for CFS,[8] the CDC group proposed one symptom (profound fatigue of at least six months duration) plus at least four out of eight different symptoms (certain types of pain, postexertional malaise, cognitive dysfunction, etc.). So, in this study, the puzzling pattern of symptoms was simplified to focus on only nine, but even with that simplification, the CDC group was forced to propose a diagnosis based a wide variation of symptoms from one case to another. Members of support groups for CFS, FM, or MCS are often struck by the variation in symptoms from one individual to another. Yes, there are some common features with, for example, MCS people often reacting to a similar array of chemicals. However, the variation is striking in the responses to these chemicals and also in the basal symptoms in the absence of known chemical exposure.

How might this play out in practice? Certain symptoms can be tied to dysfunction of different parts of the body. For example, as discussed in Chapter 3, stimulation of NMDA receptors in the amygdala of the brain will produce anxiety and panic attack symptoms. It follows that such symptoms may be forthcoming if the amygdala is impacted by this biochemistry but not otherwise. Nitric oxide increase in the vasculature may be expected to produce orthostatic intolerance due to excessive vasodilation. Increased nitric oxide/peroxynitrite and vanilloid activity in the gastrointestinal (GI) tract may be expected to produce symptoms of irritable bowel syndrome or "leaky gut syndrome," depending on that tissue distribution. So, each of these may be found in some cases but not in others.

SYSTEMIC EFFECTS

We have, then, for the first time, a plausible model to explain the stunning diversity of symptoms of these multisystem illnesses, based on localized biochemistry. Does this mean that there are no systemic influences on the etiology of these illnesses? No, it does not mean that, although it does imply that the systemic influences that may affect the body as a whole are likely to be of secondary importance in explaining the many highly variable symptoms.

There are number of systemic changes that may be expected and which may have a substantial role. For example, elevated systemic markers of oxidative stress have been reported, as discussed in Chapter 3, as well as antioxidant depletion produced by such oxidative stress. Systemic antioxidant depletion will occur whenever there is substantial oxidative stress in a substantial volume of tissue in the body, and such depletion will cause other tissues to be more susceptible to oxidant damage.

A second type of expected systemic effect will be due to the ability of nitric oxide to bind to heme in the hemoglobin of the erythrocytes (red blood cells). It has been shown that such binding makes this nitric oxide stable as long as it is so bound, therefore allowing it to circulate around the body, where it can get pumped out of the erythrocyte.[9] In this way, nitric oxide synthesized in one part of the body can be transported through the blood to parts of the body far removed from its origin. This allows a compound that would normally be too unstable to be transported widely in the body to possibly influence certain tissues away from its origin.[9]

Two other potential systemic effects may also be suggested. Some of the inflammatory cytokines can travel around the body, potentially inducing the inducible nitric oxide synthase (iNOS) at sites away from where they were synthesized and secreted. In my first paper on CFS,[10] I discussed the possible role of low cortisol caused by hypothalamic-pituitary-adrenal (HPA) axis dysfunction, and because cortisol can lower iNOS induction, low cortisol may have the effect of increasing nitric oxide synthesis systemically. In some cases of these illnesses, low thyroid function is reported, which can exacerbate the role of low mitochondrial function, given the role of thyroid hormones in regulating mitochondrial function.

Changes in neuronal function are not systemic, but they are likely to not be local either, given the role of neurons in regulating neuronal and other functions elsewhere in the body. It follows that impact of the NO/ONOO⁻ cycle in the central or peripheral nervous system may have more widespread effects due to neuronal or neuroendocrine dysfunction. I suggest a possible role of such neuronal changes in FM in Chapter 8, providing an interpretation to the widespread pain most characteristic of FM.

One needs to contrast each of the distinct systemic effects with the major, local effects suggested by most of the mechanisms of our NO/ONOO⁻ cycle. The inference to be drawn is that most, but not all, of the mechanisms are likely to be local according to this proposed etiologic mechanism.

THE CHALLENGE OF NOMENCLATURE

We humans, going back into our early prehistory, have taken to naming things as a basis for communication. Such naming is based, however, on things falling into discrete classes, allowing uniform assignment of things to different classes, with each class being given a discrete name. What do we do when there are no discrete classes, because of almost infinite variation in symptomatic patterns? Should these multisystem illnesses be viewed as one type of disease state, as four types [CFS, FM, MCS, and post-traumatic stress disorder (PTSD)], as a dozen, or a hundred? If your answer is four, what do we do with the very high comorbidities such that many cases fit the diagnosis for more than one? What do we do with Gulf War syndrome, which has elements of all four? Some have argued that CFS should be viewed as having multiple subclasses, but this may be challenged by the difficulty (impossibility?) of assigning CFS cases to discrete, distinct classes.

Each of the diagnostic criteria that have been developed for these illnesses will include somewhat different groups of patients out of this spectrum of illness. The 1988 CDC criteria for CFS will diagnose a somewhat different group of patients from the 1994 criteria, which will, in turn differ from the more recent Canadian criteria. These groups overlap each other, so which is best and why? Are the people diagnosed as having CFS really distinct from those diagnosed as having myalgic encephalomyelitis in Britain? What do you do with a patient who meets the criterion for diagnosis of FM at time T but improves to the point of no longer meeting that diagnosis while maintaining the majority of the symptoms that led to that diagnosis— does that person still have FM or not?

Some of the issues and difficulties are illustrated by the recent debate surrounding an attempt to develop a new name for CFS. Everyone agrees that the old name, chronic fatigue syndrome, should be replaced because it emphasizes one symptom, fatigue, in the name of a complex, multisymptomatic, and multisystem illness. But what group of multisystem patients should be included under the new name and what arbitrarily chosen set of symptoms or systems should be used in the new name? And what happens when a new name is proposed, neuroendocrineimmune dysfunction syndrome, which, as described in Chapter 3, should apply equally well to FM, MCS, and PTSD as it does to the currently defined CFS patients. After all, each of these four of these illnesses involves neurological, neuroendocrine, and immunological dysfunction.

My own view, which should be apparent from the earlier discussion in this chapter, is that people have been asking the wrong questions and therefore have been unable to provide satisfactory answers. These questions are based on the notion that there should be distinct subgroups of illnesses that can be objectively assigned to discrete classes. What if this notion is wrong because there are almost infinite possible variations in tissue distribution of the underlying biochemistry?

In my view, we need to recognize that groups of individuals with multisystem illnesses may well be arbitrarily defined. Each of them may be an arbitrary portion of a larger spectrum of illness.

It may still be worth comparing one such arbitrarily defined group with another to start to analyze some of the variation involved, but we should recognize that these groups may well be arbitrary and not based on one or more discrete objective and qualitative distinctions among them. Such arbitrary divisions of a spectrum are common in medical studies. For example, we often compare obese with non-obese individuals even though the division between those defined as obese and non-obese is arbitrary. Pathologists seem to be very good at determining whether a tumor is benign or malignant, despite the fact that there is a vast variation of tumor aggressiveness and invasiveness. The challenge with these multisystem illnesses is that we have a multidimensional problem in dividing those suffering from combinations of the several multisystem illnesses, rather than a largely one dimensional problem that we have with obesity or even tumor aggressiveness.

This is not the only area of the health sciences challenged by the apparent lack of well-defined, discrete classes. People talk about "autistic spectrum disorders" because of a lack of clear boundaries separating these disorders from each other. Similarly, on p. xxii of the "psychiatrist's bible," DSM-IV,[11] it is stated that "there is no assumption that each category of mental disorder is a completely discrete entity with absolute boundaries dividing it from other mental disorders or from no mental disorder." They go on to comment on the heterogeneity of individuals and the difficulty of diagnosis "in any but a probabilistic fashion." I am not suggesting here that these multisystem illnesses are primarily mental but rather that many illnesses currently classified as mental may share this profound symptomatic variation, from one case to another, with the multisystem illnesses.

The term spectrum, which has been used here, is a good one. In the classic spectrum of colors of the rainbow, there are no discrete divisions between colors—they all run into each other. The division between yellow and orange, for example, is arbitrary. Perhaps we should call CFS, MCS, FM, and PTSD multisystem spectrum diseases or even NO/ONOO⁻ cycle spectrum diseases.

DIFFERENTIAL DIAGNOSIS
AND THE BUREAUCRATIC NATURE
OF MODERN MEDICINE

Much of modern medicine is based on the notion of differential diagnosis. If you have an ill patient, it is necessary to determine if the illness is caused by infection, autoimmune disease, a nutritional deficiency disease, a hormonal dysfunction, or some other cause. If it is infectious, is it tuberculosis, influenza, malaria, AIDS, or any of many other types of infections? If it is determined to be tuberculosis, you treat with a standard antibiotic regimen, and if it turns out to be an antibiotic-resistant strain of tuberculosis, you will go to an alternative treatment. So the process is to perform a differential diagnosis and then treat based on the standard treatment for that class of illness.

The difficulty in treating multisystem illnesses is not only that there have not been enough trials testing such treatments, although that is certainly true. It is not only that treatments have not been based on a discrete, testable etiologic mechanism, although that has also been largely true. It is not only that ineffective treatments have been touted by those with vested interests in their acceptance, such as the current debate in the United Kingdom over cognitive behavioral therapy. It is, in addition, that these illnesses challenge the whole notion of differential diagnosis because they do not fit readily into discrete categories.

This is particularly important given the bureaucratic nature of modern medicine. In order to limit the growth of spending for medical care, medical care systems, whether they are health insurance or health maintenance organizations in the United States or state-supported medical care organizations in various parts of the world, many such organizations have insisted on the pattern described in the first paragraph of this section. If one cannot perform a differential diagnosis of the illness or if no effective treatment is established for a specific diagnosis, no payment may be forthcoming for treatment. We need, in my judgment, to recognize that these multisystem illnesses defy the notion of differential diagnosis and therefore are not adequately dealt with by our bureaucratic health systems.

Chapter 5

Chronic Fatigue Syndrome

TAKE-HOME LESSONS

NO/ONOO⁻ cycle etiology of chronic fatigue syndrome (CFS) is supported by the following:

- Evidence for a key role of nitric oxide in initiation of CFS cases comes from three different sources: eight distinct stressors apparently initiating cases of CFS all eight of which may act to increase nitric oxide levels; two genes influencing the incidence of CFS both of which may influence nitric oxide synthesis whereas other genes may act by increasing superoxide; and a mouse model of CFS is initiated by a bacterial extract that increases nitric oxide.
- In the chronic phase of CFS, a number of elements of the NO/ONOO⁻ cycle are reported or known to be elevated: oxidative stress and mitochondrial dysfunction are very well documented; multiple reports suggest a role for excessive nitric oxide, excessive NMDA activity and excessive inflammatory cytokines; other evidence suggests roles for excessive iNOS induction.
- Most importantly, therapy aimed at lowering nitric oxide levels, improving mitochondrial function, or decreasing oxidative stress appears to be useful in the treatment of CFS; this suggests that the NO/ONOO⁻ cycle is a useful explanatory model when it comes to the key feature of suggesting effective therapies.

I suggest a possible mechanism for the generation of postexertional malaise in CFS, probably the most characteristic symptom of CFS, a mechanism that may lead to the development of a specific biomarker for CFS.

Explaining "Unexplained Illnesses"
© 2007 by The Haworth Press, Inc. All rights reserved.
doi:10.1300/5139_05

Because the NO/ONOO⁻ cycle also provides explanations for the etiology of multiple chemical sensitivity (MCS), fibromyalgia (FM) and post-traumatic stress disorder (PTSD), we have for the first time, an explanation for the many overlaps that characterize this whole group of illnesses.

CHAPTER ORGANIZATION

This chapter is organized in a fashion similar to that of Chapters 7 to 10, each of which is focused on individual illnesses. It is divided conceptually into three major sections, aimed at determining whether three major testable features of our etiologic theory apply. The first major section will ask whether any short-term stressors initiating cases of CFS may act by increasing nitric oxide or possibly other aspects of our NO/ONOO⁻ vicious cycle such as superoxide. The second section will focus on properties of the chronic phase of CFS, asking specifically whether the properties are consistent with those predicted by the properties of our vicious cycle. The second section will also discuss some of examples of therapeutic agents that down-regulate NO/ONOO⁻ cycle biochemistry and produce CFS improvement. The third and, in this chapter the shortest, section will focus on specific properties of CFS that distinguishes it from the other multisystem illnesses and how those specific properties may be explained. I have already, in Chapter 3, provided evidence that many of the overlapping symptoms and signs of these illnesses may be explained by our NO/ONOO⁻ cycle mechanism. In this chapter, I will in addition, examine whether the symptom most characteristic of CFS can also be explained as being a consequence of this cycle. I will finish this third section by asking whether this CFS-specific symptom may lead us to develop a specific biomarker for CFS.

INITIATION OF CASES OF CFS

Infections that often initiate CFS cases have been commonly described as being flulike, but may be of diverse origins. A wide variety of infectious agents have been implicated in these infections, including coxsackie, Epstein-Barr, rubella, varicella, parvovirus, and Ross River viruses[1-8] and such bacterial agents as Lyme disease[9,10] and *Coxiella burnetii* (Q-fever).[11] One can see from these studies that the infectious agents include a variety of viruses as well as bacterial agents. It seems clear that the CFS cases appear to be initiated by such infections do not involve any specific infectious agent but may involve a common response to a variety of viral and bacterial infections. One of the obvious questions raised by the role of infection in the initiation of many cases of CFS is whether the chronic phase of the illness is caused by a chronic infection. Despite some 30 years of research searching for such a causal chronic infection, the evidence is that it does not. For example, Natelson and Lange[12] (p. 673) state in a recent review that "Thus, post viral fatigue syndrome exists, but persistence of an infectious agent has not been demonstrated." There is evidence for what appear to be opportunistic infections in CFS, discussed later, and indeed some opportunistic infections are reported in some of the other multisystem illnesses. Such infections exacerbate the symptoms of CFS and related illnesses, and may therefore be useful to treat but there is no convincing evidence that they are causal.

It is very well documented that both viral and bacterial and, indeed, other infectious agents typically produce increases in inflammatory cytokine synthesis, leading, in turn, to increased iNOS induction, producing in this way increases in nitric oxide synthesis.[13] Bacterial infectious agents act in this way and may also act more directly with a variety of bacterial substituents including bacterial lipopolysaccharides inducing increased iNOS activity.[13] A mouse model of CFS, which was discussed in Chapter 1, uses killed bacteria that are known to act as iNOS inducers to induce chronic fatigue. This iNOS induction is a common response to infection and is, therefore, an excellent candidate for an initiating event in CFS and these observations originally suggested the NO/ONOO⁻ cycle theory of CFS.[13]

The evidence discussed briefly in Chapter 1 that short-term stressors preceding cases of FM, MCS, and PTSD also lead to increased nitric oxide synthesis provides additional evidence for a pattern of action of these stressors acting via nitric oxide. That pattern is further strengthened by the reported role of other stressors in the initiation of CFS. Donnay has argued that initiation of some cases of both CFS and MCS involve carbon monoxide exposure,[14,15] and I have discussed elsewhere[16] cases of short-term carbon monoxide exposure that led to cases of chronic illness with symptoms similar to those of CFS. It is interesting, therefore, that short-term tissue exposure to carbon monoxide is reported to increase nitric oxide levels and produces increased oxidative stress.[16] One of the mechanisms involved is increased NMDA activity.[17] It follows that carbon monoxide may be a short-term stressor that acts through nitric oxide and its oxidant product, peroxynitrite. Organophosphorus pesticide exposure is also reported to initiate cases of CFS,[18,19] and such exposure can also lead to increased nitric oxide levels.[20] Organophosphorus pesticides can trigger increased NMDA activity and therefore increased nitric oxide levels (Chapter 7). An additional stressor reported to precede cases of CFS is ciguatoxin* poisoning,[21,22] and such poisoning is likely to indirectly lead to increased NMDA activity, as discussed in the next paragraph, which will in turn produce increases in nitric oxide and peroxynitrite, as discussed in Chapter 2. Approximately 5 percent of the people suffering from ciguatoxin poisoning fail to recover but go on to develop chronic CFS-like symptoms.[21] So we have an additional short-term stressor that may be able to initiate cases of CFS that may also be able produce increases in nitric oxide and peroxynitrite.

The ciguatoxin connection with NMDA activity is complex. Ciguatoxin is known to delay closing of a sodium channel in the nervous system,[23] a channel that is inhibitable by a toxin known as tetrodotoxin. Such delayed closing leads to increased sodium influx and such increased sodium influx into certain neuronal cells is known to increase NMDA activity by multiple mechanisms.[24-29] Indeed, the brevatoxins, which are very similar to ciguatoxin in both structure and toxic mechanism, are known to produce a similar sodium influx and known to produce consequent increased NMDA activity.[28,29] It seems highly likely, therefore, that ciguatoxin must produce a similar NMDA increase with consequent increases in nitric oxide levels, but that has not been directly studied, to my knowledge.

Additional short-term stressors may have roles in initiating cases of CFS. For example, in the review of De Meirleir et al.[30] a table of onset factors in "total CFS" listed infections, including upper respiratory tract, flulike illnesses, viral, bacterial, mononucleosis, pneumonia, gastrointestinal (GI) tract infections, hepatitis, CMV, toxoplasmosis (a protozoan infection, also known to produce increased nitric oxide[31-33]) and meningitis infections as preceding the majority of the CFS cases. They also list severe psychological stress/trauma in 10.6 percent of the CFS cases and physical trauma caused by a vehicle accident or surgical procedure in 9.7 percent of the cases. Other sources report a similar list of short-term stressors. For example, Bell[33] describes several CFS "trigger events" in addition to viral infections, including physical trauma from surgery, physical injury or automobile accident, emotional stress, and certain types of chemical exposures. Physical trauma and severe psychological stress are additional stressors that can act to increase nitric oxide.[16] These same stressors are common in MCS, FM, and PTSD, as we will see in Chapters 7 to 9.

---

*Ciguatoxin is a toxin found in certain tropical fish when ciguatera dinoflagellate organisms producing the toxin are found in their food chain. Poisoning due to ciguatoxin is fairly common in certain tropical areas but rare in most other parts of the world.

So we have a list of eight different short-term stressors each of which is reported to precede and presumably initiate certain cases CFS and seven of which are known to lead to increases in nitric oxide, with the eighth (ciguatoxin) likely to do so as well.

1. Viral infections
2. Bacterial infections
3. A protozoan infection, toxoplasmosis
4. Carbon monoxide exposure
5. Physical trauma
6. Organophosphorus poisoning
7. Severe psychological stress
8. Ciguatoxin poisoning

I have discussed here some of what is known about the mechanisms that may lead to increased nitric oxide in infections, ciguatoxin poisoning, and carbon monoxide poisoning. I will discuss mechanisms for the other stressors producing nitric oxide increases in Chapters 7, 8, and 9. What is striking is that we have eight stressors that are either established or proposed to initiate cases of CFS, and seven of them are documented to be able lead to increases in nitric oxide and the eighth (ciguatoxin) is expected to do so as well. The question the reader needs to ask is whether this is coincidental? If this is not the explanation for their common role in initiation of cases of CFS, what is the explanation?

I first proposed that viral and bacterial infections act to initiate CFS cases by increasing nitric oxide levels in my first CFS paper[13] published in January 2000 at the beginning of the new millennium. Since then, no one has tried to argue, to my knowledge, that this increase in nitric oxide produced by these stressors is just coincidental. As other short-term stressors apparently involved in CFS and other multisystem illnesses are shown to also increase nitric oxide levels, any argument that this pattern of evidence is just coincidental becomes progressively more difficult to make. Furthermore, if the NO/ONOO⁻ cycle mechanism is not the explanation for the chronic nature for CFS, then we need an alternative explanation, one that explains such puzzles as the diverse symptoms of signs that were discussed in Chapter 3.

Case Definitions of CFS: What Is Chronic Fatigue Syndrome?

The most commonly used case definition in studies of CFS is the 1994 CDC case definition.[35] This definition requires severe fatigue of at least six months duration with definite onset (not lifelong) together with four or more of the following:

1. Impaired memory or concentration
2. Sore throat
3. Tender lymph nodes
4. Muscle pain
5. Multijoint pain
6. Headaches
7. Unrefreshing sleep
8. Postexertional malaise

As I pointed out in Chapter 4, the substantial variation of symptoms from one case to another has produced a rationale for this consensus case definition to allow much variation in the symptoms used for inclusion of individual patients. There are also several exclusionary criteria, which exclude patients diagnosed with diseases such as untreated hypothyroidism, hepatitis infection, major depressive disorder and a number of other psychiatric disorders, malignancy, or alcohol abuse. The idea here is that if there is a known disease present that can explain the symptoms of CFS, then that disease is an exclusionary criterion. I would add, however, that it is possible that some of the patients excluded may suffer from illness essentially identical to CFS, but until we have a specific biomarker for CFS, we are unable to determine that. The problem here is that most of the symptoms of CFS also occur widely in other medical conditions and, consequently, are not individually specific diagnostic criteria.

The one apparent exception to this issue of specificity may be that of postexertional malaise, a symptom that is central to the newer Canadian[36] criteria for CFS diagnosis. These Canadian criteria are designed as diagnostic criteria in medical practice, and are distinct in this way from the CDC criteria that were designed as case definition criteria for determining possible inclusion of specific patients in clinical studies of CFS. The Canadian criteria center much more specifically on postexertional malaise as a key, perhaps *the* key diagnostic feature. Postexertional malaise is the very substantial exacerbation of symptoms of CFS patients, following exercise, typically lasting at least 24 hours. The exercise involved, can be quite modest, depending on the severity of the CFS case. I think one of the important questions that needs to be asked, and I will ask it at the end of this chapter, is whether this phenomenon of postexertional malaise may allow us to develop a specific biomarker for CFS.

CFS has often been called myalgic encephalomyelitis (ME) in the United Kingdom, and there has been considerable controversy over this illness in that country. Much of that controversy has surrounded a case definition for CFS[37] developed by a group of psychiatrists in the United Kingdom, called the Oxford case definition, which is thought to include many more patients with major depression instead of using major depression as an exclusionary criterion. Clearly, lumping in patients with major depression with others who may have "true" CFS/ME will lead to confusing results in studies of such a mixed group of patients. There have been a number of studies that have reported that the changes of hypothalamic-pituitary-adrenal (HPA) axis function in CFS cases (defined by the CDC criteria) are opposite those seen in major depression and that other properties differ between the two conditions,[38] showing that these are distinct illnesses.

The estimates of the prevalence of CFS have been highly variable and it has often been stated that the best such estimate is that of Jason et al.[39] who estimated a prevalence of about 0.42 percent among Chicago area individuals. I will argue in Chapter 11 that this figure is probably low. Only about 10 percent of diagnosed CFS cases have a complete recovery from the illness although partial recoveries are more common,[34,38] and so the impact on public health of this illness is considerable.

Evidence for the NO/ONOO⁻ Cycle Mechanism of CFS

In considering a complex illness like CFS and its possible cause by the NO/ONOO⁻ cycle mechanism, it is important to distinguish between specific observations that may support this etiology and explanations that provide a possible understanding for the puzzling features of the illness. I have already discussed explanations for many of the overlapping symptoms and signs of CFS and related illnesses in Chapter 3. Sixteen out of 17 of these symptoms and signs can be readily explained through the NO/ONOO⁻ cycle mechanism. The tremendous variation in symptoms and signs from one case to another was explained in Chapter 4. These explanations are to be distinguished from specific observations on CFS that provide evidence for this etiologic mechanism. There are 14 types of such specific observations, three of which relate to the initiation of CFS cases and the other eleven relate to what may be called the chronic phase of the illness, the only phase that can be directly studied in humans. The three on initiation (numbers 1 through 3) are discussed in this chapter. The others (numbers 4 to 14) that focus on the chronic phase have been discussed in my publications,[13,16,40-44] and I will discuss each of these here as well.

1. Of eight stressors listed earlier as apparent inducers of CFS or candidate inducers, seven appear to be able to act to produce an increase in nitric oxide and the eighth is expected to do so as well.

2. Three specific genes and one set of genes are implicated in CFS. Two of these may act by producing increases in nitric oxide, and the other two may act by producing increases in superoxide. Because the genetics provides clear evidence for a causal role, and because most cases of CFS never fully recover, these genes presumably must act to increase the frequency of initiation of CFS.

3. An animal (mouse) model of CFS has fatigue induced by a bacterial extract[45-48] reported to induce both inflammatory cytokines and also the inducible nitric oxide synthase (iNOS),[49,50] providing further evidence for a key role of excessive nitric oxide in the initiation of CFS.*

4. Two studies, the first published by the author[41] and the second by Kurup and Kurup[51] have shown that nitric oxide levels are significantly elevated in the chronic phase of CFS.

5. A number of studies have reported that inflammatory cytokines that are involved in our vicious cycle and can induce the inducible nitric oxide synthase have elevated levels in CFS.[42,52] Most of these studies show relatively modest elevation, which in some cases fail to reach statistical significance.[52] Perhaps the most elevated of those cytokines is IL-8, based on a study of changed in genetic activity in CFS.[53] It has been observed that etiology CFS is not dominated by the action of these cytokines,[54,55] since they have only modest elevations, but it seems reasonable that they may act along with other aspects of our vicious cycle to generate the symptoms of CFS.

6. Three of five studies of neopterin levels, a marker of high-level induction of iNOS, reported a statistically significant elevation in CFS versus controls.[13]

7. A series of studies from several laboratories in Europe, the United States, and Australia have reported elevated levels of markers of oxidative stress in CFS. There are two basic paradigms for the generation of oxidative stress, one involving Fenton[†] chemistry and the other involving peroxynitrite. Given the evidence from numbers 4 through 6, mentioned here, and 9 and 11, mentioned later, implicating elevated levels of nitric oxide in the chronic phase of CFS, it seems likely that

---

*Also discussed in Chapter 1.

[†]Fenton chemistry is based on the role of iron ions in generating free radicals. It is usually considered to be distinct in mechanism from that involving peroxynitrite, although they there is some overlap, because superoxide has a key role in both.

peroxynitrite is most likely to be involved, with nitric oxide acting as its precursor. I will discuss the studies of oxidative stress in some detail in the following text.

8. It is reported that cyst(e)ine levels are depleted in CFS[56] and, in addition, that glutathione levels are also depleted.[56,57] Presumably the cyst(e)ine depletion is caused by the utilization of its reduced form, cysteine, to regenerate the lost glutathione. Because glutathione depletion is thought to be a universal consequence of oxidative stress and because reduced glutathione is the most important antioxidant produced in the body, such glutathione depletion provides evidence both for oxidative stress and for the important likely biological impact of oxidative stress in CFS (see the following text).

9. Hydroxocobalamin (a form of vitamin B_{12}) injections have been used to treat CFS and CFS-like illnesses for over 60 years and have been reported to be effective in such treatment in a placebo-controlled trial (discussed in Chapter 6). Given that hydroxocobalamin is known to be a potent nitric oxide scavenger,[42] and a number of observations suggest that it is not acting primarily to allay a B_{12} deficiency, these results provide evidence supporting an important role for elevated levels of nitric oxide in CFS.

10. Mitochondrial and energy metabolism dysfunction has been reported in CFS in a series of different studies, presumably leading to lowered oxygen utilization in tissues (discussed in detail in the following). It is known that peroxynitrite can attack a number of components in mitochondria, leading to inactivation of key enzymes. In addition, nitric oxide and superoxide are also known to inhibit certain mitochondrial functions,* providing the only current plausible explanation that I am aware of for the reported mitochondrial dysfunction.

11. Placebo-controlled and other trials, described in the section on fatigue in Chapter 3, each aimed at improving mitochondrial function in CFS and CFS-like illnesses, all reported statistically significant improvements in fatigue and other symptoms of CFS, thus providing evidence for a causal role of mitochondrial dysfunction in these illnesses. There are other important observations on the therapy of CFS that support a NO/ONOO⁻ cycle mechanism and are discussed in the therapy chapter (Chapter 15).

12. The compound *cis*-aconitate and its precursor citrate are both[58,59] reported to be elevated in CFS. Both of these elevations can be explained

---

*Mitochondrial mechanisms for peroxynitrite, nitric oxide, and superoxide were discussed in Chapters 2 and 3.

by the NO/ONOO⁻ cycle mechanism. The enzyme aconitase is known to be inactivated by peroxynitrite and inhibited by both nitric oxide and superoxide (Reference 13 and Chapter 2). A lowering of its activity is expected to produce accumulations of both *cis*-aconitate and its precursor citrate. I also discussed earlier[13] two reports that another enzyme in mitochondria, succinate dehydrogenase, which is also a presumed target of peroxynitrite-mediated inactivation, also appears to be low in CFS, providing further support for predictions of the NO/ONOO⁻ cycle.

13. Clinical observations by Cheney,[60,61] Goldstein,[62] and by Kurup and Kurup[51] suggest that NMDA activity is elevated in CFS, providing some evidence for this important element of the NO/ONOO⁻ cycle mechanism. For example, Cheney is quoted as stating[60] (p. 39): "I do not know of a single drug which down-regulates NMDA receptor firing that has not been helpful in CFIDS." An important role for excessive NMDA in CFS may help explain the reported action of magnesium supplements in improving the symptoms of CFS,[63,64] given the key role of magnesium ions in modulating the activity of the NMDA receptors, as discussed in Chapter 2.

14. The arsenical drug, thiacetarsamide, has been reported by Tarello[65,66] to cure certain animal models of CFS. We have found in unpublished data that thiacetarsamide acts as a scavenger for both nitric oxide and peroxynitrite, providing evidence supporting a central role of these two compounds in the etiology of CFS.

In all complex biological systems, you have to look at the pattern of evidence available, because many different individual observations can be interpreted in alternative ways so only such a pattern may produce compelling support for a specific mechanism. Certainly, CFS qualifies as being such a complex system and the 14 types of evidence listed earlier can each be interpreted in other ways or be viewed as being just coincidental or the experimental observations themselves may be questioned. The pattern seen here is much more difficult to dismiss. When this pattern is reinforced by the set of proposed mechanisms for the overlapping symptoms and signs, discussed in Chapter 3, as well as other data from these related illnesses to be discussed below, I would argue that the pattern of evidence is quite compelling.

The pattern presented here is important not only because of its theoretical importance regarding the etiology of CFS but also because of what it suggests for effective therapy. Numbers 8, 9, and 12 through 14 have obvious implications with regard to therapy and several others suggest therapeutic approaches that may be less obvious.

Oxidative Stress in CFS

There are now at least 13 studies reporting elevated markers of oxidative stress in CFS.[43,51,63,67-76] A large number of such markers have been studied and reported to show changes indicative of oxidative stress ranging from antioxidant depletion, protein carbonyl elevation, elevation of lipid peroxides and TBARS,* increased methemoglobin levels as well as several others. This area of research has been led by the University of Newcastle group in Australia[68-70] as well as by groups in Italy, Belgium, France, and Scotland in Europe[63,67,71-75] and one group in India.[51] Ours is the only study conducted in the United States,[43] to my knowledge. It is quite possible that increased oxidative stress is the best documented marker of CFS, albeit a nonspecific one. The recent study by Jammes et al.[74] reports that oxidative stress markers are more impacted by exercise in CFS patients, as compared with controls. Given the importance of postexertional malaise in CFS, one wonders whether this may be a specific biomarker for CFS—I will discuss this issue further in the second to last section of this chapter.

Bounos and Molson suggested that depletion of the antioxidant glutathione is central to the etiology of CFS.[57] While there have been reports of glutathione depletion and there is no question of the importance of glutathione as an antioxidant, glutathione depletion alone is not a good candidate for the mechanism of CFS. For one thing, glutathione depletion occurs in any condition that generates oxidative stress, but clearly they do not all lead to CFS. In addition, glutathione depletion does not explain the chronic nature of CFS, since glutathione levels should recover over time in the absence of any other cause for oxidative stress.

I suggest that the oxidative stress is most likely generated by peroxynitrite and its breakdown products as well as by superoxide, each of which should be elevated according to the NO/ONOO$^-$ cycle. One of the questions that should be raised is whether antioxidant therapy will be useful in CFS. An animal model of CFS reports that antioxidant therapy is useful in the treatment of that model,[76] and there is one review[77] and three additional reports in humans[57,78,79] all suggesting that antioxidant therapy may be useful

---

*Protein carbonyls, lipid peroxides, and TBARS are all easily measured chemical markers of oxidative stress. TBARS stands for thiobarbituric reacting substances, which measures the amounts of certain aldehyde products of membrane oxidation.

in CFS patients. Antioxidant therapy of CFS should be increasingly studied, in my judgment, along with other approaches to down-regulate NO/ONOO⁻ cycle biochemistry.

Mitochondrial/Energy Metabolism Dysfunction in CFS

There have also been a long series of studies reporting mitochondrial and energy metabolism dysfunction in CFS. These have also been of great interest to me because of the substantial role of peroxynitrite and also both superoxide and nitric oxide on mitochondrial function.[13]* Some of these studies go back 15 years or so and they range over a wide variety of measurements that provide various types of evidence for such dysfunction.

For example, Behan et al.[80] reported that the mitochondrial ultrastructure in the muscles of people with postviral fatigue syndrome was aberrant. Plioplys and Plioplys[81] reported that serum levels of both carnitine and acylcarnitine were low in CFS, and this observation was confirmed by Kuratsune et al.[82] Given the specific roles of carnitine in mitochondria, these results provide support for the inference that mitochondrial function is aberrant in CFS. Wong et al.[83] reported that the levels of high energy phosphate compounds phosphocreatine and ATP were low in the muscle of CFS patients, using ^{31}P NMR methods for these measurements. These results provide direct evidence for energy metabolism dysfunction in the muscles of CFS patients. Barnes et al.[84] reported lowered ability to regenerate phosphocreatine in the muscles of significant number of CFS patients. McCully et al.[85] also reported lowered regeneration of phosphocreatine in muscle of CFS patients caused by reduced oxidative metabolism in the muscle, again providing evidence of energy metabolism dysfunction. Vecchiet et al.[86] reported a number of mitochondrial aberrations, including aberrations in mitochondrial ultrastructure, providing some support for the earlier study (see preceding text), as well as changes in some mitochondrial enzyme activities and a large increase in deletions occurring in the mitochondrial DNA. Deletions in mitochondrial DNA are generated by hydroxyl radical,[87] a breakdown product of peroxynitrite (Chapter 2), and so such increases in deleted mitochondrial DNA in CFS are consistent with a NO/ONOO⁻ cycle mechanism.

The inference that there is mitochondrial/energy metabolism dysfunction in CFS is further supported by a number of studies reporting lowered oxygen utilization in the tissues.[85,88,89] Because over 90 percent of the oxygen utilized in human tissues is normally used to provide oxygen for mito-

---

*Discussed earlier in Chapters 2 and 3.

chondrial cytochrome oxidase activity and subsequent ATP generation, lowered oxygen utilization provides good evidence for mitochondrial dysfunction.

These observations provide evidence for mitochondrial or energy metabolism dysfunction. Two observations specifically relate to the NO/ ONOO⁻ cycle mechanism. Peroxynitrite is known to attack a number of iron-sulfur proteins in mitochondria and elsewhere, including the enzymes aconitase and succinate dehydrogenase. There is evidence suggesting that both of these enzymes are dysfunctional in CFS. The evidence for aconitase dysfunction is the finding that both *cis*-aconitate[58] and citrate[59] appear to accumulate in CFS. Lowered succinate dehydrogenase activity was reported in two studies of mitochondrial enzymes in CFS (reviewed in Reference 13). These observations, then, provide support for a role of excessive peroxynitrite in generation of mitochondrial dysfunction in CFS. Mitochondrial dysfunction in CFS was also recently supported by a study of gene expression in CFS, suggesting both mitochondrial and neuronal dysfunction.[90]

The observations that most directly implicate mitochondrial dysfunction in generating the symptoms of CFS are the clinical studies aimed at improving mitochondrial function. There have been two types of these, one type using individual agents such as carnitine or acylcarnitine to improve mitochondrial function[91,92] and a second type using more complex combinations of agents including lipid precursors and antioxidants[93,94] to allow regeneration of the mitochondrial inner membrane (from damage presumably mainly produced by superoxide). There are clinical observations reporting that supplements of coenzyme Q10, a compound that has a key role in mitochondrial function, also lower the symptoms of CFS.[34] It should be noted that there is a substantial literature reporting that coenzyme Q10 is useful in the treatment of a number of bona fide mitochondrial dysfunction diseases. These observations suggest that therapy aimed at improving mitochondrial function should be a key element in an overall strategy for CFS therapy.

Genetic Evidence for Mechanism

Genetics is a very powerful approach to determine biological mechanism, because a demonstrated role of particular genes in a biological response is definitive in establishing a causal role of the protein produced by the gene involved. Depending on the function of that protein, such studies can help establish important aspects of the mechanisms of the biological process. Consequently, evidence for a role of specific genes in CFS should be able to provide important insights into the mechanism of CFS.

Some types of evidence for genetic involvement in CFS are of general interest but are not very useful in testing specific possible mechanisms. These include twin studies, which provide evidence for a genetic role in CFS[95,96] but do not identify the specific genes involved. A second type of study implicated one or more genes linked to the histocompatibility genes,[97] but again did not identify which specific genes are involved.

Rather, we will be looking at evidence identifying a specific gene as influencing the prevalence of CFS. Five such studies have collectively identified three specific genes[98-101] and also a set of functionally closely related genes[102] in CFS. I will consider each of these three specific genes and also the role of a set of related genes.

One gene implicated is the corticosteroid-binding globulin (CBG) gene, which is closely associated with CFS in an Australian family study.[98,99] In these Australian studies, defective function of the CBG protein was associated with CFS, and given the role of this protein in the transport and subsequent function of cortisol, it appears likely that defective cortisol function may be involved in predisposing these individuals to develop CFS. Cortisol has a key role in lowering the induction of the inducible nitric oxide synthase (iNOS), as discussed in my first paper on CFS,[13] and lowered cortisol function may be expected, therefore, to produce increased levels of nitric oxide. It may be seen from this that the role the defective CBG gene in producing CFS is consistent with a predicted central role of elevated nitric oxide in CFS. The role of this gene and the next one to be considered in the possible mechanism of CFS is outlined in Figure 5.1.

The next gene that is apparently involved in CFS is the serotonin transporter gene,[100] where forms of the gene apparently associated with in-

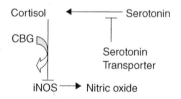

Putative Role of Two Genes in CFS:
Control of Cortisol and iNOS

FIGURE 5.1. Putative role of serotonin transporter gene and cortisol-binding globulin (CBG) gene in CFS. Cortisol inhibits the induction of iNOS and therefore may act to lower nitric oxide. Both serotonin and CBG act to stimulate this process, and therefore both the serotonin transporter gene and the CBG gene have the potential to influence nitric oxide levels by influencing cortisol activity.

creased transport and consequent lowered extracellular serotonin levels are associated with increased prevalence of CFS. This was proposed by the authors to lead to decreased HPA axis function,[100] which will lead, in turn, to lowered cortisol secretion. So here again we have a genetic influence that has been predicted to lead to lowered cortisol function and given the role of cortisol in regulating iNOS induction, may be predicted to increase nitric oxide levels. These mechanisms are also outlined in Figure 5.1.

There is a third gene to be discussed here, implicated in the prevalence of CFS, is the angiotensin converting enzyme (ACE) gene.[101] A polymorphism of this gene was studied for its association with both CFS and idiopathic chronic fatigue among Gulf War veterans and was shown to have a highly statistically significant role.[101] This study may be viewed as implicating excessive superoxide in CFS, because angiotensin II, the protein produced by the ACE protein, acts to increase superoxide, which acts, in turn, to increase vasoconstriction.[102,103] This genetic study supports the role of another element in the NO/ONOO$^-$ cycle, superoxide, in the initiation of CFS.

The fourth genetic type of genetic study to be considered here is the report from Rowe's laboratory that both orthostatic intolerance and chronic fatigue syndrome are associated with Ehlers-Danlos syndrome.[104] Ehlers Danlos syndrome is a collection of genetic diseases each caused by a mutation in a subunit of the protein collagen or an enzyme that modifies the structure of collagen.[105-107] As a consequence of the mutation, collagen, which is the predominant structural protein in the body, is dysfunctional. The most likely connection here may be with orthostatic intolerance and CFS, as I discussed in an earlier paper.[40] Ehlers-Danlos mutations often affect vasculature, leading to decreased effective perfusion of the elevated tissues of the body and therefore with tissue hypoxia in these tissues. Tissue hypoxia, as I discussed earlier[40] and in Chapter 1, can lead to increased generation of superoxide, which may then stimulate the production of peroxynitrite. It follows that the reported role of Ehlers-Danlos syndrome in CFS may also be consistent with the NO/ONOO$^-$ cycle mechanism and specifically with superoxide involvement.

I would like to say, in summarizing this genetic analysis, that the NO/ONOO$^-$ cycle mechanism for these illnesses is sufficiently complex such that quite a number of genetic mechanisms may be expected to interact with it and therefore quite a number of genetic observations may be consistent with it. Therefore, it would be a mistake to try to overstate the implications of these studies as to how strongly they support our mechanism. However, the apparent close connection of these genes to mechanisms involved in nitric oxide or superoxide synthesis do provide substantive support for the proposed mechanism, support of a type that has not been forthcoming for any alternative CFS mechanisms.

The genetic studies provide a third type of evidence implicating nitric oxide in the initiation of cases of CFS; the three types are:

1. Of the eight initiators or candidate initiators of CFS, seven are known to be able to increase nitric oxide levels and the eighth is likely to do so as well.
2. A bacterial extract that initiates cases of an animal model of CFS is known to also increase nitric oxide levels by inducing the iNOS gene.
3. Specific genes implicated in CFS initiation all may act to influence nitric oxide or superoxide levels.

Collectively, these provide very strong support for a key role of nitric oxide and possibly peroxynitrite in the initiation of cases of CFS.

Additional Biochemical Correlates: Consistent with Theory?

There are a number of additional biochemical or other measurable changes that have been reported in CFS, and one question that can be raised is whether these are consistent with the NO/ONOO⁻ cycle theory. The question raised here is in the same spirit of the similar questions raised about common symptoms and signs of these multisystem illnesses. Do we have plausible mechanisms that may provide an explanation for the observed changes? We are looking here plausible explanations, not for demonstrated mechanisms.

There are some observations for which we do not have enough information to even ask this question. For example, the University of Newcastle group in Australia reported that the level of a compound originally unidentified and called CFSUM1[58,108] and later determined to be pyroglutamate[109] was elevated in the urine of CFS patients versus controls. There is no discussion in the literature that I have been able to find on the synthesis of this compound in biological tissues, and so we have no way of assessing why its levels may be elevated in CFS. Similarly, an unidentified compound (or compounds) was measured and shown to be elevated in the sera of CFS patients as well as those with hepatitis and cancer.[110] It was assayed using an immunoassay for ciguatoxin, showing that it had an epitope similar to that of ciguatoxin. However, no structure has been determined for the compound involved and no biological activity has been established for it,[110] so its possible origin cannot be assessed.

For a number of other changes, we can, however, suggest possible mechanisms. For example, it is reported that C-reactive protein levels are elevated in CFS[111] and C-reactive protein levels are reported to be increased in response to nitric oxide[112] and possibly in response to oxidative stress and antioxidant depletion,[112] providing two plausible explanations consistent with the NO/ONOO⁻ cycle mechanism.

The polyunsaturated fatty acids in mammals are all essential fatty acids due to our inability to biosynthesize them except, in some cases, from other polyunsaturated fatty acids. These are reported to be depleted in the membranes of CFS patients.[114,115] Typically, the membranes of red blood cells have been used for these studies. These essential fatty acids are known to be 20 to 100 times more susceptible to oxidation during lipid peroxidation than are monounsaturated fatty acids. If follows that, under conditions of oxidative stress, such lipid peroxidation will lead to selective depletion of essential fatty acids. Peroxynitrite and superoxide can initiate lipid peroxidation, as discussed in Chapter 2. I suggested, therefore, in my first paper on CFS, that the depletion of essential fatty acids was probably a consequence of lipid peroxidation initiated by peroxynitrite and possibly superoxide.[13]

A number of other puzzling features of CFS also appear to be explainable by our NO/ONOO⁻ cycle mechanism. For example, Berg et al.[116,117] reported both the presence of antiphospholipid antibodies in CFS and FM and also increased blood coagulation. Phospholipids being relatively small molecules are expected to be unable to generate antibodies unless they are covalently linked to macromolecules, particularly proteins—in other words, they should act like haptens. The best-documented mechanism for the crosslinking of phospholipids to proteins is lipid peroxidation, whereby the lipid oxidation products can be cross-linked to lysine and other residues on proteins. The prediction, then, is that the formation of antiphospholipid antibodies should be correlated with lipid peroxidation, and that prediction has been confirmed.[118,119] The increased blood coagulation reported by Berg et al.[117] may also be explained through the reported role of oxidative stress on blood coagulation.[120,121]

Chaudhuri et al.[122] suggested that CFS is characterized by what they described as "channelopathies," in which ion channels and transporters are dysfunctional leading to changes in important ion concentrations, particularly potassium and calcium. Mechanisms here may involve peroxynitrite inhibition of the major potassium transporter, the Na-K-ATPase[123,124] as well as the major calcium pump in the cell (discussed in Chapter 1). In addition, a number of ion channels are reported to be blocked by peroxynitrite.[126]

One other issue: Dr. Paul Cheney has suggested that cardiomyopathy, damage to the heart muscle, may occur in some of the most severe cases of CFS,[125] possibly through mechanisms similar or identical to those of the NO/ONOO⁻ cycle. It follows that it is possible that one of the important locations of that cycle in CFS may be the heart in some of the more severe CFS cases. While there is limited data on this, this may be an exciting area of future research.

It can be seen from the above discussion, that several of the biochemical correlates of CFS appear to be consistent with our nitric oxide/peroxynitrite vicious cycle mechanism but that there are others where more information is needed, in order to make a judgment on consistency.

37 kDa RNase L

Another biochemical correlate where more information is needed to judge consistency, is the elevated levels of the 37 kDa RNase L protein found in the peripheral blood mononuclear cells* of many CFS patients. This protein was first described by Suhadolnik and colleagues and shown to be present at elevated levels in CFS patients versus controls.[127-130] While there are some CFS patients who do not show elevated levels and there are some controls who do show elevated levels, the 37 kDa RNase L appears to come closer to being a specific biomarker for CFS than are most other possible markers and may be, therefore, of substantial interest,[128,131] at least in the direct comparison of CFS patients versus normal controls. One of the important issues is whether this protein is elevated in other illnesses, and there is only one study, to my knowledge, reporting on this issue. That study reported that the 37 kDa RNase L was not substantially elevated in FM patients.[131,132] It is important, in my judgment, to repeat this study and also to look the level of this protein in a variety of other illnesses. Such studies are essential in order to make a case for specificity.

The 37 kDa RNase L is produced in the cells of the immune system by proteolytic clipping of a larger protein, the 80 kDa RNAse L.[130,133] A little over half of the 80 kDa RNAse L is removed by some protease that clips a bond connecting the two parts together, separating the 37 kDa section from the rest of the molecule. One key issue is what protease is involved in this clipping and whether its role is consistent with the NO/ONOO⁻ cycle mechanism. While the major protease involved has not been identified, a good candidate for that role is the protease calpain,[133] an intracellular calcium-

---

*These PBMCs are a particular type of cell of the immune system.

dependent protease. Because one of the mechanisms of the NO/ONOO cycle is the increase in intracellular calcium levels, which are predicted to stimulate calpain activity, it is possible that the clipping involved may be produced as a consequence of our vicious cycle in this manner. There may be other consistent mechanisms, as well. So here is an area where there may be a consistency with the NO/ONOO⁻ cycle but where more data are needed to make that judgment.

The 37 kDa RNase L may have a substantial role in generating changes in the immune system in CFS.

Opportunistic Infections

There have been a series of different studies reporting the occurrence of what are presumably opportunistic infections in CFS and related illnesses (i.e., FM and Gulf War syndrome). The infections reportedly include mycoplasma, chlamydia, the herpes virus HHV-6, as well as an enterovirus infection.[134-141] When I say these are presumably opportunistic, the evidence shows that each of these infections occurs only in some CFS patients and that they also occur in some normal controls, albeit at lower frequencies. Thus, they appear to be common infectious agents in the population, often with no obvious symptoms associated with infection, but are more common in CFS and related illnesses.

I discussed some of the evidence for immune system changes in these illnesses in Chapter 3, changes that may be generated in part by oxidants including superoxide and possibly peroxynitrite. Nitric oxide also influences the cells of the immune system. It is plausible, then, that some changes of the immune system may cause people with these illnesses to be more susceptible to these infections than are normals.

Should these infections be treated? Quite possibly. One would expect that these infections may exacerbate the symptoms of CFS and even NO/ONOO⁻ cycle mechanisms, through increased generation of inflammatory cytokines, and therefore one would expect that treatment should improve the symptoms.

Subsets in CFS

At the 2004 AACFS meeting, there was a section of the meeting dedicated to three talks on possible subsets of CFS patients. All three speakers declared their belief in subsets and all thought that the "identification" of such subsets was essential in order for the scientific studies on CFS to progress. None of the three speakers made clear what exactly the possible existence of subsets might mean.

The concept of subsets comes straight out of a mathematical theory, known as set theory. In mathematics, an unambiguous rule, or group of rules can be used to classify individual objects as being either within or without a defined set. The set of human beings or *Homo sapiens,* for example, can be identified by the rules of biological classification. That set, can in turn, be divided into discrete subsets, either overlapping or nonoverlapping by other unambiguous rules, such as divided into males and females or into children, adolescents and adults. Similarly, CFS may be defined by all those meeting the 1994 CDC case definition (the set of CFS patients) and two subsets can be defined as those either meeting or not meeting the diagnostic criteria for irritable bowel syndrome (IBS). If you wish, instead of using IBS to define subsets, you can use FM, asthma, migraine headaches, or any of a large number of other parameters to define various subsets. In this mathematical sense, there is no question that there are subsets of CFS patients, and there are thousands of them, each depending on specific, unambiguous rules to divide up the CFS patients. So, the proclaimed existence of subsets of CFS patients is a trivial point and there is no difficulty "identifying" such subsets.

What the speakers at the AACFS meeting seem to be suggesting but did not state clearly, and some others who have taken similarly unclear positions as well, is not only that there are the subsets but that these may reflect *distinct etiologic mechanisms.* Etiology is a very different issue and one that needs to be considered on its merits. In other words, they seem to be suggesting that there exist subsets of CFS patients who resemble type 1 and type 2 diabetes, where these two types of diabetes clearly reflect largely different diseases with largely different etiologic mechanisms. They may be right in suggesting this but I question that and currently, at least, we have no convincing evidence that they are right. The distinct, qualitative, and preexisting differences between type 1 and type 2 diabetes cases differs from some other types of subsets studied in medicine. For example, there are many studies comparing obese versus non-obese individuals, with obese individuals often being defined as those having body mass indexes (BMIs) above 30 (the precise meaning of this is not important here). Such studies are useful in medicine even though no one is claiming that obese people are qualitatively different from non-obese (and indeed, some individuals may move from the obese subset to the non-obese or vice versa). The cutoff of 30 is arbitrary, but it allows one to divide people into two less heterogeneous subsets and allows the study of the influence of body weight on a number of important medical problems. Subsets are often useful in decreasing the heterogeneity of groups of people to be studied and in identifying parameters that may be biologically and medically important. But they do not necessarily imply etiologic distinctions. The question that must be raised, then, is whether or not subsets of CFS patients differ from each other in terms of the basic etiology of their illnesses.

My own position, as I stated in Chapter 4, is that the tremendous heterogeneity that one sees in CFS as well as in other multisystem illnesses, is generated, in large measure, by variation in the tissue distribution of the underlying biochemistry. It follows that if this is true, then subsets of CFS patients may be useful in lowering the amount of heterogeneity within each subset but may not reflect any fundamental difference in the etiology of the subsets being studied.

What I would like to do, now, is to consider three impressive studies on the subset issue of CFS from excellent scientists, each of which appear to challenge my views on this subject. The first of these was written by Dunstan et al.[142] who clearly suggest, unlike some others, that the subsets they are studying may reflect distinct etiologic mechanisms. Dunstan et al.[142] establish their subsets by what is known as multivariate cluster analysis, using several parameters including dominant symptoms and certain aspects of urinary and lipid biochemistry to try to determine whether one can identify such covariance clusters, which *may* represent discrete, preexisting subsets of CFS patients. They provide substantive evidence for such clusters and describe them in terms of predominant features. For example, they describe three clusters, one characterized by localized pain, a second by gut dysfunction and a third by generalized pain. This is a very interesting study. I would suggest that these three clusters may represent differences in tissue distribution of the underlying biochemistry, with the first involving peripheral tissues and the spinal cord, as previously shown in hyperalgesia (Chapters 1 and 3), the second with major GI tract involvement (see Chapter 3), and the third involving central pain sensitization as has been proposed by others for FM (Chapter 8). It follows that these clusters or subsets of CFS patients may be explained by a single etiologic mechanism but with variable tissue distribution of the underlying biochemistry. I am not saying that I have proven this point, but simply that this type of analysis is insufficient to establish fundamental etiologic heterogeneity and that the variable properties may all be accounted by the tissues impacted in the different subsets.

Elsewhere in the Dunstan et al. article,[142] they report that sudden onset CFS cases could be distinguished from slow onset cases by cluster analysis as well, a distinction which I will return to shortly.

In a second cluster analysis study, Jason and Taylor[143] came up with two subsets, both showing severe postexertional malaise, emphasizing the importance of this symptom in CFS, with the two subsets distinguished by the severity of their overall symptoms. I ask whether the severity difference may be due to a quantitative higher level of the overall biochemistry or whether some specific region of the body may be responsible for generating the increased severity.

One other interesting study of subsets was published by Natelson's group,[143] where they reported that there were fairly consistent differences between sudden onset cases of CFS and slow onset cases. These results provide additional evidence for distinctions between these two subsets, when compared to the Dunstan study discussed earlier. Again, the question that needs to be raised is whether these groups of CFS patients simply differ from each other in the tissue distribution of their pathophysiology or whether they differ from each other in some more fundamental way. I would add, if there is any group of CFS individuals who do not fit the NO/ONOO⁻ cycle etiology, then the slow onset cases would be my best candidate—after all, those cases are not known to be initiated by a stressor that increases nitric oxide.

In summary, these three studies of CFS subsets do not establish that any of the described subsets are caused by distinct etiologies. They may all be explainable by variation of the tissue distribution of the underlying biochemistry.

SEARCH FOR A SPECIFIC BIOMARKER FOR CFS: POSTEXERTIONAL-MALAISE-RELATED RESPONSES

It has often been correctly observed that we are in need of specific biomarkers for each of these multisystem illnesses. Such biomarkers are valuable to verify, if that should still be necessary, that these are real physiological illnesses. Equally important, specific biomarkers for each of these illnesses would be invaluable as objectively measurable diagnostic criteria. I raise this issue elsewhere in this book, in the chapters on MCS and FM, asking where should we be looking to identify a specific biomarker for each of these illnesses.

One question that needs to be asked is why none of the changes I described here, occurring in CFS, have been developed into such a specific biomarker? The answer is that most of these changes are common changes that occur in many inflammatory diseases, including the increase in inflammatory cytokines, the increased neopterin, nitric oxide, oxidative stress, and the mitochondrial dysfunction. All of these are produced by what I have been calling inflammatory biochemistry, and all are expected to be elevated in many different inflammatory diseases. For example, they will be expected to be increased in such common medical conditions as atherosclerosis, infection, autoimmune diseases, allergies, asthma and gum inflammation. Consequently, many "normal" controls will tend to have elevated levels of these markers. Furthermore, given the wide variation of severity of these multisystem illnesses, many people fitting the case definitions for one of these illnesses, may well score in the normal range. Consequently, on average, these markers are reported to be elevated in CFS patients versus controls, but there is a wide variation within each of these groups and other inflammatory disease groups also may show similar elevation of these markers.

So where should we be looking for potential specific biomarkers for these illnesses? The obvious place to look is at consequences *directly related to the most characteristic symptom* or symptoms of each illness. In the case of CFS, the most characteristic symptom, as previously discussed, is postexertional malaise,[36] where modest exercise leads to an exacerbation of the whole spectrum of symptoms afflicting each CFS patient. My interpretation of this is that exercise leads to up-regulation of the basic biochemistry of the NO/ONOO⁻ cycle and that it is through such up-regulation that the exacerbation of symptoms occurs. This interpretation is supported by an early observation made by Dr. Melvin Ramsay in his pioneering observations of CFS,[145] who observed that those who persist in working the longest before they collapse have the poorest chance, while those who get early diagnosis and enforced bed rest have the best prognosis. From this viewpoint, one should emphasize two related questions: How might exercise lead to exacerbation of the NO/ONOO⁻ cycle biochemistry? And how might we use response to exercise in CFS patients to develop a specific biomarker for CFS?

I raised the second of these questions in a telephone conversation with Dr. Paul Cheney. I said that I thought we needed to look at aberrant responses to exercise in order to find a specific biomarker for CFS. His response was that he already had such an aberrant response in studies of his CFS patients versus controls. He finds that, when normal controls exercise, their cortisol levels increase substantially, but when his CFS patients exercise, their cortisol levels decrease. This was a fascinating response because cortisol has a general role in protecting the body from stressors. And Cheney reports that the response to the stressor exercise and in CFS patients produces a cortisol decrease rather than an increase.

Cortisol has the property that it, like other glucocorticoids, inhibits the induction of the inducible nitric oxide synthase (iNOS).[13] It follows from this that a cortisol deficiency after exercise may be expected to increase nitric oxide synthesis and therefore may be able to up-regulate the entire NO/ONOO⁻ cycle. We have here a possible interpretation for the exercise effect on postexertional malaise in CFS: Exercise in CFS as compared with controls may lead to lowered cortisol levels and therefore increases nitric oxide levels, exacerbating our vicious cycle biochemistry and therefore the whole spectrum of symptoms produced by that biochemistry. Because cortisol is a hormone secreted into the blood, its effect is expected to be systemic and the effect of its deficiency will also be systemic.

Cortisol is produced by the adrenal cortex and the adrenal cortex is controlled by what is known as the HPA axis. The control of cortisol secretion occurs as follows: several regions of the brain regulate the hypothalamus, which controls in turn the pituitary gland which controls in turn, the adrenal gland. Basically, what I am suggesting is that there is a specific region of the brain that is impacted in CFS which is responsible for the control of the hypothalamus in response to exercise. The consequent hypothamalic dysfunction after exercise produces HPA axis dysfunction and therefore lowered cortisol production following exercise.

Several types of evidence provide some support for this hypothesis. There are several studies reviewed earlier[146,147] that suggest that the HPA axis control is different in CFS than it is in FM, suggesting that there may be a specific aberration occurring in CFS. Perhaps the most relevant of the specific studies is that of Ottenweller et al.[148] who reported that the cortisol response to exercise was low in CFS, somewhat similar to the unpublished observations of Cheney, discussed above. Dinan et al.[149] reported that the adrenal glands of CFS patients were only about half the size of those of controls, a possible consequence of HPA axis dysfunction. The view expressed in this hypothesis is similar to that expressed earlier by Neeck and Crofford[150] (p. 989), who reported "abnormalities of central components of the HPA axis" in CFS. Similarities are also seen to the views of Torpy[151] (p. 1), who described "altered dynamic responses to stress, especially cortisol, to stimuli."

The relationship between postexertional malaise and hypocortisol responses in CFS has been discussed by Baschetti,[152] who recently reviewed several CFS studies on cortisol responses in CFS. Segal et al.[153] recently reported that their pediatric CFS patients showed lowered cortisol responses to low-dose synacthen tests, tests designed to monitor general HPA axis function. My own view is that it is that the cortisol response to exercise is more likely to be a specific aberration in CFS than are other more general changes in the HPA axis function. However, as Baschetti points out[152] people diagnosed as having CFS under the Oxford criteria will often not show this pattern and may be viewed, therefore, as not having true CFS.

If this lowered cortisol response to exercise leads to up-regulation of the NO/ONOO⁻ cycle, as suggested earlier in this section, this exercise-induced cycle up-regulation should lead to several predicted specific biomarkers for CFS. CFS sufferers should show increased levels of nitric oxide, oxidative stress, inflammatory cytokines, and perhaps other changes, in addition to the lowered cortisol levels after exercise. One of these predictions has already been reported. Jammes et al.[74] reported that markers of oxidative stress showed substantial increases after exercise in CFS patients but only modest increase in controls. LaManca et al.[154] reported much larger cognitive deficits after exercise in CFS patients as compared with controls.

There is one other puzzle about CFS that may be explainable through a dysfunction of exercise control of HPA axis function. Peckerman et al.[155,156] have reported on cardiac dysfunction in CFS and the control of cardiac function in response to exercise. Cheney[125] and personal communication also finds substantial cardiac dysfunction in the more severely affected CFS cases. Such cardiac dysfunction could be caused by local changes, such as the NO/ONOO⁻ cycle effects on the heart, but might also be caused by the inability to raise cortisol levels in response to exercise in CFS patients. There is a substantial literature reporting cardiac dysfunction being caused by lowered glucocorticoid levels both in humans and in animal models.[157-166] A recent study reported a particular role in the response of the heart to exercise.[157] Three studies reported specific left ventricular dysfunction in response to lowered glucocorticoid function.[159-161] Thus, it may well be the case that the cardiac dysfunction in the more severe cases of CFS may be caused by the inability to raise cortisol levels in response to exercise.*

The hypothesis that the most central dysfunction in CFS is the inability to produce normal cortisol control in response to exercise and possibly some other stressors provides some very promising leads to the possible development of specific biomarkers for CFS. Exercise is predicted to produce specific differences between CFS patients and controls, including decreased cortisol responses and increased elements of our NO/ONOO⁻ cycle, such as nitric oxide, oxidative stress markers and inflammatory cytokine levels. These are all easily testable and such tests may lead to the long-awaited establishment of specific biomarkers for CFS.

---

*In discussions with Dr. Cheney, he takes a different view. He argues that the cortisol depletion is more likely to be caused by the cardiac dysfunction, rather than the other way around. So, there is ample room for different interpretations for these observations.

PERSPECTIVE

When I started working on CFS, the mechanism I proposed was based initially on the role of nitric oxide in response to two stressors—viral infection and bacterial infection. Now, we have twelve stressors implicated to various extents in initiation of multisystem illnesses, all of which are known or predicted to lead to increased nitric oxide levels. Of these, eight are implicated in some cases of CFS. The CFS vicious cycle mechanism that I initially proposed[13] was based primarily on known biochemistry and physiology. There was essentially no consideration of the generation of symptoms and signs of CFS, no considerations of genetic evidence, and no consideration whatsoever of the other multisystem illnesses. Now, as you have seen in Chapter 3, the mechanisms of the NO/ONOO⁻ cycle mechanism fit very well with many of the diverse symptoms. Furthermore, as we shall see in subsequent chapters, the fit with the other multisystem illnesses is very good, and is especially striking in the case of MCS. This NO/ONOO⁻ cycle theory is the only detailed theory that explains this whole group of overlapping multisystem illnesses and thus provides an explanation for the overlaps and suggested etiologic similarities of this whole group of illnesses. In CFS, three of its key predictions have been confirmed—that nitric oxide levels are elevated, oxidative stress and mitochondrial dysfunction are found in CFS, and evidence has been published confirming several other predictions for the chronic phase of illness.

Having provided a proposed new paradigm for CFS, an illness that I would argue clearly needs a new paradigm in order to integrate its diverse features into one mechanism, I have been disappointed by the lack of scientific process in the field.* This is not just in response to my theory but much more generally. There is a process of debate and contention, which is an essential part of science that has been little evident in the CFS field.† For example, the first CFS meeting I attended was the 1998 AACFS meeting where there were talks in such areas as the immunology, microbiology, physiology, therapy, and psychology of CFS but no talks on how these all might fit together. In fact, there was little consideration of how to integrate these diverse observations. One thing that was striking was that there were talks supporting a somatization "mechanism" for CFS, which seemed to be

---

*Interestingly, this has not been true with MCS, in my experience, which, if anything, have been viewed as an even more challenging illness that CFS.

†An early volume on CFS[167] actually had quite a bit of interesting debate within it, but that spirit of active and spirited deliberation seems to have decreased quite substantially.

incompatible with the real, physiological measurements reported elsewhere, but there was no discussion or debate on whether these are compatible views and if not, who was right and who was wrong. This is in contrast to "hard science" areas that I have been involved in over the years, where such debate is important and evident. For example, I remember, when I was a young graduate student and went to my first major scientific meeting, two of the prominent scientists in the field having what was effect a debate on an area of contention between the two, and I remember thinking that this is what science is about. It has, at its core, the resolution of contention by presumably rational argument. This still goes on today. When I recently attended the Third International Conference on Peroxynitrite, there was a debate on the chemistry of peroxynitrite with one prominent scientist on one side and others taking a contrary position. It was all done politely, but there was no question that all of us at the meeting knew exactly what was going on and why it was important.

When I was first studying as a graduate student in the life sciences at Caltech, the faculty member in the biology division who probably was most widely respected in among that very prestigious group was Max Delbruck, who later went on to win the Nobel Prize. Max was completely unpretentious, he did not believe in hierarchy in science, and was absolutely committed to intellectual rigor. He would and often did seek people out if he thought someone knew something that he (Max) wanted to know, and it did not make any difference if that person was the greenest graduate student in the department. Conversely, if he thought an eminent seminar speaker was making a flawed presentation, he would ask pointed questions to reveal the flaw. He did not suffer fools gladly. Max also took a real joy in learning and sharing new ideas in science, even when those ideas had nothing to do with his own area of research. I still remember his being excited about the ideas of Peter Mitchell and what became known as the chemiosmotic theory, one of the two most important concepts in bioenergetics. He would go around sharing his excitement for what he called "Peter Mitchellism" because it was a new concept that made sense out of so many different puzzles of bioenergetics. We need a Max Delbruck in the CFS field.

It is my hope and expectation that, as the intellectual process of science progresses, the NO/ONOO⁻ cycle theory of CFS will triumph, but if it does not, so be it. Let the process proceed.

Chapter 6

Agents That Lower Nitric Oxide Levels Are Useful in the Treatment of Multisystem Illnesses: Hydroxocobalamin (Vitamin B_{12}) and Paroxetine

TAKE-HOME LESSONS

Long-term clinical observations and a placebo-controlled trial suggest that the hydroxocobalamin form of vitamin B_{12} is an effective treatment for chronic fatigue syndrome (CFS) but does not primarily act by allaying a B_{12} deficiency. Rather, it is known to act as a potent nitric oxide scavenger and may plausibly act in that role here. Clinical observations suggest that hydroxocobalamin is also useful in the treatment of fibromyalgia (FM) and multiple chemical sensitivity (MCS). An agent reported to be effective in the treatment of MCS and post-traumatic stress disorder (PTSD), the drug paroxetine, is reported to decrease nitric oxide synthesis via two distinct mechanisms. These observations provide support for the view that excessive nitric oxide has a central role in the etiology of these illnesses, and therefore lowering nitric oxide levels is helpful in their treatment.

THE CASE FOR HYDROXOCOBALAMIN ACTING AS A NITRIC OXIDE SCAVENGER IN THE TREATMENT OF MULTISYSTEM ILLNESSES

I first became aware of the use of vitamin B_{12} injections to treat multisystem illnesses when I was told about this by Dr. Albert G. Corrado, an elderly physician in Richland, Washington, who was collaborating with me on a pilot study on CFS. He told me that he was aware of people with unexplained chronic fatigue, presumably including CFS and FM, who had been treated with vitamin B_{12} injections going back almost 60 years. Patients treated in this way typically reported that their whole spectrum of symptoms improved, although at the time, I was unaware of any placebo-controlled trials to test the efficacy of such B_{12} injections. The injections used were typically intramuscular (IM), with doses ranging from 1 mg to as much as 20 mg. Vitamin B_{12} injections are currently being widely used to treat these illnesses in the United States, Canada, Australia, and at least six European countries. So there seems to be widespread clinical opinion that these are effective, while many have questioned whether there is a plausible mechanism for any such effectiveness.

I am aware that these injections have been used to treat CFS, FM, and MCS, although little has been published on this subject, with most publications being about CFS treatment[1-7] and some also on FM.[8-11] A survey of MCS patients found that high-dose vitamin B_{12} injections were tied with magnesium shots for the best treatment for MCS.[12] The best available study on this was published over 30 years ago by Ellis and Nasser, who performed a placebo-controlled trial on the hydroxocobalamin form of vitamin B_{12} on a group of patients with unexplained chronic fatigue.[1] CFS had not been defined at the time, and so it is uncertain whether most of the trial participants may have fit the diagnosis of CFS. In this study, they used 5 mg injections of hydroxocobalamin, twice per week, and reported two important results. The first is that the treated patients showed statistically significant improvement in their symptoms compared to those of controls. This is obviously of great importance because it provides objective evidence for the effectiveness of this treatment. The second is that there was no correlation between the pretreatment B_{12} levels in the blood and the response of the individual to B_{12} injections. That is also important because it strongly suggests that this treatment works not be allaying a B_{12} deficiency in these patients but rather primarily by some other mechanism.

There are several other types of observation suggesting that such therapy does not work primarily by allaying a B_{12} deficiency state. The classic symptoms of vitamin B_{12}, deficiency, megaloblastic anemia, and dementia, are quite distinct from those of these multisystem illnesses. Megaloblastic anemia has not been reported to be common in these illnesses although there have been studies of red blood cell morphology that would have certainly detected it. While all of these illnesses do have neurological symptoms, they appear to be distinct from those of B_{12} deficiency-induced dementia. So, if most of the symptoms of these multisystem illnesses are distinct from those of B_{12} deficiency, it is difficult to see how these could be improved by hydroxocobalamin injections if such injections act primarily by allaying a B_{12} deficiency. Two highly respected physicians treating CFS patients, Dr. Paul Cheney and Dr. Charles Lapp, have found that high-dose hydroxocobalamin injections, often 10 mg, seem to be more effective in CFS treatment than the lower doses more typically given to treat B_{12} deficiencies (typically 1 mg injections). They also report that hydroxocobalamin injections seem to be more effective than cyanocobalamin injections,[5,6] despite the fact that lower doses and the cyanocobalamin form have been widely used to treat such deficiencies. A study of lower-dose injections using the cyanocobalamin form of vitamin B_{12} in CFS patients did not show any effectiveness[13] despite the fact that the dose used should have been sufficient to allay a B_{12} deficiency, again suggesting that another mode of action is involved in the higher-dose responses reported for hydroxocobalamin therapy.

How, then, might hydroxocobalamin injections act in the treatment of multisystem illnesses? I proposed earlier that it may act because it is a known nitric oxide scavenger, thus lowering the action of excessive nitric oxide.[7] Based on our NO/ONOO$^-$ cycle mechanism, all symptoms controlled directly or indirectly by excessive nitric oxide should be improved by hydroxocobalamin treatment. Cyanocobalamin and another form of B_{12}, methylcobalamin, would be expected to be less effective than hydroxocobalamin, but not completely ineffective. Cyanocobalamin is converted to hydroxocobalamin by an enzyme found in human cells,[14] and methylcobalamin can act as a precursor of hydroxocobalamin by being used in the methylation of homocysteine. So, this is consistent with a lower effectiveness of cyanocobalamin compared with the hydroxo form.

There is considerable evidence showing that hydroxocobalamin is a potent nitric oxide scavenger both in the test tube[15-17] and inside living organisms.[18,19] This action is so well established that hydroxocobalamin has been used to specifically test whether a response involves nitric oxide—if hydroxocobalamin inhibits a particular response, this is taken as strong evidence that nitric oxide is involved.[18-23] The reported action of hydroxocobalamin in the treatment of AIDS and of migraine headaches was suggested to involve the scavenging of nitric oxide.[24-26] So I am not the only scientist to suggest that possibly important therapeutic effects of hydroxocobalamin may be caused by its scavenging of nitric oxide. Dr. Les Simpson has reported on some red blood cell abnormalities distinct from those found in vitamin B_{12} deficiency that are found in CFS patients and reported that these could be reversed overnight following hydroxocobalamin treatment.[27,28] One cannot help wondering whether these abnormalities may be caused by nitric oxide binding to hemoglobin or some other nitric oxide-dependent re-

sponse in the red blood cell; alternatively, peroxynitrite produced from nitric oxide can also interact with erythrocyte (red blood cell) membranes.[29]

One clinical trial study of B_{12} injections in CFS patients failed to produce a significant clinical response.[30] This was a study in which 0.2 mg of
cyanocobalamin was used for such injections. Note that the dosage was
only 1/25th of that used in the Ellis and Nasser study[1] and the form of B_{12}
used was not hydroxocobalamin but cyanocobalamin. If follows that, to be
active as a nitric oxide scavenger, it would have to be efficiently converted
to hydroxocobalamin. The failure to see a clinical response here provides
further support for the notion that hydroxocobalamin acts primarily as a nitric oxide scavenger and that higher doses are needed for an optimal clinical
response with CFS than are needed to treat a B_{12} deficiency.

When I wrote my paper on hydroxocobalamin and CFS and related illnesses, I did it for two reasons. One was to provide some observational support for the proposal that excessive nitric oxide has an important role in
these illnesses. The second was to provide a rationale for physicians pre-
scribing hydroxocobalamin in patients showing no vitamin B_{12} deficiency.
It has had some success in both of these areas.

Before leaving this topic, it is important to point out that, although the
main effect of hydroxocobalamin here may be by acting as a nitric oxide
scavenger, that inference does not imply that these illnesses may not also
tend to lower vitamin B_{12} levels in the body. There are known mechanisms
by which other reactive nitrogen species can deplete B_{12}, and so this may
well occur in the presence of nitric oxide and peroxynitrite. Such lowered
B_{12} levels have been reported in both CFS and MCS.[31]

Hydroxocobalamin injections have been reported to produce objectively
measurable improvements in a series of mental patients with normal vitamin B_{12} levels,[32] suggesting that such mental dysfunction may be related to
excessive nitric oxide levels. I noted in Chapter 3 that excessive nitric oxide
appears to be an important causal element in depression and elevated nitric
oxide is implicated in several psychiatric disorders.[33]

THE DRUG PAROXETINE REPORTED EFFECTIVE
IN THE TREATMENT OF PTSD AND MCS

The drug paroxetine is a "selective serotonin reuptake inhibitor" (SSRI),
a group of pharmacological agents widely used to treat depression. It was
reported by Finkel et al. to lower nitric oxide synthesis,[34] and further observations supporting this inference were reported by two other research
groups.[35,36] This has led others to suggest the use of this drug to treat other

medical conditions involving excessive nitric oxide.[37] There appear to be two distinct mechanisms by which paroxetine lowers nitric oxide synthesis. One is that it inhibits the nitric oxide synthase enzyme activity in in vitro assays,[34] and two, it also decreases the level of nNOS enzyme.[35] Paroxetine is reported to be an effective treatment of PTSD.[38-40] A recent review discussing the use of this drug in the treatment of PTSD stated that[38] "Paroxetine is especially well studied in this regard, with demonstrated efficacy in men and women, in both short-term and long-term studies, and in combat veterans and civilians" (p. 76). Interestingly, paroxetine has been reported in two studies to be effective in the treatment of MCS, at least in individual patients.[41,42] A third study reported that another SSRI, citalopram, was also effective in the treatment of a case of MCS,[43] and citalopram was also reported to lower nitric oxide synthesis.[36]

Let me make clear that, although paroxetine was developed as a drug because of its activity as a serotonin reuptake inhibitor, its effects lowering nitric oxide synthesis must be partly or wholly separate from this SSRI effect. In any case, we have evidence that a second agent that lowers nitric oxide levels appears to be useful in the treatment of this group of illnesses.

OVERALL CONCLUSIONS

These studies provide support for the inference that elevated levels of nitric oxide have important etiologic roles in these illnesses and that these agents act to lower nitric oxide levels. Having said that, I must add that the evidence supporting this inference is not completely convincing. The data do not rule out the possibility that the correlation between lowering nitric oxide and the reported physiological response with these illnesses may not be coincidental. Still, these observations add substantially to the pattern of evidence supporting the proposed etiologic mechanism that is the central focus of this book and show that different agents producing decreased nitric oxide levels may be useful in the treatment of multisystem illnesses. Perhaps the most important inference to be drawn from this chapter is that the NO/ONOO⁻ cycle mechanism makes useful predictions on what therapeutic agents may be useful in therapy.

Chapter 7

Multiple Chemical Sensitivity

No se puede mirar.	One cannot look at this.
Yo lo vi.	I saw it.
Esto es lo verdadero.	This is the truth.

Francisco Goya

TAKE-HOME LESSONS

The many puzzling features of MCS have created great challenges to attempts to describe a comprehensive but plausible causal mechanism for this illness. The sensitivity to many distinct types of chemicals, on the order of 1000-fold increase in sensitivity as compared to normal controls, the initiation by previous chemical exposure, the chronic nature of MCS, and the role of both central (brain) and peripheral sensitivity have all created great challenges to those trying to understand the mechanism of MCS. However, we now have a detailed model of MCS, supported by 40 distinct types of observations, that provides plausible explanations for all 11 of the most challenging puzzles about this illness.

The model fuses the insights of the NO/ONOO⁻ cycle with those on neural sensitization (Bell), on peripheral sensitivity (Meggs) and the role of vanilloid receptor (Anderson), the many insights of Miller, and many others. The fusion of the NO/ONOO⁻ cycle biochemistry with the presumed mechanism neural sensitization (long-term potentiation) provides a fusion model that suggests six distinct mechanisms for central sensitivity. Each of these six involves peroxynitrite, nitric oxide, or superoxide and other oxidants, with each acting synergistically with the others to provide the very-high-level sen-

Explaining "Unexplained Illnesses"
© 2007 by The Haworth Press, Inc. All rights reserved.
doi:10.1300/5139_07

sitivity shown in MCS. Related mechanisms and others such as neurogenic inflammation and mast cell activation may explain the peripheral sensitivities seen in the lower lungs, upper respiratory tract, and regions of the skin.

The four main classes of chemicals involved in MCS, three classes of pesticides and volatile organic solvents, each act according to this model to indirectly produce increased NMDA stimulation, followed by increased nitric oxide and peroxynitrite. It is this common response to these four classes of chemicals, each acting through known pathways, which allow each of them to initiate sensitivity and to produce sensitivity responses in those suffering from MCS.

The NO/ONOO$^-$ cycle model provides us with explanations for 11 challenging puzzles for MCS, only one of which was previously explained. Given the many challenges that face those of us trying to understand the mechanism of MCS, the fit of this model to the complex properties of the illness is truly extraordinary.

INTRODUCTION

Multiple chemical sensitivity has often been viewed as the most controversial of these multisystem illnesses, and there is no question that there is a large number of puzzling features of this illness that have challenged explanation. As such, it may be viewed as the highest mountain to be scaled in this group of illnesses—if we can understand MCS, we should be able to understand them all. I am going to write this chapter, unlike the others in this book, partially as a voyage of discovery, paralleling my own search for understanding of MCS. I am doing this because I think it should make more sense to you when written this way, and I apologize for the ego trip here. Specifically, I will introduce, as we go along, certain puzzles about MCS before providing solutions to those puzzles as well as the evidence supporting those solutions. By the time we are finished, it is my hope and expectation that you will be convinced that we have a detailed and compelling set of mechanisms that explain all of the most puzzling features about MCS, a set of mechanisms that are supported by over three dozen different types of observations. I also hope to convince you that, having come up with a compelling set of mechanisms for MCS, centered on excessive levels of nitric oxide, peroxynitrite and NMDA activity, that it helps to strengthen the arguments for similar mechanisms in these other multisystem illnesses.

One other thing I will do in this chapter is to refer to my six papers on MCS, published and in press,[1-6] for many citation references rather than provide citations for all of the evidence that I will discuss. These papers are recent, with two having been written recently, and so they include most of the relevant references supporting this discussion.

All of our progress in understanding of MCS is dependent on the studies of dedicated physicians, committed to trying to understand this illness as well as treat it, physicians who include Theron Randolph and Mark Cullen, who started our whole understanding of MCS. Many of these physicians have labored ceaselessly in order to try to improve the lives of their MCS patients as well as to help with our understanding of the science, trying to do so despite great difficulty. I will, later in this chapter, borrow shamelessly from several of these. I do so with no apologies—science always progresses on the shoulders of pioneers who came earlier.

The courage and integrity of these physician scientists is emphasized by the fact that they have had to labor in these fields with almost no financial support from health funding agencies. In one of my papers,[2] I estimated that the prevalence of MCS from epidemiological studies is similar to that of diabetes, but the funding available for its study has been only about 1/1000th as much. Why is this? It is largely because MCS has been repeatedly described as controversial, and while some of that controversy has been based on real science or the lack of it, most of it has been due to the effective role of organizations and individuals who have a financial interest in its being viewed as controversial. This can be quite effective in preventing research funding. When a research proposal comes before a National Institutes of Health (NIH) study section, it is always in competition with many other proposals from many areas that are already well understood and thus viewed as noncontroversial. If one or two members of that study section are very skeptical about whether the proposal is in a legitimate area of study, it is very difficult to obtain funding for it, and so a widespread perception of controversy can be very effective in allowing that perception to continue. This perception, as well as the lack of funding, has led to other consequences. It is not unusual for a faculty member of a medical school to be "advised" to get out of this area of study for the sake of his or her professional career. Rosenthal[7] over a decade ago commented that "In trying to research MCS . . . we are in a Catch-22 situation. It is difficult to attract research money for a controversial condition and it is difficult to resolve the controversy without the necessary research" (p. 624). Ironically, despite the lack of funding for MCS research, there is very substantial evidence supporting the mechanism developed in this chapter, and while much of this evidence comes from studies not focused on MCS but still providing key information about the proposed mechanisms for MCS, other studies have come from the dedicated physicians studying this illness.

When I first became aware of the overlaps between MCS and CFS, as a consequence of this perceived "controversy," I had a feeling of considerable trepidation in considering whether I should try to approach the MCS field with the biochemical approach I had previously used for CFS. However, I have always felt that the best scientists have the courage and integrity to follow the science wherever it leads, and so I have tried to do likewise. I hope that you will feel, as I do, that this was the best decision I have ever made.

MCS PUZZLES

Cases of MCS typically start with either one high-level exposure or several lower-level ones to chemicals, and the chemicals involved are usually either volatile organic solvents or certain pesticides, most commonly organophosphorus or carbamate pesticides,[8,9] although two other groups of pesticides, pyrethroids and organochlorine pesticides and mold toxins, are implicated as well.[6,8-10] This leads to a very-high-level sensitivity to the same classes of chemicals with individuals typically reporting sensitivity to gasoline and other organic solvent fumes, diesel exhaust, jet exhaust, cleaning materials, perfumes, the so-called air fresheners, unpolymerized components of plastics including foams, products of incomplete combustion including tobacco smoke, and the outgassing of chemicals in certain buildings (typically from building materials or carpeting), as well as pesticides. I estimated based on both, anecdotal reports and a controlled exposure study, that MCS sufferers are at least 100 times more sensitive than normals and are probably more on the order of 1000 times more sensitive.[2] MCS sufferers have not been reported to fully recover, although those who carefully avoid further chemical exposure sometimes report long-term decreases in sensitivity. Many of the symptoms in common with CFS are reported to be induced by chemical exposure in MCS.[8,9] Many of these symptoms involve the brain or neuroendocrine system dysfunction, but others involving sensitivity in other organs of the body (peripheral sensitivity) are also commonly found (Chapter 3). The symptoms of MCS are quite diverse and quite variable from one individual to another, and Sorg, in her review lists over 40 such symptoms (Table 1, Reference 9).

The pattern of properties reported in MCS clearly raises certain questions:

1. Why are these certain classes of chemicals involved but not others? Specifically, what is the mode of action of the volatile organic sol-

vents and of the organophosphorus/carbamate pesticides? How might the two other classes of pesticides, organochlorine pesticides, and pyrethroids be involved?

2. How does previous chemical exposure act to produce high-level sensitivity?
3. Why is MCS chronic?
4. Why are there high levels of comorbidity with CFS and FM?
5. Why are the symptoms and signs of MCS similar to those of CFS, FM, and PTSD (Chapter 3), except that in MCS they are typically either induced by or exacerbated by low-level chemical exposure?
6. How can the exquisite sensitivity reported in MCS be generated?
7. Why do some of the symptoms appear to involve the brain and others the peripheral parts of the body?
8. Why are there so many variations in symptoms from one individual to another?

You can probably already see possible answers to some, but not to others, of these questions from information derived from earlier chapters.

There are other puzzling features in MCS. Several research groups have reported that several of the enzymes of porphyrin biosynthesis are low in MCS, producing accumulation of several intermediate compounds in that biosynthetic pathway,[3] leading to the question of what might be the cause in these multiple changes in porphyrin synthesis. Meggs and others have reported on peripheral sensitivity responses,[11-15] and Meggs has reported that the process of neurogenic inflammation is involved in peripheral sensitivity.[11-14] This raises the question of what mechanisms may generate this neurogenic inflammation and what role it may have in peripheral sensitivity mechanisms.

These many puzzles about MCS have led Miller[16] to propose that we were in need of a new paradigm of human disease in order to explain this illness, a paradigm that might take years before its outlines could become clear. Many other scientists also supported this view (cited in Reference 2), suggesting that despite the important insights obtained by Bell, Meggs, Anderson, Miller herself, Millqvist, and others, we were still some considerable distance from an overall etiologic theory of MCS.

So, there is a daunting list of the puzzling questions that should be answered by any etiologic mechanism for MCS. They set the standards for what is needed. I am going to tackle the questions numbered 1 to 6 first, as listed previously, and then return to several other difficult questions that also need to be answered.

EVIDENCE FOR A NO/ONOO⁻ CYCLE THEORY OF MCS

My own approach to MCS started, as you might guess, with the proposal that excessive levels of nitric oxide and peroxynitrite are central to its etiology.[1] In a subsequent paper, I listed 10 different types of observations about MCS that provided support for this view.[2] These 10 and an 11th are listed in Exhibit 7.1. You can see from this exhibit that there is evidence for a possible nitric oxide role in the initiation of MCS, with both organic solvents and organophosphorus pesticides producing increases in nitric oxide[1-3,6] and therefore possibly initiating cases of MCS through that mechanism. There are also nine other types of evidence consistent with an elevated nitric oxide/peroxynitrite role in the chronic phase of MCS. Having said that, the most puzzling questions about MCS were not answered by an elevated nitric oxide/peroxynitrite theory. Specifically, there was no answer as to how the exquisite chemical sensitivity, on the order of 1000-fold higher than normals, could be generated in MCS. There was evidence that organic solvents could increase nitric oxide levels, but there was no evidence known to me, supporting any specific mechanism for this to occur.[1-3] There was evidence for oxidative stress in MCS, and studies of an animal model provided evidence for a key role of nitric oxide in the MCS.[2] One question that was answered by this proposal was how organophosphorus and carbamate pesticides may act in initiating cases of MCS,[1-3] and I will discuss this answer subsequently.

So while we have 11 different types of observations providing support for a nitric oxide/peroxynitrite role in MCS, that in and of itself does not provide an etiologic explanation for this illness.

Putative Common Response Mechanism for Each of the Four Classes of Chemicals

Each of the three classes of pesticides[1,2,6] and also the volatile organic solvents[5] are proposed to act to stimulate a common end point, as diagrammed in Figure 7.1. Each of the three groups of pesticides are proposed to act through distinct but well-documented pathways to activate NMDA receptor activity, and the volatile organic solvents are thought to act via stimulation of the vanilloid receptor[5] to produce the same final end point—increased NMDA activity and consequent increased levels of nitric oxide and peroxynitrite. The pesticides each act through their major neurotoxicant response mechanisms to indirectly produce the increase in NMDA activity.[1,2,6,22-25] They also are reported, as would be ex-

EXHIBIT 7.1. Types of Evidence Implicating
Nitric Oxide/Peroxynitrite in MCS

1. Several organic solvents thought to be able to induce MCS, formaldehyde, benzene, carbon tetrachloride, and certain organochlorine pesticides all induce increases in nitric oxide levels.

2. A sequence of action of organophosphate and carbamate insecticides is suggested, whereby they may induce MCS by inactivating acetylcholinesterase and thus produce increased stimulation of muscarinic receptors, which are known to produce increases in nitric oxide.

3. Evidence for induction of inflammatory cytokines by organic solvents, which induce the inducible nitric oxide synthase (iNOS). Elevated cytokines are an integral part of the proposed feedback mechanism of the elevated nitric oxide/peroxynitrite theory.

4. Neopterin, a marker of the induction of the iNOS, is reported to be elevated in more severe cases of MCS.

5. Increased oxidative stress has been reported in MCS,[17] and antioxidant therapy may produce improvements in symptoms, as expected if the levels of the oxidant peroxynitrite are elevated. The concept of a possible central role of oxidative stress in MCS was first explored by Levine over 20 years ago.[18-20]

6. In a series of studies of a mouse model of MCS, involving partial and complete kindling, both excessive NMDA activity and excessive nitric oxide synthesis were convincingly shown to be required to produce the characteristic biological response.

7. The symptoms exacerbated on chemical exposure are very similar to the chronic symptoms of CFS,[1] and these may be explained by several known properties of nitric oxide, peroxynitrite, and inflammatory cytokines, each of which has a role in the proposed mechanism.

8. These conditions (CFS, MCS, FM, and PTSD) are often treated through intramuscular injections of vitamin B_{12} and B_{12} in the form of hydroxocobalamin is a potent nitric oxide scavenger, both in vitro and in vivo.

9 and 10. As discussed later, peroxynitrite is known to induce increased permeabilization of the blood brain barrier and such increased permeabilization is reported in a rat model of MCS. It has also been reported to be permeabilized in human MCS patients.[21]

11. As discussed later, several types of evidence implicate excessive NMDA activity in MCS, an activity known to increase nitric oxide and peroxynitrite levels.

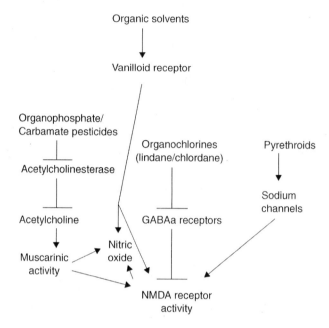

FIGURE 7.1. Action of four classes of chemicals on NMDA receptor activity. Each of the four classes of chemicals implicated in MCS can act via a distinct receptor target to produce increased NMDA activity. The sequence of action of the pyrethroid and the organic solvents involves only stimulatory interactions, indicated by the arrows, leading the increased NMDA activity. The organo-phophorus and carbamate pesticides and the organochlorine pesticides both have two inhibitory steps, with the double negative sequence also leading to a stimulation of NMDA receptors. This diagram shows how all four classes of chemicals, each acting through known sequences, can lead to a common response—stimulation of NMDA receptor activity and consequent increases in nitric oxide and peroxynitrite.

pected from the NMDA response, to lead to increases in nitric oxide levels. [1,2,6,26-29]*

I had proposed earlier that volatile organic solvents might act through three other pathways,[2] not through the vanilloid receptor, but there was no available evidence either supporting or refuting those three potential pathways. It was Dr. Julius Anderson's idea that the vanilloid receptor** was

*As was noted in Chapter 2, stimulation of 3 out of 5 muscarinic receptors and also the vanilloid receptor will directly lead to increased nitric oxide synthesis.

**The vanilloid receptor, the receptor for capsaicin, the "heat" in hot capsicum peppers, is sometime designated TRPV1.

the probable major target for organic solvents, and the two of us worked on that idea for six months or so before convincing ourselves that it had considerable merit and then wrote a paper making the case for that view.[5] The 12 types of evidence supporting this view were discussed in that paper.[5] The vanilloid receptor may not only be the major target for organic solvents in MCS; it may also be the target for the actions of such oxidants as chlorine gas[5] and of certain mold toxins (mycotoxins) as well.[5] Vanilloid receptor stimulation is known to be able to lead to increased NMDA activity,[5] as indicated in Figure 7.1. Pesticides are usually sprayed as solutions in organic solvents so that pesticide toxicity may be produced through both the major target of the pesticide itself as well as through vanilloid stimulation by the solvent. These solvents are usually described as "inert ingredients" even though they are not inert to the human body.

It is proposed that the same putative response pathways act both in the initiation phase of MCS sensitization in response to chemical exposure as well as in the chronic phase, where chemical exposure produces sensitivity responses. Thus, the two phases described by Ashford and Miller,[8] the initial "elicitation" phase and the subsequent "triggering" of symptoms may both involve these same pathways.

The putative patterns of action diagrammed in Figure 7.1 are important for at least three reasons. Firstly, they show that diverse chemicals of at least four different classes can produce a common response. This is important because MCS skeptics have argued that the diversity of chemicals reported to be involved in sensitivity responses in MCS is so great that there cannot be a common response to all of them. Clearly, what I have presented here shows that they are wrong about that key issue.

Secondly, they provide evidence for a common elevation of nitric oxide and peroxynitrite, both of which are known responses to NMDA stimulation, as was discussed in Chapter 2. Thus, they provide evidence that the NO/ONOO$^-$ cycle mechanism,is a viable one for MCS. Nitric oxide increases are predicted and reported to be produced by exposure to any of these four classes of chemicals.[2-6]

Thirdly, all four of these pathways come to a common end point with elevation of NMDA activity, raising the issue of whether such NMDA elevation may be have a key role in MCS that may be distinct from its role in increasing nitric oxide and peroxynitrite.

BELL'S NEURAL SENSITIZATION THEORY
AND DEVELOPMENT OF A "FUSION THEORY"

It may be seen, from the preceding, that the nitric oxide/peroxynitrite theory is consistent with some important aspects of MCS but does not explain the very-high-level sensitivity responses induced by previous chemical exposure and seen on subsequent exposure to a wide range of chemicals. It is this high-level sensitivity to many chemicals that is the most intriguing and challenging aspect of MCS. I looked, therefore, at previously developed theories of MCS that might provide further enlightenment and specifically at the neural sensitization theory developed by Iris Bell, MD, PhD, professor at the University of Arizona. Basically, what Bell's neural sensitization theory posits is that MCS centers on the role of chemicals increasing the sensitivity of neuronal synapses, the sites at which different neurons (nerve cells) communicate with each other, with neural sensitization involving increased synaptic sensitivity such that one neuron (the presynaptic one) has a greatly increased chance of triggering what is known as an action potential in a second neuron (the postsynaptic one). Neural sensitization normally occurs on a highly selective basis in learning and memory such that only certain specific synapses become sensitized, with this selectivity leading to the high level of specificity in learning and memory. Essentially, what is being proposed is that chemical exposure may be able to massively stimulate this process of neural sensitization so that, instead of being a very selective process, it is very nonselective. Because much of this neural sensi-tization in the brain occurs in the limbic system and specifically in the hippocampus, the sensitization process proposed here has been called limbic kindling or partial limbic kindling.[30-34] Bell and coworkers have published a series of interesting papers on this theory and have published specifically on several important parallels between MCS and neural sensitization.[30-34] There is very substantial experimental support for Bell's theory,[30-34] and Ashford and Miller[8] list 10 different striking similarities between time dependent neural sensitization and MCS.

The presumed mechanism of neural sensitization, known as long-term potentiation (LTP), involves the stimulation of the NMDA receptors in the brain, particularly in regions of the hippocampus, which has an important role in learning and memory.[2] This mechanism is thought to be important in the whole process of learning and memory, selectively strengthening specific synapses through which neurons may trigger electrical responses in one another.[2] What happens if chemical exposure produces a massive stimulation of LTP,* as opposed to the highly selective stimulation that is thought to be involved in learning and memory?

The answer to that may be diagrammed in Figure 7.2. LTP involves stimulation of NMDA receptors,[2] which, as we discussed in Chapter 2, leads to increases in production of nitric oxide and its oxidant product peroxynitrite.

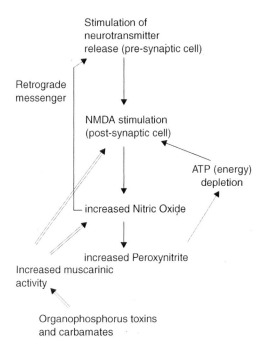

FIGURE 7.2. Chemical stimulation of long-term potentiation mechanism cycle. The upper three quarters of the figure diagrams the cycle of stimulation that may be expected on excessive stimulation of long-term potentiation mechanisms. Nitric oxide produced by excessive NMDA stimulation acts as a retrograde messenger, stimulating increased glutamate release by the presynaptic cell, leading to still more NMDA activity. Peroxynitrite, acting to inhibit mitochondrial (energy metabolism), leads to ATP depletion and therefore to increase NMDA sensitivity to stimulation. The organophosphorus pesticides (lower part of figure) are shown feeding into this mechanism. Other chemical classes should also feed into this mechanism, as outlined in Figure 7.1.

---

*The process of long-term potentiation is a very complex one in which over 100 different components have been implicated. I will discuss here only the few that appear to have direct relevance to MCS.

Nitric oxide serves as what is known as a retrograde messenger, diffusing back to the presynaptic cell and stimulating the release of the neurotransmitter glutamate, thus producing increased NMDA stimulation.[2] So, one has here a potential vicious cycle mechanism involving some of the mechanisms outlined in our overall NO/ONOO⁻ cycle that was outlined in Chapters 1 and 2—excessive NMDA activity leading to increased nitric oxide, leading, in turn, to excessive NMDA activity (Figure 7.2). Peroxynitrite may also act via two distinct mechanisms, as also shown in the figure, because of its ability to attack elements of the mitochondrion and also stimulate ADP-ribosylation, thus decreasing the levels of energy in the form of ATP (mechanisms discussed in Chapter 2, Chapter 3, and Chapter 5). It is known that, when cells containing NMDA receptors are depleted of ATP, those NMDA receptors become hypersensitive to stimulation, thus leading to further increases in NMDA activity, and so the excessive peroxynitrite levels* may also be expected to contribute to the vicious cycle in the brain.[2] Furthermore, the neurotransmitter glutamate that activates the NMDA receptors has its levels lowered by being transported into glial cells in the brain, an energy-dependent process that is predicted to be inhibited by peroxynitrite damage to mitochondria.[35,36†]

The idea that one or more of these neurotransmitter receptor systems stimulated by chemicals may influence NMDA activity, LTP, and learning and memory in the hippocampus in the brain has been studied and confirmed in a number of studies involving the muscarinic receptors.[37,38] These studies help confirm the involvement of the processes outlined earlier in this section in the process of learning and memory, starting with muscarinic receptor activity, which is stimulated through the action of organophosphorus/carbamate pesticides. The way in which organophosporus/carbamate pesticides may feed into the mechanisms of LTP is diagrammed in Figure 7.2.

If you put together what has been presented in this and the previous section of this chapter, including Figure 7.1 and Figure 7.2, you should be able to see how central chemical sensitivity appears to fit together. Each of the four classes of chemicals converges on a common response, centered on

---

*I am focusing here on the role of peroxynitrite in producing mitochondrial/energy metabolism dysfunction, although both nitric oxide and superoxide also have roles in this as well (Chapter 2). The reason for my focus here is that the probable peroxynitrite role appears to be the most important.

†The role of energy metabolism in controlling excessive NMDA stimulation through glutamate transport was not suggested to be linked to MCS previously, but should have been.

elevated levels of NMDA activity, nitric oxide, and peroxynitrite.* This response, acting through vicious cycle mechanisms, including mechanisms normally involved in LTP, produces elevated chemical sensitivity. Thus, we have a convergence of the NO/ONOO⁻ cycle theory with the neural sensitization theory to form a fusion theory that appears to answer key questions about MCS. We also have a convergence of action of the four classes of chemicals to produce this common response. I hope that this double convergence makes sense to you and produces the long-awaited "aha" experience in your understanding of MCS. This is the key conceptual focus for our understanding of the central nervous system action of chemicals in MCS— how chemicals can both initiate chronic chemical sensitivity in the brain by triggering a vicious cycle, which is itself focused on the mechanism of LTP, and also produce sensitive responses to subsequent chemical exposure through the action of these same pathways.

ADDITIONAL "ACCESSORY" MECHANISMS IN CHEMICAL SENSITIVITY

I proposed other, what might be called accessory, mechanisms that may be expected to act both individually and collectively to produce still higher levels of chemical sensitivity. Each of these is based on well-described biochemical and physiological mechanisms, but their role in MCS needs to be further studied. Three such mechanisms are described here—two that were proposed earlier in my *FASEB Journal* paper on MCS[2] and one additional that was described in our vanilloid paper.[5] Each of them involves either nitric oxide, superoxide, or peroxynitrite, and thus are predicted to be involved as part of the overall mechanism. They are as follows:

- Peroxynitrite-mediated permeabilization of the blood-brain barrier (BBB). This will be expected to produce increased chemical exposure to the brain.[2,3]
- Inhibition of solvent and possibly other chemical metabolism by cytochrome P450s produced by excessive nitric oxide.[2,3] In this way, nitric oxide may be expected to lower chemical metabolism, thus leading to increased chemical exposure.

---

*One of the questions raised by the proposed roles of peroxynitrite in Figure 7.2 is whether peroxynitrite has a role in "normal" LTP. The answer to that is unclear, but there are number of studies that have implicated superoxide (the other precursor of peroxynitrite) in LTP, consistent with this possibility.

- Increased vanilloid activity produced by oxidants including super-oxide.[39,40] This will be expected to produce increased sensitivity to organic solvents and other chemicals whose activity is mediated by the vanilloid receptor but not to pesticides. The probable mechanism for such oxidant effect is through the known role of oxidants in stimulating protein kinase C activity,[41-43] leading in turn to increased vanilloid activity.[5,44,45]

Of these three mechanisms, the breakdown of the BBB was reported to occur both in MCS patients[21] and in an animal model of MCS.[46] Increased vanilloid activity also is reported to occur in MCS.[5] The predicted lowering of cytochrome P450 activity in MCS has not been studied and is relatively difficult to study. It must be studied in intact tissue because tissue preparation, as might be possible in an animal model, will not detect the predicted change, given the instability of nitric oxide and the consequent rapid reversal of any inhibition following tissue disruption.

NMDA receptors have a central role in LTP, and there are six distinct types of evidence implicating NMDA receptors in MCS[2]:

1. Clinical observations supporting a critical role for NMDA activity in responses to chemicals in MCS
2. Animal model data implicating excessive NMDA activity in the animal model response
3. Data from a single animal model implicating NMDA-stimulated nitric oxide and the nNOS enzyme activity in the sensitivity response
4. Genetic evidence from studies showing that the CCK-B receptor has a role in MCS, a receptor known to regulate NMDA activity
5. Evidence that certain organic solvents implicated in MCS can produce, presumably indirectly, increased NMDA activity
6. Of course, the evidence, discussed earlier, showing that each of the four classes of chemicals reported to often initiate cases of MCS each produce increases in NMDA activity

Summary: Mechanisms in Fusion Theory That Help Explain High-Level Chemical Sensitivity

In summary, then, there are six distinct mechanisms that may contribute to the high-level chemical sensitivity reported in MCS:

1. Role of nitric oxide as a retrograde messenger, increasing release of glutamate by presynaptic neurons
2. Role of peroxynitrite and subsequent energy metabolism dysfunction in sensitizing neurons containing NMDA receptors to such receptor stimulation
3. Role of peroxynitrite and subsequent energy metabolism dysfunction in lowering the action of glial cells in transporting and therefore lowering the extracellular concentrations of glutamate, thus leading to increased NMDA stimulation
4. Role of peroxynitrite in the permeabilization of the BBB, leading to increased chemical exposure in the brain
5. Role of nitric oxide in inhibiting cytochrome P450 metabolism of chemicals, leading to increased chemical accumulation
6. Role of superoxide and other oxidants in increasing the vanilloid receptor activity, leading to increased response to volatile organic solvents and certain other chemicals

The combination of all six of these mechanisms may be expected to act to produce increased sensitivity, with each acting at a different level. It is the expected synergism among these six levels that is expected to produce the exquisite, high-level sensitivity seen in MCS. Because all four classes of chemicals should be able to produce convergent responses, such convergence also provides an explanation for the diverse types of chemicals reported to initiate chemical sensitivity and trigger sensitivity responses in MCS.

SICK BUILDING SYNDROME AND A COMPARISON OF THE ACTION OF ORGANOPHOSPHORUS PESTICIDES WITH THOSE OF VOLATILE ORGANIC SOLVENTS

"Sick building syndrome" is a situation in which many people in a particular building become ill, typically coming down with symptoms of MCS.[5,8,9] There are two types of sick building syndrome situations—those where new or recently remodeled buildings that presumably have high levels of volatile organic solvents outgassed from building materials are the apparent cause,[5,8,9] and mold-infested buildings caused by water condensation and subsequent mold growth. Both of these "sick building situations" are associated with initiation of MCS cases.[5,8-10] The toxins involved with these mold-associated cases have not been identified, but we have recently reviewed evidence that some dialdehyde mold toxins are volatile vanilloid agonists, possibly acting along with some volatile organic solvents also produced by molds to stimulate the vanilloid receptors.[5] Thus, the initiation of MCS cases by mold-infested buildings may follow the same pathway of action as that thought to be stimulated by volatile organic solvents. Mold infestations in buildings are also reported to be an important risk factor in the initiation of asthma cases,[5] and given the similarities between asthma and MCS, which are discussed subsequently, this should not be surprising.

One of the interesting studies on MCS was published by Miller and Mitzel,[47] comparing MCS cases initiated by volatile organic solvents from building remodeling (sick buildings) with cases apparently produced by pesticide exposure, most of the latter involving organophosphorus pesticides. This is an interesting study because it compares MCS cases initiated by two distinct classes of initiators. The symptomatic patterns of these two classes were similar but not identical. The organophosphorus pesticide cases tended on average to be somewhat more severe, and there were also some differences in symptoms, with some being more severe in one class but some others being somewhat more severe in the other class. Overall, then, the pattern reported by Miller and Mitzel[47] is that there are great similarities between the two classes of MCS cases, however with some distinctions as well. One question that may be raised here concerns the distinct pathways of apparent action of these two classes of compounds, with one acting as an acetylcholinesterase inhibitor and the other presumably acting as vanilloid agonists. The similarities suggest that there is considerable overlap in the NMDA receptors that are indirectly activated by each pathway, but because there are some differences, the overlap is not complete.

ANOTHER PUZZLE POSSIBLY EXPLAINED BY VANILLOID RECEPTOR INVOLVEMENT

Low-level repeated or prolonged exposures of MCS patients to volatile organic solvents has been observed to lead to lessened sensitivity responses.[8,9,48] This phenomenon has been called masking or desensitization, and has been an additional puzzling and previously unexplained feature of MCS. It is known that low-level sustained or repeated exposures to many but not all vanilloid agonists leads to lowered vanilloid receptor responsiveness, and this may provide a cogent explanation for the masking/desensitization observations.[5]

RESOLUTION OF AN ADDITIONAL MCS PUZZLE: CHANGES IN PORPHYRIN METABOLISM

Four different research groups have reported accumulation of certain intermediates in the porphyrin biosynthetic pathway in MCS,[3] accumulation that involves lowered synthesis of more than one enzyme in that pathway. This is an unusual type of change in the porphyrin pathway. Classical porphyria typically involves low levels of only one enzyme in the pathway and is usually caused by a mutation in one of genes that encode the enzyme involved. What could be the mechanism of this unusual change in porphyrin metabolism? It is reported that nitric oxide lowers the synthesis of several enzymes in the porphyrin pathway,[3] so I proposed that increased nitric oxide may produce the observed changes in this pathway.[3] Furthermore the last enzyme in the porphyrin pathway is probable inactivated by peroxynitrite.[3] Thus, yet another MCS puzzle appears to be resolved by this NO/ONOO⁻ cycle mechanism.

GENETIC EVIDENCE AND MCS

There are three genetic studies that have important implications for the mechanism of MCS. One is the CCK-B receptor study,[49] mentioned previously, and the other two both implicated the *PON1* gene.[50,51] The last of these[51] implicated several other genes that each produce an enzyme that metabolize the chemicals implicated in initiating and producing sensitivity symptoms in MCS.

The CCK-B study,[49] as discussed earlier, provides evidence implicating NMDA receptors in MCS, because of the known role of the CCK-B receptor in controlling NMDA activity.[2] The second paper[50] discussed here is a paper from Haley's group, reporting that Gulf War veterans carrying *PON1* genes producing protein less able to metabolize the organophosphorus toxicant sarin had greater prevalence of neurological symptoms including chemical sensitivity symptoms. This leads to the inference that sarin gas had a key role in producing the neurological symptoms in the Gulf War veterans, with symptoms of MCS being important aspects of these neurological symptoms, with those less able to metabolize sarin gas being more susceptible, therefore, to its neurotoxicological effects. In the third study recently reported by a Toronto research group studying civilian MCS patients,[51] it was shown again that the *PON1* gene had a somewhat similar role to that reported earlier by Haley. The Toronto study also showed that four other genes that all help determine the rates of metabolism of organic solvents or organophosphorus pesticides also influenced the prevalence of MCS.[51] It may be inferred from this that the chemical forms of both organophosphorus toxins and organic solvents are important in determining their activities in MCS and that they act, therefore, as toxicants due to their specific chemical structures. Specifically, the organophosphorus toxins must be in their original neurotoxic form in order to trigger MCS. This is exactly what would be expected from the pathway of action proposed earlier in this chapter, where organophosphorus toxins act as acetylcholinesterase inhibitors. The Toronto study[51] also implicates the volatile organic solvents as toxicants in MCS because their chemical structure as determined by their metabolism may also be inferred to have a critical role, based on this genetic study.

There is another, much broader context in which the genetic evidence should be considered. Genes act to produce specific proteins that can act, in turn, either within or outside the cells of the human body. Genes also act to determine the structure of those specific proteins. They act then to influence the biology by determining the chemical structure of human cells and the extracellular environment. But there has been much unsupported speculation that MCS is some kind of psychiatric illness with skeptics arguing that MCS may be some kind of belief system rather than a real biological illness. These arguments are based on an assumed dualism between the psychological/psychiatric/mental and the biological/physiological/physical, with the advocates of this point of view arguing that MCS is entirely on the psychological side of the line. This dualism has been long rejected by modern science, as I will discuss in Chapter 13. The point I want to emphasize here, given the amount of nonsensical psychological speculation about MCS, is that those who argue for some kind of "psychogenic mechanism" of MCS are simply wrong and the genetic studies show that they are wrong. Genetics clearly influences the biology of organisms; so any speculation arguing that MCS is entirely on the psychological side of such a dualism is incompatible with any genetic role. The fact that the genetic studies provide further support chemicals acting as toxicants and for a role for NMDA receptors is just the icing on the cake, in this context.

PERIPHERAL SENSITIVITY MECHANISMS IN MCS

The mechanisms outlined earlier on neural sensitization, NMDA receptors, nitric oxide, and peroxynitrite involvement in MCS focus on the dysfunction in the brain. However, Meggs and others[11-15] have discussed the role of what may be described as peripheral sensitivity mechanisms in MCS.

Specifically, Meggs has discussed the role of reactive airways dysfunctions syndrome (RADS) in MCS, reactive upper airways dysfunction syndrome (RUDS), and other peripheral sensitivities including skin sensitivity. There is even a local chemical sensitivity in the intestine called reactive intestinal dysfunction syndrome (RIDS).[15] Each of these are sensitivities initiated by previous chemical exposure, with the range of chemicals reported to be involved being similar to those involved in producing central sensitivity in MCS. RADS is a form of asthma initiated by chemical exposure, and RUDS involves upper airways inflammation including rhinitis, which again is initiated by previous chemical exposure.

Dr. Anderson and I have argued that each of these involves vanilloid receptors because, first of all, well-documented vanilloid agonists such as capasaicin, eugenol, toluene diisocyanate, and formaldehyde are all reported to be active in inducing these sensitivity responses.[5] In addition, pharmacological studies have implicated the vanilloid receptor itself in these sensitivity responses. These are all overt inflammatory responses, and not surprisingly, they all involve increases in nitric oxide and peroxynitrite. It is also known that peripheral vanilloid stimulation can lead to stimulation of NMDA receptors, another part of the NO/ONOO$^-$ cycle.

So how does this all fit into our view of MCS? Meggs argues that, because asthma is reported to be initiated by chemical exposure and because most asthmatics show chemical sensitivity responses in the lungs, asthmatics who also have chemical sensitivities in one additional organ meet the Cullen case definition for MCS.[11]

Clearly, there are some striking similarities between the central neural sensitization sensitivity we discussed earlier in this chapter and the peripheral sensitivities, and some of those similarities may be explained through a role of the vanilloid receptors apparently acting in both as the major target of organic solvents and certain other chemicals. What about the NMDA receptors—do they have a role in these peripheral sensitivity mechanisms? They are reported to be involved in skin sensitivity reactions.[52-54] They are reported to have a role in an animal model of asthma,[55] and the reported effectiveness of magnesium in the treatment of asthma[56,57] is consistent with an NMDA role but may be explained by other mechanisms also. The clinical observations that an NMDA antagonist, dextromethorphan, stops all of the standard sensitivity responses in MCS[2] suggests that excessive NMDA activity may have a role in such peripheral sensitivity responses. The Miller and Mitzel study[47] compared the symptomatic patterns of MCS people presumably initiated by organic solvents with those initiated by organophosphorus pesticides. They reported that both groups reported similar sensitivities to monosodium glutamate, and glutamate acts, in part, as an

NMDA agonist. In addition, both groups showed similar patterns of peripheral sensitivities, suggesting a similar response to both sets of chemicals. In summary, there is some evidence suggesting a role for elevated NMDA activity in peripheral sensitivity responses, but this evidence must still be considered to be weak, and so this aspect clearly needs more study.

Nitric oxide and peroxynitrite are also widely reported to have roles in peripheral sensitivity, not surprising given their overt inflammatory nature.

So, what can we say about the probable mechanisms involved in these peripheral sensitivity responses? We can say that these are overt inflammatory responses involving excessive vanilloid sensitivity, nitric oxide, peroxynitrite, and probably NMDA activity. It seems likely that the well-described influence of both inflammation and specifically oxidants including superoxide have roles in the vanilloid elevation and that vanilloid elevation is likely to be one of the important mechanisms in producing the increased chemical sensitivity. In addition to this, there are other inflammatory mechanisms that are implicated. Meggs and coworkers[14] have reported that neurogenic inflammation is involved in these peripheral sensitivities, a process that would be expected to maintain and exacerbate the chronic inflammation. It is known that neurogenic inflammation is stimulated by both vanilloid receptor stimulation[5] and also by nitric oxide.[3] Thus, neurogenic inflammation may respond to both vanilloid activity and nitric oxide, and by increasing the inflammation, it may increase vanilloid activity, nitric oxide, and other aspects of NO/ONOO⁻ cycle biochemistry. Another inflammatory influence may be expected to come from the stimulation of mast cells, which are some of the few non-neural cell types known to have vanilloid receptors. Mast cell degranulation is reported to be stimulated by both vanilloid stimulation[5] and by nitric oxide,[2,3] thus again potentially exacerbating the inflammatory response. It is likely that other inflammatory regulatory responses are involved as well.

In general, then, it may be argued that we are less able to explain in detail the properties of peripheral chemical sensitivity but that they involve some of the same aspects of central sensitivity (probable vanilloid role, nitric oxide and peroxynitrite, inflammatory biochemistry, and a possible NMDA role). The peripheral sensitivity may be very good examples of the local nature of the NO/ONOO⁻ cycle mechanisms, as discussed in Chapter 4. All of the available evidence suggests that these are primarily local responses to previous local chemical exposure and certainly skin sensitization is produced in the regions of the skin that were previously chemically exposed.

There is one other aspect that should be mentioned. Sensitivity in general may often be basically *sensitivity to excessive nitric oxide*. In asthma, for example, the lungs are sensitive to antigens, which are reported to produce nitric oxide increases when reacting with antibodies.[58-62] Asthmatics are sensitive to cold as well, and while the target involved in this cold response has not been identified, there are two cold-responsive receptors, one in the vanilloid family of receptors[63] and the second a very distant vanilloid relative;[64] both of these receptors, when stimulated, open channels that allow calcium influx into the cell and will presumably produce, as a consequence of this, increased nitric oxide. So, it is possible that cold works via nitric oxide. In skin sensitivity, heat sensitivity is known to be transduced by the vanilloid receptor and so will produce increases in nitric oxide. Central sensitivity may also, to some extent, be a sensitivity to excessive nitric oxide. For example, many MCS patients report sensitivity to electromagnetic fields (EMFs),[8,65] and such fields are reported to produce increases in nitric oxide.[66-70]

IS ASTHMA CAUSED BY AN ELEVATED NITRIC OXIDE/PEROXYNITRITE MECHANISM CENTERED ON THE NO/ONOO⁻ CYCLE?

The role of asthma in MCS, and the similarities between the sensitivity mechanisms in asthma and those that appear to be involved in sensitivity in other regions of the body in MCS, suggests that one should look for a similarity in etiology between the two illnesses. Specifically, is asthma caused by the NO/ONOO⁻ cycle localized to certain regions of the lung? It has been widely reported that asthma is comorbid with CFS and FM, and even in PTSD, which is classified as a psychiatric illness, asthma has often been reported to be a comorbid condition.[71-75] It is interesting that asthmatics are reported to have elevated nitric oxide levels in the air coming from their lungs and that nitric oxide levels increase to much higher levels during asthmatic attacks.[76-80]

From the principles developed in Chapter 1, one would argue that one needs three types of evidence to support the view that asthma may be caused by the NO/ONOO⁻ cycle. There should be evidence for initiation of disease by short-term stressors that may act by increasing nitric oxide levels. There should be evidence for a chronic phase of the illness characterized by elevated levels of the various elements involved in the vicious cycle. There should be evidence that the characteristic symptoms and signs of the illness may be generated by elements of the cycle. We have already provided in the preceding section of this chapter some evidence to the last of these three—that sensitivity symptoms of asthma may be generated by elements of our vicious cycle. There is also extensive evidence that nitric oxide, peroxynitrite, oxidative stress, NF-κB activity, inflammatory cytokines, intracellular calcium, and vanilloid activity are all elevated in asthma, and there is also evidence that some of these, notably nitric oxide and NF-κB activity, have important causal roles in the disease. The evidence for these is so extensive that it would take a whole chapter to review them, but any reader can identify this literature through the PubMed database.

So, we are left with the first of these three—is it possible that short-term stressors that may initiate cases of asthma act by increasing nitric oxide? Stressors implicated in initiation of cases of asthma include infections of the lung, including both viral and bacterial, a variety of chemical exposures including occupational sensitizers and tobacco smoke, allergies, and mold (presumbly mycotoxin) exposure.[5,81-85] Each of these may be able to act via increases in nitric oxide, as argued in Chapter 5 and elsewhere in this chapter. Of these stressors, the proposed mechanism for mycotoxin action leading to nitric oxide and subsequent initiation of asthma is speculative, but the actions of the other stressors in increasing nitric oxide are all very well documented. The observations here also provide support for the view that these stressors act locally in the lung, because initiation of asthma cases are reported to involve lung infections or chemicals or antigens breathed into the lung.[11,81-85] So, the overall evidence is substantial that asthma may be a NO/ONOO⁻ cycle lung disease.

LACK OF AN ESSENTIAL OLFACTORY ROLE IN MCS

MCS is often described as sensitivity to odors, but you may have noticed that the mechanism outlined earlier does not predict an essential role for the sense of smell, the olfactory system, in MCS. It has long seemed unlikely that the pesticides might act by an olfactory mechanism, given how often they are reported to be involved in the initiation of MCS cases and given the lack of any strong odor of these pesticides themselves. Rather, the common involvement of pesticides suggests that they act through their known neurotoxicological mechanisms. Similarly, the putative role of the vanilloid receptor as the major target of volatile organic solvents argues against any key role of the olfactory system.

There were other studies reported earlier (reviewed in References 8 and 86) that also argued against an important olfactory role. For example, people with nasal congestion due to colds or other upper respiratory tract infections, or whose nasal passages have been clipped off to prevent any sense of smell, can still show chemical sensitivity responses. In addition, acosmic individuals, those with no apparent sense of smell, are reported to suffer from MCS.[8] While none of these observations argue against any possible accessory role of the olfactory system in MCS, they do argue against any essential role. Because of this, we should stop referring to MCS as sensitivity to odors, in my judgment, and this caution should extend both to those advocating a physiological explanation for MCS and to the psychogenic advocates, where the latter may still exist. Individuals with MCS may well have NO/ONOO$^-$ cycle-caused changes in their olfactory organs and may therefore experience changes in olfactory sensitivity, but that is not the causal mechanism of MCS.

USEFUL WAYS TO LOOK AT MCS

Some of you may be convinced that I am onto something very important with this presentation but may also feel overwhelmed by the detail and the many complex interactions that have been presented here. The evidence always lies in these details, but what are the important perspectives that may give one an overview of MCS?

Sensitivity is local. The local nature of the NO/ONOO$^-$ cycle mechanism means that initiation of sensitivity in different organs can occur independently of each other.

Sensitivity is to stressors that increase nitric oxide/peroxynitrite, not just chemicals. In peripheral sensitivity, we see sensitivity to antigen–antibody reactions, especially in asthma and rhinitis, to cold and to oxidant stress induced by excessive exercise. In central sensitization, many cases of MCS also show properties of sensitivity to EMFs. Exposure to EMFs has been reported to increase nitric oxide synthesis,[6] and so it is possible that the mechanisms of EMF sensitivity may be similar or identical to those seen in MCS.

The NO/ONOO$^-$ cycle theory has allowed for a seamless fusion of the views of Dr. Iris Bell on neural sensitization, of Dr. Julius Anderson on a vanilloid receptor role, and of Dr. William Meggs on peripheral sensitization. As such, it may be viewed as a *conceptual keystone* in producing a consistent model for MCS and related processes. Central (brain) sensitization is what happens when there is a *massive stimulation of the normal process involved in learning and memory.*

Multiple mechanisms are involved, both centrally and peripherally, *producing the exquisite sensitivity found in MCS.* It is only through the action of these multiple mechanisms, which act synergistically with each other, that one can get the circa 1000-fold increase in sensitivity seen in many MCS patients.

SUMMARY OF THE EVIDENCE

Given the lack of funding for research on MCS, there is a surprising number of different types of observations that provide support for the mechanism of MCS presented in this chapter. Eleven types of evidence were published supporting a nitric oxide/peroxynitrite role in MCS (Exhibit 7.1). In addition to this, Ashford and Miller (pp. 258, 259, Reference 8) list 10 distinct striking similarities between MCS and neural sensitization, providing support for the proposed role of neural sensitivity in MCS. Anderson and I list 12 types of evidence supporting a role for the vanilloid receptor as the major target of volatile organic solvents and certain other compounds in MCS.[5] So these three publications provide a total of at least 33 different types of support. There are others.

The convergence of *both* organochlorine pesticides and pyrethroid pesticides, discussed earlier in this chapter and elsewhere,[6] onto the NMDA/ nitric oxide/peroxynitrite mechanism provides two additional types of support. This NMDA response was previously proposed to be central to both the actions of organophosphorus/carbamate pesticides[2,3] and to that of vanilloid activation,[5] thus providing a convergence of all four classes of chemicals.

The reported role of the CCK-B receptor in MCS based on genetic evidence provides support for a role of NMDA receptors, given the known role of CCK-B in the regulation of NMDA receptors.[2,49]

Clinical observations with dextromethorphan, a known NMDA antagonist, in blocking chemical sensitivity responses provide evidence for this receptor activity in MCS.[2]

BBB permeabilization was reported to occur in MCS patients,[21] providing evidence for a possible peroxynitrite BBB role.

Kuklinski, who published the BBB study mentioned here, also sent me as yet unpublished evidence that citrulline levels are elevated in sera of MCS patients; citrulline is the co-product with nitric oxide of nitric oxide synthases, and so this provides evidence for increased nitric oxide synthesis in MCS.[87]

Miller and Mitzel[47] reported that MCS patients are hypersensitive to monosodium glutamate; because glutamate acts as an excitotoxin to a substantial extent by stimulating NMDA receptors, this provides further evidence that MCS patients are hypersensitive to NMDA stimulation.

If you add up each of these individual observations that provide support for this model of MCS, you come up with 40. While there is no doubt that many of these require further study and all of them can be individually interpreted in other ways, the total number of observations providing support is, nonetheless, quite impressive. The case is even more impressive if one adds to these, all of the cogent explanations for the many previously puzzling features of MCS.

THE NO/ONOO⁻ CYCLE
AS AN EXPLANATORY MODEL OF MCS

The NO/ONOO⁻ cycle excels as an explanatory model of MCS. After all, it was the many unexplained puzzles about MCS that led many to conclude that we needed a new paradigm to explain it. And it was those unexplained puzzles that allowed psychogenic advocates to argue that it must be psychological, arguing falsely that if we do not understand something, it must be psychological. Because the NO/ONOO⁻ cycle explains each of these challenging puzzles, it is a most compelling as explanatory model. Let us review each of these puzzles and briefly describe our explanation.

1. How can so· many diverse chemicals initiate a common sensitivity mechanism and trigger sensitivity responses? Each of the four classes of chemicals, the three classes of pesticides and the volatile organic solvents, can stimulate a distinct receptor with each receptor producing stimulation of the NMDA receptors and consequently increasing nitric oxide and peroxynitrite. It is the convergence of these pathways that allows for a common response to these diverse chemicals.

2. Why is MCS chronic? Because, the NO/ONOO⁻ cycle is a vicious cycle that propagates itself over time. It should be noted that the chronic nature of the central sensitivity mechanisms was previously explained by the changes in the synapses in the brain in the neural sensitization mechanism and this is part of our explanation here as well. Howeve neural sensitization did not explain the chronic nature of peripheral sensitivity, but the NO/ONOO⁻ cycle does.

3. How can MCS sufferers be so exquisitely sensitive to chemicals, on the order of a thousand times more sensitive than normals? The central sensitivity is explained by six distinct sensitivity mechanisms, five of which involve either peroxynitrite or nitric oxide and the sixth involving oxidants. It is the combination of these six mechanisms, each acting synergistically with the others, that can generate this high-level sensitivity in regions of the brain. One of these six mechanisms, peroxynitrite-mediated permeabilization of BBB, cannot be involved in peripheral sensitivity. A second such mechanism, nitric oxide acting as a retrograde messenger, may also not be involved in peripheral sensitivity. But other peripheral mechanisms includ-

ing neurogenic inflammation and mast cell activation may be expected to add to the peripheral sensitivity. Thus, we can explain both central sensitivity and peripheral sensitivity through a NO/ONOO⁻ cycle mechanism.

4. How can diverse volatile organic solvents initiate and trigger sensitivity responses? Probably through the action of the vanilloid receptor that appears to be stimulated by diverse solvents and other irritants.

5. Why are the symptoms of MCS patients so diverse? Because, variation in the tissues impacted by the NO/ONOO⁻ cycle biochemistry from one patient to another leads to distinct symptomatic patters. The local nature of most of the cycle mechanisms causes this pattern in a particular patient to propagate itself over time.

6. Why is MCS comorbid with CFS and FM and why is it part of Gulf War syndrome? Because, they are all NO/ONOO⁻ cycle illnesses. Their common biochemistry is often triggered in tissues producing symptoms characteristic of more than one of these illnesses.

7. How can MCS patients show desensitization/masking in response to repeated or chronic low-level chemical exposure? The day-to-day chemical exposures involved are to volatile organic solvents where sensitivity is apparently mediated by the vanilloid receptor. It is known that many vanilloid agonists (chemicals that stimulate the vanilloid receptor) have the property that chronic or repeated low-level exposure leads to lowered vanilloid receptor sensitivity. It is this lowered vanilloid sensitivity that explains the desensitization/masking response in MCS patients.

8. How can molds in some "sick building syndrome" situations produce MCS? Probably through volatile mold toxins (mycotoxins) that stimulate the vanilloid receptor. In this way, mycotoxins may act to initiate cases of MCS and also to trigger subsequent sensitivity responses in those already sensitive, acting through the same pathway as do volatile organic solvents.

9. Why is neurogenic inflammation found in peripheral chemically sensitive tissues? Because neurogenic inflammation is stimulated by both nitric oxide and vanilloid receptor activity, both elements of the NO/ONOO⁻ cycle. The chronic nature of the cycle means that neurogenic inflammation will also be chronic, adding an additional component to the peripheral sensitivity mechanism.

10. How can mast cell activation be involved? Mast cells are also activated by nitric oxide and by vanilloid activity and may be expected to be stimulated, therefore, by the NO/ONOO⁻ cycle.

11. How can the reported changes in the porphyrin biosynthetic pathway be produced? Mostly by nitric oxide, which is reported to down-regulate the activity of several porphyrin biosynthetic enzymes.

The NO/ONOO⁻ cycle mechanism provides us with explanations for eleven challenging puzzles for MCS. Of these puzzles, we previously had only a partial explanation for only one of them (the chronic nature). It was the challenging nature of these puzzles that made MCS so controversial. The NO/ONOO⁻ cycle, as a powerful explanatory model, should put much of this controversy to rest.

SEARCH FOR SPECIFIC BIOMARKERS FOR MCS

The search for specific markers for each of these multisystem illnesses is made more difficult because so many of the reported changes are simply caused by their inflammatory biochemistry and will be shared, therefore, with many inflammatory illnesses. The specificity needed for a biomarker must come from whatever specific tissue or tissues is most characteristically impacted in a particular multisystem illness. In MCS the most obvious thing to do is look at the response to low level chemical exposure, because the *chemical sensitivity of certain tissues is the most characteristic feature of MCS*. It is only in the response to these chemicals that the needed specificity of a biomarker for this illness is likely to be found.

There are already some reports that may suggest such a specific response to low-level chemical exposure. For example, Bell and her colleagues[33] reported that certain EEG changes were seen in response to low-level chemical exposure in MCS patients. In a recent example, Kimata[88] reported that substance P levels were elevated in MCS patients and that further elevation was produced by low-level chemical exposure. Because substance P is released on vanilloid stimulation, this may help confirm a role of the vanilloid receptor in response to chemicals in MCS and also suggests that this may be useful as a specific biomarker. Kimata also looked at two additional responses to chemicals that may both be related to vanilloid stimulation, and found increased responses of both on chemical exposure of MCS cases. One of these, histamine release, may be explained by the activation of mast cells produced by both nitric oxide and vanilloid stimulation and the other, nerve growth factor increase, may also be a consequence of vanilloid stimulation. Recently, Millqvist and coworkers confirmed the results of Kimata on nerve growth factor increases in response to chemical exposure[89] in MCS cases, in this study using the chemical capsaicin, a classic vanilloid agonist. This may indeed be a useful specific biomarker for MCS and that is due to hyperresponsiveness of the vanilloid receptor.There are other apparent specific responses of MCS patients to low-level chemical exposures.

Shinohara et al.[90] reported hypersensitive reactions of MCS patients to low-level chemical exposures.

There is one apparent nonlocalized response to chemicals, that reported by Joffres et al.[91] They found MCS-related increases in skin conductivity in response to low-level chemical exposure. This is probably an involuntary reaction to brain sensitization, producing a skin response similar to that seen in lie-detector tests when someone is lying.

The approach that I would like to see, given my understanding MCS, would be to measure nitric oxide levels (directly or indirectly) before and after low-level chemical exposure, predicting that increases in nitric oxide should be much greater in MCS patients compared to controls. Interestingly, an increase in nitric oxide after exposure to treatments producing sensitivity responses has now been very well documented in asthma, where measurements of nitric oxide levels coming from the lungs show substantial increases accompanying an asthmatic attack. It should be noted that nitric oxide is stable in the gas phase, unlike in biological fluids, and so it can be measured directly in the air coming from the lungs.

I am optimistic that we are probably on the verge of developing several responses to low-level chemical exposure as specific biomarkers of MCS, biomarkers that can be used as objective measures of diagnosis and can also be used to demonstrate aspects of the disease mechanism.

Chapter 8

Fibromyalgia

TAKE-HOME LESSONS

Cases of fibromyalgia (FM) are most commonly initiated by physical trauma, particularly head and neck trauma, or by viral or bacterial infection, stressors known to be capable of increasing nitric oxide levels. Severe psychological stress, another stressor that can act to increase nitric oxide levels, is also reported to be involved in initiation of some FM cases. Secondary FM in persons suffering from autoimmune disease may also involve nitric oxide and other inflammatory aspects of NO/ONOO$^-$ cycle biochemistry.

Many of the elements of the NO/ONOO$^-$ cycle are reported to be elevated in the chronic phase of FM, including oxidative stress, mitochondrial dysfunction, nitric oxide, inflammatory cytokines, NMDA activity, and vanilloid activity. Some studies of therapy of FM are also consistent with a NO/ONOO$^-$ cycle etiology. Perhaps the most puzzling question about FM is how the widespread pain that is its most characteristic feature is generated. I suggest a hypothesis that the widespread pain is generated by the impact of NO/ONOO$^-$ cycle biochemistry on the thalamus, producing lessened down-regulation of pain processing in the spinal cord and therefore excessive widespread pain sensitivity. A number of agents that down-regulate elements of the NO/ONOO$^-$ cycle are reported to produce improvements in FM patients, and I will discuss in Chapter 15 how combinations of these agents may provide an effective treatment protocol.

INTRODUCTION

Fibromylagia, like the other three multisystem illnesses, has many of symptoms and signs shared with these illnesses, which may be explained by

Explaining "Unexplained Illnesses"
© 2007 by The Haworth Press, Inc. All rights reserved.
doi:10.1300/5139_08

our NO/ONOO⁻ cycle mechanism, as discussed in Chapter 3. As with the other illnesses, it is important to consider in some detail the evidence for such a mechanism, and this will entail considering both the initiation by reported stressors increasing nitric oxide levels and the properties of the chronic phase of the illness to determine whether the properties of that phase are consistent with those predicted by our mechanism.

POSSIBLE INITIATION VIA NITRIC OXIDE

Four distinct types of short-term stressors are reported to precede and presumably induce cases of FM. Two of these are similar to those most commonly preceding many cases of chronic fatigue syndrome (CFS), notably viral and bacterial infections,[1-7] and as discussed in Chapter 5, these are established to produce increases in nitric oxide levels. In addition, physical trauma, typically a bad fall, automobile accident, or operation often precede cases of FM.[1,8-13] In one study, it was reported that the types of trauma most commonly leading to cases of FM was head and neck trauma.[9] Physical trauma, in general, has been reported to produce increases in nitric oxide in both humans[14-16] and in a rat model,[17,18] and is also reported to produce oxidative stress;[18] so it is possible for physical trauma to act through nitric oxide increases. In addition, head trauma, producing traumatic head/brain injury, has been shown in many studies to lead to increases in NMDA activity and consequent increases in nitric oxide levels (see, for example, References 19-24). The relationship between head injury and nitric oxide level increases has been extensively studied, and there are multiple mechanisms involved but with each acting to increase NMDA activity. The fourth type of stressor reported to initiate cases of FM is severe psychological stress,[25-29] and the way this may act to increase nitric oxide levels will be discussed in Chapter 9.

There are cases of FM that have been considered "secondary" to previous cases of other diseases, particularly the autoimmune diseases rheumatoid arthritis and lupus.[30,31] These autoimmune diseases, as was discussed in Chapter 2, are characterized by elevated nitric oxide and peroxynitrite in the tissue being attacked, with such tissue also showing evidence for many other inflammatory biochemical changes. So, how might such inflammatory changes be causally linked to the initiation of FM? Possibly through the action of the systemic (as opposed to the local changes) that may be expected to occur as a function of this biochemistry and possibly, in the case of lupus, through direct attack on the tissue most centrally involved in producing the symptoms of FM. Such systemic changes were discussed in

Chapter 4, and may include transport of nitric oxide in the red blood cells to other parts of the body, depletion of antioxidants by oxidative stress, and possibly the transport of inflammatory cytokines to other tissues. The argument here, and the inference cannot be taken as established, is that the inflammatory biochemistry produced by the autoimmune response may have a role in the initiation of cases of FM.

The important take-home lesson is that each of the five types of stressor, viral or bacterial infection, physical trauma, severe psychological stress, and autoimmune inflammation, commonly reported to initiate cases of FM, may well act via their ability to increase nitric oxide levels and other aspects of NO/ONOO⁻ cycle biochemistry.

CHRONIC-PHASE CORRELATES OF FM

Most of the aspects of our proposed vicious cycle mechanism have been studied in the chronic phase of FM and have been shown to be elevated as predicted. For example, there are six studies of markers of oxidative stress that have been reported, and each of these provides evidence for elevated oxidative damage in this illness.[32-37] These are consistent with the interpretation of Ali and coworkers, who suggested that FM is an illness of oxidative stress.[38,39] Certain other observations about FM may be produced by an etiology involving oxidative chain reactions. For example, Klein and Berg reported that both antiphospholipid and antiganglioside antibodies were often present in FM;[40] because such antibody formation presumably requires covalent cross-linking of these haptenic groups to proteins and such cross-linking can occur by lipid peroxidation chain reactions in membranes, formation of such antibodies can be interpreted as being due to oxidative stress initiated chain reactions. Four clinical studies with agents with substantial antioxidant activity[41-44] provide some support for the view that oxidative stress may contribute to the symptoms of FM.

Another prediction of our vicious cycle is that inflammatory cytokine levels will tend to be elevated, and this prediction has also been supported by several studies of FM.[45-50]

There are two studies that have reported evidence that nitric oxide levels appear to be elevated in FM. One of them is the study of Larson et al., in which the levels of citrulline, a marker of the synthesis of nitric oxide, is elevated in the cerebrospinal fluid of FM patients.[51] A second was a study of Bradley et al.[52] reporting that nitrate/nitrite levels in the blood of FM patients were elevated. Because nitric oxide and peroxynitrite break down to produce nitrate/nitrite, this provides additional evidence for elevated nitric oxide synthesis in this illness. However, a third study inferred that nitric oxide synthesis was low in FM.[36] This was based on measurements of S-nitrosothiols in proteins of FM patients, a marker that may be questioned on whether it is a reliable marker for nitric oxide levels when studied in the presence of high levels of oxidants. S-nitrosothiols react with both superoxide and peroxynitrite, destroying their structures, and therefore both superoxide and peroxynitrite may be expected to lower the levels of S-nitrosothiols (Chapter 2). It follows that the low reported levels of S-nitrosothiols in FM may reflect high levels of superoxide and/or peroxynitrite, rather than low levels of nitric oxide. There are three reasons to raise some doubts about the interpretation of this third study: One is that there are two other studies that support the opposite conclusion. A second is that there are some reasons to doubt the specificity of the marker being studied, as was discussed in Chapter 3. The third is that both inflammatory cytokines (see the preceding text) and NMDA activity (see the following text) are reported to be elevated in FM, and both of these are known to be able to raise nitric oxide levels. Based on all of these studies, the predominant evidence suggests that nitric oxide levels are elevated in FM.

Mitochondrial/energy metabolism dysfunction in FM was reported in 11 studies (cited in Chapter 3). These may be consistent with the known mechanisms by which peroxynitrite, nitric oxide, and superoxide can produce such dysfunction (discussed in Chapter 2). Is there any evidence suggesting that the particular types of mitochondrial dysfunction produced by peroxynitrite may occur in FM? There is one type of study that this may be true. Ali[38,39] has reported that citric acid levels are elevated in the vast majority of FM patients, and citric acid will accumulate due to peroxynitrite inactivation of the aconitase enzyme, as was discussed in Chapter 5. This provides some evidence consistent with a possible role of peroxynitrite in producing the mitochondrial/energy metabolism dysfunction in FM.

Another aspect of our vicious cycle mechanism is the elevation of vanilloid activity. Such elevation has been reported in three studies of FM,[53-55] providing some support for this inference.

EXCESSIVE NMDA ACTIVITY IN FIBROMYLAGIA

There are three distinct types of evidence that provide support for the inference that excessive NMDA activity has an important causal role in the generation of FM symptoms. The first of these comes from a series of studies from various laboratories reporting that drugs that act as NMDA antagonists improve the symptoms of FM patients.[56-64] These results not only suggest that one of the predictions of our proposed vicious cycle—that NMDA activity is elevated in FM—but also that lowering this parameter leads to substantial improvement in symptoms.

The second is the evidence, reported by Larson et al.[51] and similar evidence reported by Peres et al.[65] that the glutamate levels in the cerebrospinal fluid of FM patients are elevated when compared with controls. It follows that, since glutamate acts to stimulate NMDA activity, this provides evidence for a particular mechanism of NMDA stimulation.

The third study is that of Smith et al.[66] in which they report that certain FM patients show a cessation of symptoms when placed on a diet devoid of monosodium glutamate and aspartame. Glutamate is an excitotoxin, acting in part through NMDA stimulation and aspartame is degraded (hydrolyzed) to release aspartic acid, another excitotoxin known to stimulate NMDA activity. The authors inferred from these results that excitotoxic activity of these two food additives may act to exacerbate the symptoms of and possibly the basic mechanism of FM.[66] These results suggest that, in these FM patients, the action of any vicious cycle mechanism is insufficient to maintain an elevated pain response and other symptoms of FM without continued stimulation of the FM mechanism, in this case, by these excitotoxins. These results are similar in concept to the observations of some multiple chemical sensitivity (MCS) patients who have reported improved MCS symptoms when they were able to carefully avoid chemical exposure (Chapter 7). However, the improvement in FM symptoms in these FM patients reported by Smith et al.[66] was much more rapid. In any case, these results provide a third type of evidence implicating elevated NMDA activity in FM.

Let me just remind you again, as was discussed in Chapter 2 and Chapter 3, excessive NMDA activity is known to produce excessive nitric oxide and peroxynitrite levels, and thus can exacerbate the basic biochemistry most central to our vicious cycle mechanism.

WHAT IS THE CORE MECHANISM OF EXCESSIVE PAIN IN FM?

Mechanisms have consequences, and you have already seen how the primarily local nature of our NO/ONOO⁻ cycle mechanism leads to understandings of many aspects of these illnesses. It leads to understandings of the overlapping and variable symptoms and signs of these illnesses, as discussed in Chapters 3 and 4, and of the properties of both CFS and MCS as discussed in Chapters 5 and 7. In FM, however, the cardinal symptom is the widespread excessive pain seen in this illness, and the question must be raised about how such widespread excessive pain can be generated as a function of the possible impact of our NO/ONOO⁻ cycle on a particular tissue? FM pain is distinct from the usual pain of hyperalgesia, in that hyperalgesia pain is usually localized to one or possibly several specific regions of the body, whereas FM pain is characteristically, consistently and widely dispersed. The most common approach to diagnosis of FM is centered on large numbers of tender points, but it is well documented that excessive pain in FM is much more widely present and that the tender points are just a convenient method of assessing this pain. This widespread pain produces a challenge for the NO/ONOO⁻ cycle mechanism because that mechanism ascribes the characteristic symptoms of each illness to the impact of the cycle on one or perhaps a few tissues. So, the question that needs to be raised is whether there is a mechanism by which our proposed vicious cycle may be able to generate such widespread excessive pain through its impact on a single tissue.

A series of studies have suggested that the basic mechanism in FM is central[67-73]—that is derived from a change in the central nervous system, but that leaves open the question of what region of region of brain and/or spinal cord causes the increased pain perception in FM.

While hyperalgesia is usually distinct from the widespread pain in FM, the pain mechanisms involved in hyperalgesia may, nevertheless, be important in understanding the excessive pain in FM. You may recall that hyperalgesia pain involves all of the elements of our vicious cycle (Chapter 2) but that they are involved in two distinct regions of the body. Such elements as excessive vanilloid activity and the whole pattern of inflammatory biochemistry are involved in the initial tissue impacted by such excessive pain in what is called primary hyperalgesia. However, these initial changes influence the pain data processing in the dorsal horn regions of the spinal cord, with changes in NMDA activity and nitric oxide being particularly important there, leading to changes in the synapses in this part of the central nervous system (Chapter 2). The changes in the dorsal horn may produce, in turn, changes in the peripheral tissues, impacting somewhat broader tissue regions than were initially impacted, through such mechanisms as neurogenic inflammation, leading to a more widespread inflammatory response in the peripheral tissues. It is the combination of the changes in the dorsal horn and the inflammatory response in the peripheral tissues that are responsible for what is known as secondary hyperalgesia.

There are two potentially important consequences of the mechanisms outlined in the preceding paragraph. One is that any mechanism that impacts a specific dorsal horn region will produce a pain response in only a limited region of the body. The dorsal horn regions on many different vertebrae must be impacted if there is to be widespread pain, such as that seen in FM. The second consequence is that the intercommunication of two regions of the body through the nervous system can cause an initial pain response involving one limited tissue to impact additional tissue regions, in this case the dorsal horn, impacting back on a wider region of peripheral tissue. It follows from this that a mechanism that is essentially local may have wider impact through the action of the nervous system. The basic question that I am raising here is whether there is a particular part of the brain involved in the processing of pain information, which, if impacted, may be expected to lead to the widespread changes in both pain perception and also real peripheral tissue changes that have been reported in FM? In other words, is the initial mechanism a local one starting in a specific region of the brain, but one in which, because of the action of the nervous system, the initial change may lead to the widespread pain response we view as most characteristic of FM?

Staud and coworkers have documented changes in what is called wind-up pain processing in FM, processing that involves changes in each of the many dorsal horn regions of the spinal column.[72] These studies imply that many dorsal horn regions are changed in FM, not just a few, showing changes characteristic of those found in other hyperalgesia situations.

So, which brain region may be involved in producing such multiple changes in the dorsal horn regions? The proposal here, and I am drawing on previous insights published by Larson and Kovacs,[74] by Henriksson,[75] and also by Staud,[76] is that the critical region of the brain may be the thalamus.

The thalamus is stimulated by neurons ascending from the dorsal horns to the thalamus, known as the spinothalamic tract[77,78] (Figure 8.1), with the spinothalamic tract carrying much of the information about pain from the spinal column into the brain, where it can be interpreted. Most importantly, the thalamus also has descending neurons, known as lamina I neurons, which modulate the activity, primarily negatively, of the dorsal horns[79-81] (Figure 8.1). The dorsal horns, in turn, may modulate the activity of the peripheral nociceptors, the receptors that produce the perception of pain (Figure 8.1). In this way, changed activity in a single part of the brain in FM, the *thalamus,* may be expected to produce the widespread excessive pain perception seen as the cardinal symptom of FM. Through changed activity of the descending neurons, it may increase the sensitivity through induced changes in the various dorsal horn regions. A deficiency in descending pain inhibitory activity in FM patients was recently reported by a group in Quebec,[82] providing one type of support for this viewpoint.

Changes in the thalamus have been reported to occur in several brain scan studies of FM patients,[83-86] providing some support that it may be the

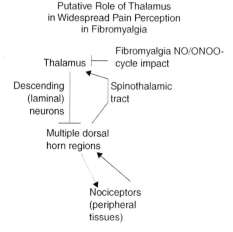

FIGURE 8.1. How impact on the thalamus may lead to widespread pain in FM. The thalamus has largely inhibitory neurons, called descending lamina I neurons, which inhibit pain processing in the dorsal horn regions of the spinal cord. Putative impact of the NO/ONOO⁻ cycle on the thalamus may be expected to lower this inhibitory activity, thus greatly increasing pain processing at the different dorsal horn regions of the spinal cord, leading to the widespread pain that is the cardinal symptom of FM.

critical tissue initially impacted in FM. A central role for the thalamus in FM is also suggested by the observations of Larson et al.[87] providing support for the view that mast cell activation in the thalamus may have an important role in FM. As was noted in Chapter 8, mast cell activation is stimulated by both vanilloid receptor stimulation and by nitric oxide, both elements of our vicious cycle mechanism.

There is one other observation that makes the thalamus an attractive candidate for the most important tissue involved in producing the widespread pain in FM—its location in the anatomy of the body (Figure 8.2). You may recall that a potentially important study reported that FM was often initiated specifically by head and neck trauma.[9] Given the location of the thalamus in the brain, a direct extension of the spinal column and pons, it may be expected to be susceptible to impact by such head and neck trauma, with such trauma possibly pulling on the upper spinal column, leading to damage in the nearby thalamus. So, the reported role of such head and neck trauma in many cases of FM appears to be consistent with the suggested role of the thalamus in FM.

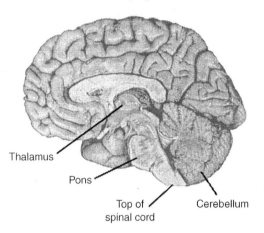

Thalamus

Pons

Top of
spinal cord

Cerebellum

FIGURE 8.2. Location of thalamus, leading to sensitivity to head and neck physical trauma. The thalamus is a roughly egg-shaped part of the brain, directly above the spinal cord and pons. Because of its location and the fact that neurons connect the thalamus with the spinal cord, head and neck physical trauma may be expected to lead to physical stress in the thalamus, possibly leading to excessive NMDA activity in the thalamus. This is a reasonable supposition on how head and neck trauma may lead to NO/ONOO⁻ cycle biochemistry in the thalamus and consequently the widespread excessive pain of FM. *Source:* This brain section was prepared by the Digital Anatomist Project of the University of Washington and is used with permission; the role of that project and of Dr. Kate Mulligan are both gratefully acknowledged.

The notion here is not that the thalamus is the only tissue impacted but rather that a variety of other tissues are impacted in part because of the changes in the thalamus, including dorsal horns, peripheral tissues, and other pain centers in the brain, including the anterior cingulate cortex.[88] Furthermore, as appears to be the case with each of these illnesses, additional tissues may also be independently impacted by the same NO/ONOO⁻ cycle inflammatory biochemistry, with such impact leading to additional symptoms, with both the tissues involved and the symptoms generated varying considerably from one patient to another.

In a study of a rat model of this type of process, a possible rat model for FM[89] showed changes in the thalamus involving serotonin, NMDA activity, and nitric oxide. Changes in serotonin control have been implicated in FM[90-95] as well as NMDA receptor activity and nitric oxide, as discussed earlier in this chapter, with the latter two also being of central importance in our model.

The notion that the thalamus is most centrally responsible for the excessive pain in FM has to be viewed as a hypothesis less well established than many other parts of our overall etiologic theory. It is nevertheless important, because it shows how the local impact on one part of the brain may be able to generate the widespread pain sensitivity seen in FM. That, in turn, is important because it shows how the mainly local nature of our basic mechanism may be compatible with the cardinal symptom of FM—widespread pain.

REACTIONS OF PAIN CENTERS
IN THE BRAIN IN FM

In the discussion of MCS (Chapter 7), it was suggested that the only way in which a specific biomarker of MCS might be developed was in terms a specific response to chemical exposure. One may be tempted to make a parallel argument for FM—that the most likely approach to developing a specific biomarker for FM would be in measuring a specific response to what, in normals, would be modest stimuli. There have been a number of studies reporting that measurable changes in brain responses to such stimuli, where the responses in FM are distinctive enough to often be distinguishable from those of normal controls.[96-98] These studies suggest an approach to develop a specific biomarker for FM, one that can be used as an objective criterion for diagnosis. These scan studies use specialized and expensive equipment, and so this may prevent there being used routinely for standard diagnostic tests.

Chapter 9

Post-Traumatic Stress Disorder

TAKE-HOME LESSONS

A number of the elements of the NO/ONOO⁻ cycle are reported to be elevated in post-traumatic stress disorder (PTSD). The severe psychological stress that commonly initiates cases of PTSD acts in animal models through increased NMDA activity and the consequent nitric oxide increase is also reported to have a role. There are plausible mechanisms by which severe psychological stress may produce a similar NMDA/nitric oxide response in humans. Head trauma, which is considered a paradoxical initiator of PTSD, also produces large increases in NMDA activity. Several elements of the NO/ONOO⁻ cycle are reported to be elevated in PTSD animal models and in humans, but further study is needed in this area.

The generation of some of the psychiatric symptoms of PTSD was already discussed in Chapter 3, while potential mechanisms for others, most characteristic of PTSD, are discussed in this chapter. The concept of allostatic load may be explained, in part, as being a direct consequence of NO/ONOO⁻ cycle biochemistry in regions of the hippocampus. PTSD may simply be another NO/ONOO⁻ cycle illness, whose most characteristic symptoms are classified as psychiatric. In the other multisystem illnesses, we have studies of therapy reporting that agents predicted to lower NO/ONOO⁻ cycle biochemistry produce improvement. However, in PTSD, we have no similar studies.

INTRODUCTION

Why, some have asked, have you included PTSD? After all, is it not a psychiatric disease? And, does including it not just give increasing fodder to those who argue that these other illnesses are "all in your head"?

Explaining "Unexplained Illnesses"
© 2007 by The Haworth Press, Inc. All rights reserved.
doi:10.1300/5139_09

My own view is that this just shows that many medical categories are arbitrary, based mainly on the most characteristic symptoms rather than on any basic differences in etiology. And those categories ignore the many similarities and overlaps seen among these illnesses, similarities and overlaps whose mechanisms were explored in Chapter 3. Most importantly, one needs to keep in mind that the earlier dualism between the mental/psychiatric/psychological and the physical/biological/physiological has been firmly rejected by modern science. For example,[1] and I will quote this again in Chapter 13:

> the term mental disorder unfortunately implies a distinction between "mental" disorders and "physical" disorders that is a reductionist anachronism of mind/body dualism. A compelling literature documents that there is much "physical" in "mental" disorders and much "mental" in "physical" disorders. (p. xxi)

So if the American Psychiatric Association in their most important publication (Reference 1) rejects this dualism, should we have any hesitation in doing likewise?

We have already seen in Chapter 3 that 14 or 15 of the 17 symptoms and signs shared among these multisystem illnesses occur in PTSD sufferers, showing that PTSD shares many similarities with the other multisystem illnesses. These shared properties include elevated levels of inflammatory cytokines, low natural killer (NK) cell function, irritable bowel syndrome, circulatory dysfunction including orthostatic intolerance, hypothalamic-pituitary-adrenal (HPA) axis dysfunction, as well as positron emission tomography (PET) scan and single-photon emission computed tomography (SPECT) scan changes. So there is much that is physiological in PTSD, as much as there is in these other multisystem illnesses. It follows that we should consider the possibility of a similar etiologic mechanism in PTSD to that of these other multisystem illnesses, as has been previously suggested.[2-5]

Does PTSD fit our NO/ONOO$^-$ cycle paradigm or not? In order to answer that question, we need to look at the same types of criteria that we have with these other illnesses. I have already discussed three types of evidence for the cycle in PTSD along with the other multisystem illnesses:

1. Evidence from animals models implicating excessive NMDA activity and nitric oxide in the etiology of PTSD (Chapter 1)
2. Evidence that common PTSD symptoms and signs, shared with chronic fatigue syndrome (CFS), multiple chemical sensitivity (MCS),

and fibromyalgia (FM), can be explained by a NO/ONOO⁻ cycle mechanism (Chapter 3)
3. Evidence that psychological stress is involved in initiating a minority of cases of FM, CFS, and MCS (Chapter 1)

Now, it is time to look at other aspects of PTSD.

INITIATION OF CASES OF PTSD

Cases of PTSD are typically preceded by severe psychological stress, and the such stress is often included as an essential criterion for the diagnosis of PTSD. For example, the *Diagnostic and Statistical Manual of Mental Disorders*,[1] fourth edition (DSM-IV), states that PTSD must occur after an "event or events that involve actual or threatened death or serious injury, or threat to the physical integrity of self or others" (p. 424). Thus, there can be no doubt that the psychiatric literature on PTSD considers the short-term stressor of severe psychological stress to be causal in the initiation of cases of PTSD. So we have a short-term stressor followed by a chronic illness, what may be viewed as the classic pattern of case initiation according to the vicious cycle model of these illnesses. Can this short-term stressor act via nitric oxide?

The best evidence that it may act in this way comes from studies of the initiation of PTSD-like responses in animal models, where such mechanisms can be most easily analyzed. The initiation of animal models of PTSD has been shown to require excessive NMDA activity, with such responses being blocked by NMDA antagonists,[6-10] agents that lower NMDA activity. It is well-known that excessive NMDA activity leads to increases in both nitric oxide and its oxidant product, peroxynitrite, as was discussed in Chapter 2. It follows that, in animal models, severe psychological stress in the initiation of PTSD-like responses may act via increased nitric oxide.

It has been suggested in several reviews that excessive NMDA activity and other glutamate-stimulated receptors are involved in PTSD in humans,[11-19] as well as in animal models, but these observations may be more relevant to the chronic phase of illness.

What mechanisms may be expected to lead from severe psychological stress to excessive NMDA stimulation? There are two such mechanisms thatm ay be suggested. One is that such severe psychological stress can generate high levels of glucocorticoid secretion.* Glucocorticoid stimula-

---

*The glucocorticoid secreted in humans is cortisol.

tion is reported to have an important role in the generation of PTSD-like responses in animal models[20-22] and is thought to be involved in PTSD initiation in humans as well. It is well documented that there is elevated glucocorticoid release in response to severe psychological stress and that such high levels glucocorticoid stimulation produce, in turn, increased NMDA stimulation.[23-30,*] A possible mechanism that may be involved in producing such NMDA stimulation by glucocorticoids is the inhibition of energy metabolism by glucocorticoids that occurs in the hippocampus.[26] I have discussed in both Chapter 3 and Chapter 7 the mechanisms by which lowered energy metabolism leads to increased NMDA activity.

A second mechanism that may be involved in the generation of excessive NMDA activity during severe psychological stress may be the high-level stimulation of processes involved in learning and memory. It is well established that memories of events surrounding severe psychological stress are typically vivid and detailed, suggesting that the processes involved in learning and memory are elevated under such conditions. People recalling stressful events often recall detailed, second-to-second accounts of what occurred. The processes establishing such memories, presumably centered on the mechanism of long-term potentiation (LTP), were discussed in Chapter 7 because of their apparent role in MCS. These processes involve both NMDA receptor activity as well as nitric oxide, so it may be inferred that both elevated NMDA activity and nitric oxide levels may be expected in the vivid and detailed memory processing associated with severe psychological stress.

So, both the role of excessive glucocorticoids and the mechanisms of LTP may help explain how excessive NMDA activity and consequent nitric oxide and peroxynitrite may be involved in the initiation of PTSD in response to severe psychological stress.

Role of Head Trauma in Initiation of Some Cases of PTSD

Harvey and coworkers[31] discuss evidence from a number of studies where cases of PTSD or PTSD-like illness are initiated not by severe psychological

---

*It should be noted that the effect of high levels glucocorticoid here is to increase NMDA activity and consequent nitric oxide levels, and that glucocorticoids can also lower the induction of the inducible nitric oxide synthase (iNOS) and so may have the opposite effect on nitric oxide levels under other conditions. Given the importance of both NMDA receptors and nNOS in the brain and particularly in the hippocampus, the increased nitric oxide may be expected to be the predominant effect in the initiation of PTSD.

stress but rather by traumatic head/brain injury. This conflicts with what they describe as the "widely held belief . . . that an individual who has sustained a traumatic brain injury (TBI) during a traumatic event of sufficient severity to involve coma, loss of consciousness, or severe amnesia cannot subsequently develop posttraumatic stress disorder" (p. 663). Examples of such responses include individuals in motor vehicle accidents who may have no recollection of the accident or even where the accident was sufficiently rapid and unanticipated such that not only is there no recall of psychological stress but it is difficult to see how such stress could have occurred. Such cases of PTSD are considered paradoxical[31] because they occur without any apparent severe psychological stress and therefore occur in the apparent absence of one of the key criteria for PTSD diagnosis required by DSM-IV.[1]

You have already seen in Chapter 8, that there is extensive evidence that traumatic head/brain injury can produce major increases in NMDA activity that will be expected to produce increases in nitric oxide and its oxidant product peroxynitrite. It follows that the expected biochemical/physiological consequence of traumatic head/brain injury appears to closely resemble that discussed for severe psychological stress, described in the previous section of this chapter. It follows that both of these types of stressors may act primarily via excessive NMDA/nitric oxide/peroxynitrite activity, possibly producing similar neurological and behavioral changes. The overall model, which is the focus of this chapter, as a possible mechanism for PTSD is outlined in Figure 9.1.

In this figure, three types of mechanisms producing a common response starting with NMDA receptor activity in regions of the hippocampus, the amygdala, and elsewhere lead to initiation of a vicious cycle responsible for the chronic symptoms of PTSD. While all of the elements of the NO/ONOO$^-$ cycle are not detailed in Figure 9.1, those elements may well be implicated here, and evidence for them should be looked for in the chronic phase of PTSD in humans and in animal models.

NO/ONOO$^-$ Cycle Elements in the Chronic Phase of PTSD

As with the other three multisystem illnesses, it is important to ask whether there are elements of the NO/ONOO$^-$ cycle mechanism known or reported to occur in the chronic phase of PTSD. Here, we will discuss both cases of PTSD and also animal models. Let me remind you that this vicious cycle involves nitric oxide, peroxynitrite, superoxide, oxidative stress, inflammatory cytokines, NF-κB, NMDA receptor activity, and vanilloid receptor activity. Of these, there is some evidence for elevation of five of the

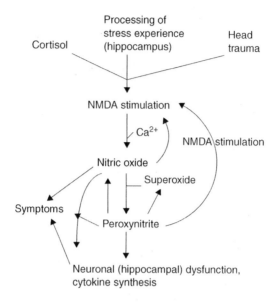

FIGURE 9.1. PTSD stressors leading to increased NMDA activity and subsequent NO/ONOO⁻ cycle interactions. Processing of the stress experience, cortisol elevation, and, in some cases, head/brain trauma all lead to increased NMDA activity. The NMDA activity produces excessive levels of nitric oxide and its oxidant product peroxynitrite, which directly or indirectly lead to hippocampal and other brain changes, elevated inflammatory cytokine levels, and a variety of symptoms of PTSD. The upward pointing arrows diagram the actions of proposed positive feedback loops that collectively make up a NO/ONOO⁻ cycle mechanism, responsible in part for the chronic nature of this disorder.

eight. One of these, documented in Chapter 3, is oxidative stress, where there is evidence for elevation in animal models, but the one study in humans was mixed, suggesting perhaps only a modest elevation. It should be noted that the SPECT scan studies of PTSD patients also suggests some oxidative stress (Chapter 3). The elevated NMDA activity in PTSD is discussed in several reviews.[23-30] Some clinical studies provide support for an elevated NMDA role including a report of improved symptoms on treatment with gabapentin,[32] a drug that indirectly lowers NMDA activity and also with the NMDA partial agonist D-cycloserine.[33] A possible role for excessive glutamate stimulation is also supported by a study implicating excessive activity of the AMPA receptors as well.[34]

A key nitric oxide role was reported in an animal model study where a nitric oxide synthase inhibitor was found to block the development of certain symptoms characteristic of the response to stress in this animal model.[35] In a similar animal model, elevated oxidative stress was also reported,[36] and two previous animal model studies also reported elevated levels of oxidative stress.[37,38] An important nitric oxide role as well as key roles of several other elements of our vicious cycle model were reported in recent animal model studies.[39-41] In these recent studies, evidence was reported of supporting roles of NMDA activity, NF-κB activity, and both increased nNOS and iNOS activity. Hippocampal nitric oxide levels were measured and shown to be elevated in this model.[41] These studies alone implicate several of the elements of our vicious cycle model in PTSD.

In general, then, where we have data on the elements of the NO/OONO-cycle in the chronic phase of PTSD, either in humans or in animal models, the data seems to be consistent with the predictions of the vicious cycle. Still, as is the case with all multisytem illnesses, there are substantial areas where adequate data are lacking.

Possible Damage to the Hippocampus and Amygdala

One of the topics that we have not discussed much in this book is the possible lethal and other long-term damage that may occur to cells as a consequence of NO/ONOO⁻ cycle action. Such damage may occur as a consequence of peroxynitrite-induced apoptotic cell death, as was discussed in Chapter 2. Apoptosis, as you may recall, is a process of programmed cell death that can be induced by a number of stressors on cells. High peroxynitrite levels are known to induce apoptosis in many cell types. Nitric oxide can also have long-lasting effects on the brain through its influence on neuronal cell differentiation.[42-44] Not surprisingly, NMDA activity is also reported to influence such neuronal differentiation.[45,46] It is possible that these effects, and possibly other consequences the NO/ONOO⁻ cycle, may produce long-lasting damage to regions of the brain that are impacted by them.

Does such damage occur in PTSD and does it help us make sense out of the some of the symptoms of PTSD? It has long been proposed that there is hippocampal degeneration in PTSD,[47-50] and such degeneration has been reported in certain animal models.[50] It is reported that people with PTSD tend to have small hippocampi, leading one to question whether these may have effects on their neurophysiology and behavior. A recent study of twins, where one twin had PTSD but the co-twin did not, showed that these pairs of twins tended to have small hippocampi, suggesting that such small hippocampi may have a role in susceptibility to PTSD. But the PTSD-affected twins did not have smaller hippocampi than did their co-twins.[51] This study tends to argue against a hippocampal degeneration process in PTSD, and I am unsure whether this should be considered definitive or not, given all of the other evidence on this issue. Even if there is no change in hippocampal size due to PTSD in humans, there may possibly be damage at the cellular level without any evident overall change in size of the organ involved.

There are some observations coming from some animal model studies suggesting such induced damage in PTSD in the amygdala rather than in the hippocampus. These studies involve NMDA activity in an animal model, both of which were published by Davis and coworkers. In the first of these,[52] Miserendino et al., reported that NMDA antagonists diffused into the amygdala shortly after stress prevented the acquisition of the fear-potentiated startle response, a characteristic response in PTSD. It may be inferred that NMDA activity in the amygdala is essential for the "learning" of this response. However, in the second, it was also reported that NMDA antagonists diffusing subsequently into the amygdala prevented the extinction of this same response.[53] Thus, it appears that NMDA activity is required for both phases of this learned response—the acquisition phase and the extinction phase. PTSD sufferers behave as if the first phase is hyperactive and the second phase is hypoactive, thus leading to a prolonged and potentiated startle reaction. It is tempting to suggest that the first phase of NMDA hyperactivity may, possibly through peroxynitrite-induced apoptosis or other chronic damage, produce the subsequent second-phase NMDA hypoactivity in PTSD. Interestingly, an exaggerated startle response has also been reported to occur in some cases of MCS and FM,[54,55] suggesting that a similar process may be occurring in some cases of those illnesses.

Learning from experience can often be viewed as a two-phase process. The first phase is remembering the actual experience, which, as we have discussed earlier in this chapter, leads to particularly detailed and vivid recollections when it occurs under stress. The second phase is putting the experience into a context: Where is this experience relevant and what is the "take home lesson" that the individual should learn from it? This second phase seems to be defective in PTSD, and so the individual often repeatedly relives his or her trauma, under conditions where such reliving may be viewed as dysfunctional. So I cannot help suggesting that perhaps the second learning phase may be ineffective because of the damage created by the first phase, possibly by the excessive peroxynitrite produced in association with the first phase. It should be noted that learning and memory dysfunction is a common feature in PTSD,[39,56,57] consistent with hippocampal dysfunction.

Clearly, much of what I am saying here is speculative, but it may help us to see how the NO/ONOO⁻ cycle mechanism may lead to some of the symptoms of PTSD. Let me remind you at this point that three of the psychiatric symptoms of these illnesses that are common in PTSD, anxiety, depression, and rage, are all explicable in terms of the NO/ONOO⁻ cycle mechanism, as was discussed in Chapter 3. So there may be a number of what are classified as psychiatric symptoms of PTSD that may be explicable by a NO/ONOO⁻ cycle mechanism.

Reported Blood-Brain Barrier Permeabilization

It has been reported that PTSD victims have substantial permeabilization of their blood-brain barrier (BBB),[58,59] a change that was also reported in two animal models[60-62] but not in a third[63] animal model. Such BBB permeabilization may be produced by elevated levels of peroxynitrite, and I cited 14 studies in one of my papers reporting such a peroxynitrite role.[64] It follows from this that these observations may be viewed as being consistent with our model and as providing some evidence in support of the model.

OVERVIEW

If one does a search of PTSD research in the PubMed database, one finds that the vast majority of studies, over 95 percent of them, have focused on the psychological/psychiatric aspects of PTSD rather than searching for any physiological underpinnings of this illness. Despite this, there has been some very insightful research on the physiology of PTSD, and this work provides substantial evidence supporting our NO/ONOO⁻ cycle mechanism. Short-term stressors initiating cases of PTSD may well work via elevated NMDA activity and consequent nitric oxide and peroxynitrite production. There is evidence for elevation of five different correlates of the NO/OONO⁻ cycle in the chronic phase of the illness. The many overlapping symptoms and signs of PTSD with those of the other three multisystem illnesses, discussed in Chapter 3, provide suggestive evidence for a common etiology, and that etiology may well be our nitric oxide/peroxynitrite cycle mechanism. Clearly, I am relying much more heavily on animal model data in this analysis of PTSD than I did with the other multisystem illnesses, and this must be viewed as a significant limitation in the supporting data. I would argue, however, that the PTSD animal models are often strikingly similar to the human condition and are, in my judgment at least, more convincing as potentially relevant models than are many other animal models discussed elsewhere in this book.

It seems to me that the perspective underlying this chapter is compatible with the views of many who have wrestled with the possible physiological mechanisms involved in the etiology of PTSD, including Sapolsky, McEwen, Bremner, the two Harvey's, Friedman, Yehuda, Antelman, Buskila, and others. Certainly, the proposed role of neural sensitization in PTSD[13,65] is consistent with our proposed mechanism because of the role of NMDA receptors and nitric oxide in such sensitization. Of course, these thinkers will have to weigh in on whether they see such compatibility or not.

I would like to finish by discussing the possible parallels between the mechanisms proposed in this chapter and those of McEwen. McEwen has developed the concept of allostatic load of repeated or chronic stress to describe the cumulative damage to the brain, particularly to the hippocampus.[66] The mechanisms involved in allostatic load include glucocorticoid stimulation, excitatory amino acid (glutamate) stimulation, increased NMDA activity, and, at least in some cases, inflammatory cytokine activity.[66] The similarities between these mechanisms and the mechanisms of the NO/ONOO$^-$ cycle raise the issue of whether part of the physical basis of allostatic load is none other than the action of NO/OONO$^-$ cycle.

Chapter 10

Gulf War Syndrome: A Combination of All Four (CFS, MCS, FM, and PTSD)

TAKE-HOME LESSONS

Veterans were exposed to as many as 18 short-term stressors during the Gulf War, with at least 14 having the potential to increase nitric oxide levels. These include individual stressors often associated with initiation of multiple chemical sensitivity (MCS), chronic fatigue syndrome (CFS), fibromyalgia (FM), or post-traumatic stress disorder (PTSD). It should not be surprising, therefore, that people suffering from what is often called Gulf War syndrome often meet the diagnostic criteria for two, three, or all four of these illnesses. With these large numbers of possible stressors, it is difficult to determine the role of each of them in initiating cases of Gulf War syndrome. However, organophosphorus/carbamate toxins and vaccine components are the stressors most likely to be involved. Some very interesting animal models of Gulf War syndrome have been studied, and some of these are reported to have elevated elements of the NO/ONOO$^-$ cycle. However, there have been few physiological studies of the Gulf War veterans; so unlike the four multisystem illnesses, we have essentially no data on whether the NO/ONOO$^-$ cycle biochemistry is elevated.

Whereas other postconflict syndromes may be predominantly PTSD-like, Gulf War syndrome appears to be a much broader multisystem illness. This is not surprising, given the number of stressors that are similar or identical to those initiating cases of MCS, FM, or CFS. Because the ground war in the Gulf War was only four days long, psychological trauma may have been relatively muted in the veterans.

Explaining "Unexplained Illnesses"
© 2007 by The Haworth Press, Inc. All rights reserved.
doi:10.1300/5139_10

The proposal that Gulf War syndrome is a multisystem illness mixture of MCS, CFS, FM, and PTSD suggests interesting approaches to study its biochemistry and physiology. It also suggests interesting approaches to therapy and to avoidance of similar syndromes in future conflicts. Unfortunately, there has been no research to investigate these approaches.

INTRODUCTION

One of the things that helps confirm that a scientific theory is on the right track is when it allows one to look at what has been viewed as a very different and previously puzzling area and immediately gives one important insights. That is decidedly the case of the $NO/OONO^-$ cycle when it comes to what has been called Gulf War syndrome.

The military personnel who participated in the 1991 Gulf War were exposed not to one short-term stressor but to over a dozen distinct stressors, most of which have the potential to produce increases in nitric oxide via mechanisms discussed elsewhere in this book. So, one has here the same pattern of short-term stressor followed by a chronic condition that one has with the other multisystem illnesses, except that there are many possible stressors potentially involved, such that identification of the specific important initiating stressors may be quite difficult. One also has the potential of the multiple stressors acting synergistically with each other, something that has been supported in certain animal model studies that I will discuss in the following text.

Studies of what has sometimes been called Gulf War syndrome or Gulf War illness have shown that all four of our multisystem illnesses are implicated in this syndrome. Specifically, studies have reported that Gulf War personnel suffering from previously unexplained chronic symptoms have elements of CFS, MCS, FM, and PTSD.[1-18] I have argued in an earlier publication[19] that Gulf War syndrome is a complex combination of all four of these, with illnesses initiated by several short-term stressors presumably acting by increasing nitric oxide. This chapter is an expansion of that argument. One part of the argument here is that because so many distinct stressors may have been involved in case initiation, the tissues impacted by them, and therefore the tissues impacted by the subsequent vicious cycle, in most cases are sufficiently broad that most Gulf War sufferers of these chronic symptoms meet the diagnosis for more than one of the four multisystem illnesses.

Certainly the pattern of short-term stressors, followed by chronic illness that is explained by the $NO/ONOO^-$ cycle in the four multisystem illnesses, can also be seen in Gulf War syndrome, which is a combination of these four.

Several other diseases are reported to be elevated in Gulf War personnel including migraine headache,[1,9,10,17,22] asthma,[1,17,20-22] and gastrointestinal (GI) tract dysfunction[17,23] each of which is also known to be comorbid with the other multisystem illnesses (Chapter 2).

Perhaps the most interesting example of comorbidity with Gulf War syndrome is that of amyotrophic lateral sclerosis (ALS, or Lou Gehrig's disease), a progressive fatal disease producing motor neuron dysfunction. Substantial increases in the prevalence of ALS among Gulf War veterans were reported[24,25] and associated with Gulf War syndrome symptoms.[25] ALS has been widely been shown to involve excessive NMDA activity, nitric oxide, and peroxynitrite, so the comorbidity here may be caused by common factors in the etiology. A number of brain scan studies reviewed recently[26] have confirmed brain neurological dysfunction associations with Gulf War syndrome.

This chapter is intended to explore the relevance of the NO/ONOO⁻ cycle mechanism to Gulf War syndrome and is not intended as a general review of that syndrome. I acknowledge, however, the value of the recent review produced by The Research Advisory Committee of Gulf War Veteran's Illnesses.[26] In that document, evidence is reviewed showing that chronic, multisymptomatic illness in Gulf War veterans occurs at a prevalence 26 to 32 percent higher than with nondeployed veterans groups.[26]

The NO/ONOO⁻ cycle mechanism for Gulf War syndrome provides an overall understanding for this illness and conflicts with the notion of overall confusion about its likely etiology that seems to dominate the view in many quarters. An example of such confusion may be seen in the views of psychiatrist Simon Wessely of King's College London, who stated at an October 18, 2004, news conference,[58] in referring to the Gulf War veterans, "There is no shadow of a doubt that something has happened, something has gone wrong. There are huge areas that remain unclear and I am afraid I suspect will always remain unclear."

STRESSORS THAT MAY BE IMPLICATED IN GULF WAR SYNDROME

Some of the possible stressors that Gulf War military personnel were exposed to[26] are listed in Exhibit 10.1.

Among these stressors most of them may potentially act by increasing nitric oxide, based on evidence presented in the earlier chapters. These include infections (Chapter 5), physical trauma (Chapter 8), and psychological stress (Chapter 9). They include multiple chemicals similar or identical

EXHIBIT 10.1. Partial List of Possible Stressors Related to Gulf War Involvement

Infectious diseases

Physical trauma

Psychological stress

Neurotoxins including:

    Sarin and cyclosarin chemical warfare agents (organophosphates)

    Pyridostigmine bromide (used as an experimental drug; carbamate)

    Organophosphate pesticides

    Organochlorine pesticides

    Pyrethroid pesticides

Oil well fire incomplete combustion products

Tent heater fumes

Diesel fuel and gasoline

Gasoline and petroleum (from water carried in petroleum trucks)

DEET (insect repellant)

Depleted uranium

Vaccine components including but not limited to:

    Anthrax vaccine

    Vaccine adjuvants including aluminum hydroxide, squalene, pertussis

    Preservatives including benzethonium and thimerosal

Antibiotics and antimalarials

to those implicated in MCS, including the organophosphorus toxins (both chemical warfare agents and pesticides), carbamates (both pyridostigmine bromide, used as an investigational drug, and also carbamate pesticides), organochlorine pesticides and pyrethroid pesticides. Exposures to each of these toxins/pesticides occurred during the Gulf War, and each have probable or established mechanisms for increasing nitric oxide, as discussed in Chapter 7. The various organic solvents and incomplete combustion products including gasoline, diesel fuel, and other petroleum products and the products of the oil well fires and tent heaters may all possibly act via the vanilloid receptor to increase nitric oxide. When you look at this group of chemicals, including both these solvents and the pesticides and other organophosphorus toxins/carbamates, it should not be surprising that MCS appears to be a major component of Gulf War syndrome, given the role of these chemicals (including both pesticides and organic solvents) in initiating cases of MCS.

Some of the other stressors listed in Exhibit 10.1 are less clear candidates as possibly acting via increased nitric oxide. The insect repellant, DEET, is reported to be an irritant,[27-30] and in one study was reported in induce inflammatory cytokines that induce iNOS,[30] and so it may act via this pathway to increase nitric oxide. Many irritants act in part or in whole by stimulating the vanilloid receptor, a mechanism that will produce increases in nitric oxide, and so it is possible but not established that DEET may act to increase nitric oxide levels. The radioactivity from depleted uranium may act to increase nitric oxide; it is known that ionizing radiation activates NF-κB activity,[31-33] which is known to act both directly and indirectly to induce iNOS, as was discussed in Chapter 1. It should not be surprising, then, that ionizing radiation is known to be able to induce increases in nitric oxide.[33-35] So it is possible that depleted uranium may act to increase nitric oxide and iNOS activity[36] by this pathway. An animal model study showed that depleted uranium exposure produced increases in both short- and long-term lipid peroxidation in the brain, a marker of oxidative stress;[37] this is consistent with a NO/ONOO⁻ cycle mechanism.

The vaccine components are more problematic, however. It is known that a number of bacterial extracts can induce iNOS, but I am unaware of any studies asking whether this is true of the anthrax vaccine components. The anthrax bacterium, *Bacillus anthracis,* shares with other gram-positive bacteria two components, peptidoglycan and lipoteichoic acid, both of which are reported to induce iNOS.[38] So it seems reasonable that the anthrax vaccine, in one or more of its variations, might increase nitric oxide levels, but this has not been directly tested, to my knowledge. Pertussis, which was used as an adjuvant with vaccines, is known to induce inflammatory cytokine production, particularly that of IL-1β,[39] and through that mechanism, can increase nitric oxide levels. Of the other vaccine components, the only one that, to my knowledge, has been tested for effects on nitric oxide is the preservative thimerosal, where there is extensive evidence that it does increase nitric oxide.[40-45]

Which if Any of These May Be Involved in the Initiation of Gulf War Syndrome?

When there are many different stressors that may be involved in the initiation of Gulf War syndrome, this makes it much more difficult to obtain convincing evidence implicating individual stressors. Still, there is evidence implicating individual stressors, particularly vaccines and their components and the acetylcholinesterase inhibitors, organophosphorus/carbamate toxicants (Exhibit 10.1; reviewed in Reference 26). Reference 26 provides the following statement of apparent linkage between vaccines and Gulf-War-associated symptoms (p. 68): "Information concerning a possible link between vaccines and chronic symptoms in Gulf veterans comes from multiple sources. Population-based studies have consistently found that immunizations reported to be received by Gulf veterans are associated with higher rates of multisymptom illness," citing seven different studies. "These include findings of excess illness in Gulf War veterans associated with particular types of vaccines, the number of vaccines received, and the number of vaccines received after veterans' arrival in theater." Reference 26 goes on discuss particular concerns about the anthrax vaccine.

With the exception of the organophosphorus/carbamate toxicants, discussed subsequently, the possible linkage of the other stressors to Gulf War syndrome symptoms is still uncertain. For example, Reference 26 states (p. 69): "Scientific reviews commissioned by federal agencies have often indicated that there is insufficient scientific evidence to determine whether exposures encountered in the Persian Gulf theater are likely to be associated with chronic health problems such as those experienced by Gulf War veterans. The majority of exposures investigated thus far have been neither conclusively ruled in nor ruled out as having contributed to veterans' chronic symptoms." I would simply add that, if these various exposures contributed individually in only a relatively minor way to the generation of Gulf War syndrome, the difficulty in determining their individual causal roles is very substantial.

The most convincing evidence for a group of stressors in Gulf War syndrome focuses on the role of organophosphorus and carbamate compounds. As was discussed in Chapter 7, these act as acetylcholinesterase and will all consequently act both relatively directly, through acetylcholine stimulation of muscarinic receptors, and indirectly, through the NMDA receptors to increase nitric oxide levels.

In a discussion of epidemiological evidence on organophosphorus toxins/carbamates, it is stated that:[26]

> Epidemiologic studies have assessed both ill health and wartime exposures among Gulf War veterans in different ways. As shown in Table 10 [Reference 26], however, these studies have consistently identified AChEis [acetylcholinesterase inhibitors] to be significantly associated with higher rates of symptoms and illnesses in Gulf War

veterans. The uniformity of these results contrasts with a lack of consistent findings in multivariable analyses for such wartime experiences as participation in combat, exposure to oil fire smoke, and exposure to depleted uranium. Limitations in epidemiologic studies that rely on self-reported exposures always require a cautious interpretation of findings. (pp. 62-63)

In Table 10, Reference 26, are listed eight studies linking self-reported exposure to chemical weapons, presumably sarin and/or cyclosarin organophosphorus toxins, to veterans' illnesses; 10 studies linking the taking of the carbamate experimental drug pyridostigmine bromide to illnesses; and 10 studies linking the use of pesticides, many but not all of which fall into category of organophosphorus/carbamates, with Gulf War veterans' illness. It goes on to state that "However, the overall consistency of epidemiologic findings indicating higher rates of ill health in association with AChEis exposures, as reported by multiple studies using different methods and different populations, provides compelling support for a role of AChEis in the development of Gulf War veterans' illnesses" (pp. 62-63).

The role of these compounds in the initiation of Gulf War syndrome is greatly strengthened by the genetic evidence. This is particularly true of Haley and coworkers evidence linking a particular polymorphism of the *PON1* gene with neurological symptoms among Gulf War veterans.[46] *PON1* encodes an enzyme that degrades organophosphorus toxins, and this study reported that those carrying a form of that gene such that they are less able to metabolize these compounds are at substantially greater risk of Gulf War syndrome symptoms. The activity of the enzyme encoded by the *PON1* gene was also implicated in a British study of Gulf War syndrome.[47] Other genetic studies also suggesting an important role for acetylcholinesterase inhibitors have implicated the related enzyme butyrylcholinesterase in some cases of Gulf War syndrome or related illnesses.[48,49] The genetic and biochemical studies implicating these enzymes is particularly important because the veterans involved do not have any idea what their enzyme activities or related genotype is likely to be. They are simply reporting their symptoms; both the genetics and the biochemistry are studied by objective means, and so the association cannot be due to any psychiatric bias on the part of the veterans involved.

Let me add that the evidence supporting a key role for organophosphorus/carbamate compounds in the initiation of Gulf War syndrome should not be viewed in isolation from the similar evidence supporting a similar role in civilian cases of MCS, as discussed in Chapter 7. The similar patterns of evidence suggesting important roles for these compounds in both, Gulf War syndrome and in civilian MCS cases, strengthens the inference that these compounds have important causal roles in the initiation of both of these closely related illnesses.

Before leaving this discussion, it is important to review the careful study of Miller and Prihoda comparing the chemical sensitivity symptoms of MCS patients with those of Gulf War veteran sufferers.[50] In that study, Miller and Prihoda documented the chemical sensitivity of those Gulf War veterans, with the veterans showing similar but somewhat lower sensitivity reactions to those of civilian MCS patients. This pattern should not be surprising, because many of the stressors to which the Gulf War personnel were exposed, including organophosphorus and carbamate compounds and various organic solvents, were similar or identical to those previously reported to initiate MCS cases.

ANIMAL MODEL EVIDENCE FOR POSSIBLE SYNERGISM OF STRESSOR ACTION

There have been many distinct studies of possible synergism among the stressors that Gulf War veterans were exposed to. In Reference 26 (Table 9, pp. 60-61), some 28 different mammalian studies were summarized, most of which provided evidence of synergism. In addition to these mammalian studies, even amphibia have been reported to show such synergism. The effects of groups of chemicals and other stressors may be much larger than predicted from the possible additivity of individual effects. Some of these studies can be interpreted in terms of increased absorption of one chemical after skin exposure to others or, alternatively, increased brain exposure due to partial breakdown of the blood–brain barrier induced by stress or chemical exposure.

Several of the studies reported synergistic effects on major findings that may be due to consequences of NO/ONOO⁻ cycle. For example, two studies reported synergistic effects on oxidative stress[51,52] and a third on blood-brain barrier permeabilization,[53] with both of these possibly a consequence of increased peroxynitrite levels. The first two of these studies[51,52] are of particular significance because they measured increased levels of 3-nitrotyrosine, thought to be a specific consequence of increased levels of peroxynitrite, thus providing evidence for a elevated peroxynitrite role in these animal models. Four studies reported increased mitochondrial release of cytochrome C[54] or increased neuronal cell death[53,55] and other cell degeneration[56] and apoptosis,[57] all possibly due to increased peroxynitrite-induced apoptosis (discussed in Chapter 2).

While there is substantial evidence possibly linking these animal models with predicted changes in chronic-phase biochemistry and physiology predicted by the NO/ONOO$^-$ cycle mechanism, there is essentially no such data on human sufferers from the Gulf War. That may be because so many of the human studies have focused on possible psychiatric issues to the exclusion of biochemistry or physiology. At this time, the only substantial linkage of our predicted changes to Gulf War syndrome sufferers is from the brain scan studies discussed briefly in the preceding text and through the fact that they also often meet diagnostic criteria for CFS, MCS, FM, and PTSD. For each of these four illnesses, there is much published evidence that they show several of the features predicted by our vicious cycle, as discussed earlier in this book.

RELATIONSHIP TO CHRONIC ILLNESSES FOLLOWING OTHER WARS

Other wars have been characterized by chronic illnesses in a substantial fraction of military personnel with such illnesses often being described by different names, as listed in Exhibit 10.2. These have usually been viewed as being due to PTSD. The point raised here as well as in Chapter 9 is that neither PTSD nor these various postconflict illnesses should be viewed as strictly psychiatric, both because they may have significant elements of CFS, MCS, and FM and because all four of these multisystem illnesses have important biochemical and physiological elements that need to be treated for their aberrant biochemistry in addition to treatment for any psychiatric symptoms.

Still, there is a substantial quantitative difference between Gulf War syndrome and these other postconflict illnesses. The evidence in the case of Gulf War syndrome suggests that PTSD is a substantially smaller component of

EXHIBIT 10.2. Some Other Postconflict Syndromes

Specific war	Name(s) of postconflict syndrome
U.S. Civil War	DaCosta's syndrome
World War I	Soldier's heart, Shell shock
World War II	Effort syndrome, Battle fatigue
Korean War	Battle fatigue
Vietnam War	In country syndrome, usually referred to as PTSD

that illness than it is of most other postconflict illnesses. This should not be surprising because the 1991 ground war conflict was limited to four days and many of the non-Iraqi military personnel were exposed to limited psychological stress as a consequence of the conflict. From the stressors involved in the 1991 Gulf War, one can see that the one stressor most associated with initiation of PTSD, severe psychological stress, may have affected only a limited number of military personnel, whereas the stressors most associated with the initiation other multisystem illnesses, particularly those associated with MCS, may have impacted all such personnel. It should not be surprising, then, that Gulf War syndrome is characterized less by PTSD and more by MCS-, CFS-, and FM-like symptoms. The stressors apparently involved predict exactly such a symptom shift. Still, these are quantitative differences, not qualitative differences, and other previous postconflict illnesses may well have also had combinations of these multisystem illnesses comprising components of them.

PREVENTION IN FUTURE CONFLICTS

There are, two large "icebergs" reflected in the studies of Gulf War syndrome and other postconflict illnesses. One is that, in the 1991 Gulf War, most of the true casualties among the allied military personnel came from those afflicted by Gulf War syndrome and these are not counted among the official casualties of that conflict. I refer to this as an iceberg because, as with icebergs, most of the mass is hidden under the sea, and most of the true casualties of the 1991 Gulf War are largely hidden under the still questioned category of this syndrome. This pattern may well be true in other future conflicts as well. The issue of prevention of similar future postconflict illnesses is very important in minimizing the true casualty costs associated with warfare.

There is a second iceberg, a potentially larger one relating to the true civilian costs of warfare. If civilians caught up in warfare are also afflicted by conflict-associated multisystem illnesses, the true costs to the lives and health of such civilians may be much larger than most have been willing to acknowledge. Certainly, future tests allowing for objective diagnostic measures of these multisystem illnesses may allow the measurement of such civilian casualties of warfare. Clearly, some of the stressors listed earlier for the 1991 Gulf War (in Exhibit 10.1) may have been expected to affect civilians but others would not have been, and so it is impossible to predict the size of this second iceberg from that conflict. Minimizing such civilian casualties in future conflicts will require minimizing civilian exposure to these various stressors.

Similarly, minimizing such military casualties in future conflicts should focus, in part, on minimizing chemical exposures and vaccine exposures that may have been involved in producing the 1991 Gulf War syndrome victims. For example, exposure to pesticides and DEET should be considered as having potential hazards associated with them, as should exposure to depleted uranium. Pyridostigmine bromide, used as an experimental drug, should also be considered to have potential long-term hazards associated with its use. Decisions previously made on the assumption of no significant hazard should be reconsidered in the future in the light of the possible key roles of these stressors. The vaccine preservative thimerosal should be avoided, and the use of inadequately tested vaccines such as the anthrax vaccine and the use of pertussis as a vaccine adjuvant should be questioned on the basis of possible long-term hazards. It may be prudent to spread out over time the vaccination protocol of future military personnel so that the individuals being vaccinated may have time to physiologically adjust to the individual stressors of such multiple vaccinations.

One of the most important concepts derived from the NO/ONOO⁻ cycle mechanism is that there is now a plausible mechanism linking a variety of short-term stressors to chronic illnesses. It has been common to dismiss possible linkages between such stressors and chronic illnesses in the past, based on the lack of any plausible mechanism for such linkage.* Indeed, it may be argued that one of the largest barriers to acceptance of this etiologic mechanism may well be from those who have a vested interested in continuing to deny any linkage between specific stressors and resulting chronic illness.

Avoidance of some stressors in a wartime situation may, in many cases, be completely impractical, but other disease avoidance strategies may be suggested. Many of the therapeutic agents I will discuss in Chapter 15 may well be more effective in avoidance of these illnesses than they may be in therapy. I think that there should be consideration of placebo-controlled trials of military personnel to test the possible influence of such agents in avoiding future postconflict illnesses. Such agents as magnesium supplements, which minimize NMDA hyperactivity as well as a variety of antioxidants and possibly the use of dextromethorphan and folic acid supplements, all of which are well tolerated, are some of the possible agents that should be considered for such prevention trials, in my view. Additional preventive agents may be suggested in the light of discussions in Chapter 15.

---

*There are some situations where a short-term stressor can initiate an autoimmune response. However, in the absence of any data supporting an autoimmune etiology, the possibility of a linkage between stressors and chronic illness has often been dismissed.

Chapter 11

The Toll of Multisystem Illnesses

TAKE-HOME LESSONS

The prevalence of substantial suffering from one or more of these multisystem illnesses is estimated to be about 7.4 percent in the U.S. population. World prevalences are much more difficult to estimate but may well be roughly similar. The U.S. prevalence calculation does not include those moderately affected by multiple chemical sensitivity (MCS), nor those affected by illnesses possibly similar to fibromyalgia (FM) or chronic fatigue syndrome (CFS) such as widespread chronic pain or other chronic pain syndromes or unexplained chronic fatigue.

An economic calculation of loss, based on loss of paid employment, leaves out the many additional losses suffered by people afflicted by the multisystem illnesses. The rough calculation of these economic losses is $444 billion per year in the United States alone and perhaps four times that amount for world losses. These figures are rough estimates, but they provide a gage of the staggering economic losses produced by these illnesses. Such an economic estimate only estimates a part of the human toll caused by multisystem illnesses.

INTRODUCTION

To estimate the toll of the four multisystem illnesses on human health, we need to estimate the prevalence of each of the four illnesses in different national populations. We need then also assess the toll on the average sufferer.

Explaining "Unexplained Illnesses"
© 2007 by The Haworth Press, Inc. All rights reserved.
doi:10.1300/5139_11

PREVALENCE OF FM

The most extensive and consistent data on the prevalence of these four illnesses are found on FM. FM prevalences commonly range from about 1 to 5 percent of populations, with many individual figures clustering around 2 to 2.5 percent, as reported in several reviews.[1-3] The figures are consistently higher in women than in men and are somewhat higher in adult populations and somewhat lower in pediatric populations. I would like to give you several examples of specific studies to give you a feeling for the variation of these figures and the extent of the available data.

- Bennett estimated the overall prevalence of FM in the United States at about 2.2 percent.[4]
- Wolfe et al.[5] estimated the FM prevalence in the United States at 2.0 percent.
- White et al.[6] measured the FM prevalence in a Canadian city among noninstitutionalized adults at 3.3 percent.
- An Israeli review[7] found the prevalence of chronic widespread pain to be 9.9 percent, with FM being about 25 percent of these cases, for an overall prevalence of 2.5 percent. Other studies also reported that chronic widespread pain has about four times the prevalence of FM.
- A Spanish study[8] found the prevalence of FM to be 2.4 percent.
- The two lowest recent estimates of FM prevalence I have found were from two Scandinavian studies. A Danish study reported a "minimum estimate" of FM in Danish adults to be 0.66 percent (p. 233, Reference 9), A Finnish study that expressed skepticism about FM reported a prevalence in the Finnish population of 0.75 percent with the authors adding (p. 216, Reference 10) that "The prevalence of fibromyalgia was sensitive to even minor modifications of the definition."
- There have been a number of studies of FM prevalence in Third World countries. For example, three Mexican studies all came up with similar prevalence figures. A study of FM prevalence in adults in southern Mexico estimated a prevalence of 1.3 percent.[11] An overall community estimate in Mexico City came up with a figure of 1.4 percent.[12] An estimate of FM prevalence among Mexican children came up with a 1.2 percent prevalence figure.[13]
- A study of adults in Bangladesh measured three FM prevalences: 4.4 percent among rural, 3.2 percent among urban slum, and 3.3 percent among urban affluent populations.[14]
- The overall prevalence in Brazil was reported to be 2.5 percent.[15]

- The prevalence of FM among women in Turkey was reported to be 3.6 percent,[16] quite similar to many of the figures for women in the United States and Europe.
- A few specific populations have FM prevalences outside of the 1 to 5 percent common range. For example, a study of FM among the Amish in Canada showed a prevalence of 7.3 percent.[17]

From the aforementioned studies and reviews, it appears that the best FM estimate of overall population prevalence of FM in the United States and also the world is probably close to 2.1 percent. With a population in the United States of almost exactly 300 million, the U.S. number of FM patients is about 6.3 million and a world estimate may be estimated to be roughly 140 million.

PREVALENCE
OF MULTIPLE CHEMICAL SENSITIVITY

There are fewer population prevalence studies for MCS than there are for FM. Most of these have studied U.S. populations. Sorg[18] (p 284) in reviewing several epidemiological studies of MCS, concluded that the "prevalence of severe MCS in the United States is approximately 4 percent with greatly reduced quality of life for the patient." She further states[18] that "Less severe problems with chemical exposures have been reported in approximately 15-30 percent of the population." Similar figures have been obtained in several more recent U.S. studies.[19-23] I would estimate that, from all of these studies, a best estimate for the prevalence of severe MCS may be about 3.5 percent, slightly lower than the figure that Sorg used. Prevalence studies in Canada[24] and in Germany[25] came up with prevalences of about half to two-thirds of the U. S. figures. One cannot help wondering whether there is more care taken in chemical usage in those countries than in the United States.

PREVALENCE
OF POST-TRAUMATIC STRESS DISORDER

The vast majority of studies of prevalences of post-traumatic stress disorder (PTSD) have been of populations at special risk-survivors of war, sexual or physical abuse, military veterans, natural disasters such as hurricanes, earthquakes, or major floods, or other groups at special risk. We have relatively few general population studies, and even those often involve studies of populations at special risk such in Bosnia, Afghanistan, Israel, or Palestine.

Population prevalences have been estimated as being from 1 to 9 percent[26-29] with a few higher ones among the specially-at-risk national populations going as high as 40 percent.[30]

The best U.S. prevalence study was that of Kessler et al.[31] who came up with a lifetime prevalence of PTSD of 7.8 percent. In order to compare this "lifetime prevalence" figure with the other prevalence figures, it is necessary to define what this means and then relate it to the properties of PTSD. People who have suffered from PTSD at any time in their lives, up to the present, will be counted in the lifetime prevalence figure. Because PTSD has a much higher recovery rate than do the other multisystem illnesses, with about 60 percent recovering usually within the first two years of becoming ill, the actual prevalence rate is only about 46 percent of the lifetime prevalence rate. This figure comes from the approximately 40 percent who will never recover and the 6 percent who will recover but have not yet done so (the other 54 percent having already recovered). It follows that the 7.8 percent lifetime prevalence rate corresponds to current prevalence rate of 3.6 percent. So, this is more than 50 percent higher than the best prevalence estimate for FM and is close to that for severe MCS.

Some other countries have PTSD prevalence figures similar to those of the United States with Canadian and Swedish figures somewhat lower,[32,33] but Spanish and Portuguese figures are somewhat higher.[34,35] An Israeli population prevalence of 9.4 percent, more than 2.5 times the U.S. figure, was elevated presumably due to experiences with terrorism.[36]

CFS PREVALENCE

One of the disturbing features of the CFS literature is the huge range of prevalence estimates that have been published over the years. In a recent review,[37] prevalence estimates ranging from 0.006 to 3.0 percent were discussed depending on setting and definitions used. This is a 500-fold variation in prevalence, about two orders of magnitude higher than the variation one seen in the FM literature. It has been generally been argued that the prevalence study of Jason et al.[38] is the best available such study. They studied the CFS prevalence in a group of random households in Chicago, trying to avoid the problems caused by the failure of many CFS patients to seek medical care because of their frustration with the lack of responsiveness they see in many medical care providers. Jason and coworkers estimated the CFS prevalence at 0.42 percent from this study.[38]

I have great respect for Jason's study, but my feeling is that the CFS prevalence is actually substantially higher than this, perhaps more similar to the prevalences reported for CFS-like illnesses[39,40] in the Netherlands (3.6 percent) and in Sweden (2.36 percent). Let me explain my views on this. The symptoms that are used to determine CFS in individuals in the 1994 CDC case definition, the most commonly used case definition, requires fatigue and at least four of the other eight symptoms.

1. Impaired memory or concentration
2. Sore throat
3. Tender lymph nodes
4. Muscle pain
5. Multijoint pain
6. Headaches
7. Unrefreshing sleep
8. Postexertional malaise

With the exception of the postexertional malaise, these are all fairly common symptoms, where it is difficult if not impossible to objectively divide those suffering from these symptoms from normals. When one is doing a large, population-based study, this is made much more difficult because one is dealing with thousands of people, each with distinct observations. It may be possible for a physician or other person to divide more consistently CFS patients from controls when dealing with a few dozen patients, but to do so with thousands is a daunting task. In comparing the variation in estimated prevalence of CFS with that of FM, the FM case definition appears to be more straightforward and therefore may lead to less variation in estimated prevalence.

So, how might that help us? It is possible to *calculate the CFS prevalence from the FM prevalence and the comorbidity between CFS and FM*. FM prevalence figures and also the comorbidity figures are vastly more consistent than are the CFS prevalence figures. What happens when we try to make such a calculation? FM has a prevalence in the United States of about 2.1 percent, as discussed earlier. In their review, Aaron, Burke, and Buchwald[41] (p. 221) state that "it has been estimated that between 20 percent and 70 percent of patients with FM meet the criteria for CFS and, conversely, 35 percent to 70 percent of those with CFS also have FM." Those ranges still hold, although there are three more recent studies providing independent estimates that have since been published.[42-44]

The average the different studies for each you get an estimated number of FM patients who meet the criterion for CFS at 49.7 percent. If we use this estimate and multiply this by the best prevalence estimate for FM, one gets a CFS prevalence of 2.1 percent times 0.497 = 1.04 percent, or about 2.5 times the Jason figure. And this only includes the CFS patients who also have

FM. We can estimate the total CFS prevalence from the fraction of CFS patient who also have FM (and therefore the fraction who do not have FM). The average estimate for that figure, averaging the estimates from the different studies, is 53 percent. This gives an overall estimated prevalence 1.97 percent or almost 5 times the Jason estimate. These figures could easily be off by perhaps 10 to 30 percent or so, given the variations in the comorbidity figures from the different studies, but they clearly provide strong support for the view that the CFS prevalence is much closer to the FM prevalence figure than they are to the 0.42 percent from the Jason study. Because both the FM prevalence figures and the two comorbidity figures involved are *much more consistent than are the CFS prevalence figures,* it is plausible that the calculated prevalence may be more reliable than is the measured CFS prevalence estimate.

OVERALL PREVALENCE
OF MULTISYSTEM ILLNESSES

So, what may a best guess for the overall prevalence of these four multisystem illnesses? In doing this calculation, I am going to include only the severe MCS patients, those most likely to have major impact on their employment, ability to live in an easily found apartment or house, and those most likely to have to have to strictly limit their social interactions, travel and shopping in order to minimize chemical exposure. I am also not going to include the larger number of people who have chronic widespread pain but do not meet the diagnostic criterion for FM. The total, based on the aforementioned consideration, *if you just add the prevalences,* is $2.1 + 3.5 + 3.6 + 2.0 = 11.2$ percent. But, you will correctly point out to me that, because of the comorbidities among these illnesses, you cannot just add them because, in so doing, you are counting individuals meeting the criteria for more than one illness more than once. That is correct. One needs to do a complex calculation based on the estimated comorbidities to correct for this error. When you do that, you get an estimated overall prevalence of 7.4 percent. In a U.S. population of almost exactly 300 million, that gives an estimate of about 22.2 million people substantially afflicted by one or more of these multisystem illnesses.

How Can One Estimate the Illness Toll
for These 22.2 Million?

Now, we are getting to the core question. The usual way to measure overall toll is to simply calculate economic losses. I am going to try to do that, but I want to point out that economics is not a very good way to measure the toll on people with multisystem illnesses. It does not measure the numbers of families stressed, divorces that result, the number of premature deaths, the impact on people's social lives, the long-term friendships that disintegrate, and the limitations on travel and many other freedoms that we so cherish. We take most of our pleasures from either mental or physical activities, activities that often become impossible when one suffers from both cognitive dysfunction and fatigue, both very common symptoms in these illnesses. When you add the intrusive nature of chronic pain, the losses become manifest. The MCS sufferers have many additional restrictions, in foods, places in which they can shop, public events that cannot be attended, and so forth. PTSD sufferers typically suffer from the psychiatric symptoms, which impact, in turn, their family and other social interactions. Sufferers can add an additional detailed perspective on the losses they have felt most poignantly. So, while economics is one way of putting a number on the toll, it leaves out many important impacts.

So, we will do our calculation based on economic losses while acknowledging that we are leaving out many important losses that cannot be easily quantified. The only economic measure that I am aware of is the study published by Reynolds et al.[45] on the economic impact of CFS in the United States. They calculated the economic loss per CFS patient due to lowered pay from employment as being $20,000.

Are there comparable losses in employment pay for the other multisystem illnesses? Assefi et al.[46] compared employments losses between FM and CFS and found that FM patients had slightly greater losses, with those afflicted by both FM and CFS having still greater losses than those suffering from FM alone or CFS alone. Other studies of FM unemployment and underemployment also reported substantial losses,[47-50] but are more difficult to compare with the CFS figures. In general, FM employment losses are probably similar to those from CFS, so it is probably not unreasonable to use the same $20,000 figure for FM.

MCS employment losses are still harder to estimate. Two studies of highly selected patients reported that over two-thirds of them claimed disability based on the chemical sensitivity status.[51,52] Perhaps a better overall assessment may be that of Caress and Steinemann, who reported that 1.8 percent of the entire population they studied lost their jobs because of chemical hypersensitivity.[22] While some of these may have obtained other employment, often at lower pay, this suggests that, among those severely affected by MCS, the loss of paid employment per person is roughly similar to that of CFS patients.

Finally, a number of studies of PTSD reported losses of paid employment similar to those of CFS and FM,[55-59] suggesting the $20,000 per person figure may again roughly approximate the losses in PTSD.

The simple calculation, then, is that with 22.2 million people in the United States suffering from one or more of these illnesses at a loss of employment of about $20,000 per person, the total economic loss from employment loss alone may be roughly $444 billion dollars per year. This is a staggering amount, and while it is a rough measure and could well be off by 10, 20, or 30 percent (either up or down), it gives one a feeling for the staggering cost of these illnesses, based solely on economic losses due to loss of employment. Let me add that I am not including other real economic losses such as the increased medical care costs associated with these illnesses nor, of course, the noneconomic losses.

One can even try to make a much rougher estimate of economic losses for the entire world. Only FM prevalences can be said to be similar internationally. The data on the other multisystem illnesses, as you have already seen, are distinctly limited, but what data is available suggests that PTSD prevalences may be higher and MCS prevalences lower in some other countries. Perhaps, overall multisystem illness prevalence on a world basis may be similar to the U.S. estimate. Because the United States is responsible for about quarter of the world economic output, one might estimate that the world economic losses may be on the order to four times the U.S. losses, or perhaps 1.776 trillion dollars.

I would encourage others who may see better ways to do these estimations to go ahead and do them. They are not easy to do, and I am sure that others can come up with more reliable estimates than I have. Still, I doubt that my U.S. estimates are off by as much as a factor of two, although the world estimate may well be off by that or perhaps more than that.

I would encourage the reader to consider, when reading Chapter 15, the chapter on therapy, the consequences of cutting these losses by 50 percent or perhaps an even a greater percentage with an effective therapy. The improvement on both human health and on economic health would be tremendous.

Chapter 12

Overall Evidence,
and What Else Is Needed?

TAKE-HOME LESSONS

The goal of this chapter is not to discuss all areas in which further study of multisystem illnesses is needed. It is, rather, to outline several areas where specific future focus is needed:

- The search for *specific biomarkers* is important both because they reflect on etiologic mechanism and because they should provide objectively measurable diagnostic markers.
- Brain scan studies are needed to attempt to correlate changes in specific regions of the brain with the occurrence of specific symptoms. The goal here is to determine to what extent specific regions of the brain are involved in producing specific symptoms of these illnesses.
- Animal model studies are needed to more definitively test biological mechanism.
- Several *MCS-specific* studies are needed both in humans and animal models. Some of these should focus on the roles of both the NMDA receptor and the vanilloid receptor.
- The possible role of *nitric oxide synthase uncoupling* in the initiation of these illnesses can be probed in animal models and in studies of therapeutic agents that lower uncoupling in humans.
- More *genetic studies* are needed, testing the role of specific genes in determining the prevalence of these illnesses. Such genetic studies are important in testing biological mechanism in humans.
- The NO/ONOO$^-$ cycle predicts that *therapy should focus on the down-regulation of NO/ONOO$^-$ cycle biochemistry.* More clinical

Explaining "Unexplained Illnesses"
© 2007 by The Haworth Press, Inc. All rights reserved.
doi:10.1300/5139_12

trial studies are needed to probe this area, both because of its theoretical importance in our understanding of these illnesses and because of the practical importance to the treatment of sufferers. *Prevention* of these illnesses, including post-traumatic stress disorder (PTSD) and Gulf War–syndrome-like illnesses, via agents minimizing NO/ONOO⁻ cycle biochemistry also needs to be studied.

INTRODUCTION

I have outlined earlier in this book a pattern of evidence and interpretation supporting the NO/ONOO⁻ cycle etiology of these multisystem illnesses. This evidence and interpretation may be summarized as follows:

- Evidence that a dozen short-term stressors, reported to initiate cases of these illnesses, can all act by increasing nitric oxide.
- Evidence that known and reported biochemical and physiological mechanisms may be able to constitute the NO/ONOO⁻ cycle, providing an explanation for the chronic nature of these illnesses.
- Evidence from studies of the chronic phase of these illnesses for elevation of multiple elements of the NO/ONOO⁻ cycle.
- Evidence that most of the elements of that cycle act locally, providing support for the view that the local nature explains the profound variations one sees in comparing cases of these illnesses with each other.
- Evidence that many of the overlapping and also the specific symptoms and signs of these illnesses may be explained as being produced as a consequence of the elements of the NO/ONOO⁻ cycle.
- Evidence from animal models of these illnesses, implicating nitric oxide, NMDA activity, oxidative stress, and other elements of the cycle.
- Evidence from genetic studies of chronic fatigue syndrome (CFS) and multiple chemical sensitivity (MCS), providing support for several features of the proposed cycle model.

So while it can be argued we have a fairly compelling pattern of supportive evidence, we also have here an interesting conundrum. On the one hand, we have a pattern of evidence supporting the NO/ONOO⁻ cycle explanatory model. And that model provides answers to the most previously puzzling questions about these multisystem illnesses—answers that argue that the claims that these are unexplained illnesses are false.

However, there are many areas where the evidence is relatively weak, and therefore, studies to test this etiology are certainly needed. How many such studies are needed is a question that I will leave largely to others. This is a question that is very difficult to answer with conviction, given the complexity and interactive nature of the NO/ONOO⁻ cycle. My primary goal, in this chapter, is to outline some of the areas where I think much of the needed study should focus, rather than trying to state how much such study is needed.

Certainly, you, the reader, can look at the evidence cited in Chapter 1, Chapter 3 and Chapter 5 to Chapter 10 to see where some of the evidence is weak and where it is relatively strong. An example of an area of weakness is the set of plausible mechanisms presented in Chapter 3 that provide explanations for many of the shared symptoms and signs of the multisystem illnesses. These are largely untested explanations *as they may apply to these illnesses* and clearly need to be tested in these multisystem illnesses.

Many of the challenges in assessing the strength or weakness of the data are caused by the fact that so much of the basic nature of these illnesses has been contested. Let me give you an example where I see considerable difficulty in assessing the strengths and weaknesses. There is evidence supporting the view that excessive NMDA activity occurs in the chronic phase of each of these illnesses. Being a potentially important element of the cycle, this is certainly an important point to be assessed. However, the strength of the evidence supporting this is strongest in fibromyalgia (FM) and weakest in CFS. To what extent can one lump all of that evidence together in making the case? This depends on how certain one is that these illnesses share a common etiology and that depends, in turn, on one's point of view. So, how important is it that we study this further in CFS? My own view is that it is important but perhaps not as important as it would be if the CFS data were to stand on its own. One can make similar arguments about mitochondrial dysfunction, which have been studied in CFS and FM but not in MCS or PTSD. Oxidative stress is best documented in CFS and least documented in MCS and PTSD—how much further study is needed in the latter two illnesses? These are difficult questions to answer.

For the most part, I am not going to go over such specific weaknesses in detail. What I am going to do in this chapter is to focus on a few specific areas where particular emphasis is needed.

SEARCH FOR SPECIFIC BIOMARKERS

Probably the most important area of future research is to search for specific biomarkers for each of these illnesses that are consistent with the overall NO/ONOO⁻ cycle etiology. I have pointed to what I consider to be the most fruitful places for such searches for CFS, MCS, and FM. In CFS, it is the possible role of the brain in controlling hypothalamic-pituitary-adrenal (HPA) axis response to exercise and possibly some other stressors. In MCS, multiple regions of the body are often involved whereby organic solvents and certain pesticides can lead to increased NMDA stimulation and increased nitric oxide and peroxynitrite. In FM, the best guess may be the impact on the thalamus and the consequent predicted effect on pain processing up and down the spinal cord. Each of these must be viewed as hypotheses not sufficiently supported to be incorporated into the core theory. Each of these will require substantial future work to determine whether these predictions are borne out or not. These are of special importance because, if correct, they will provide objective markers for diagnosis, as well as confirming important aspects of their etiology. My own view, then, is that the search for specific biomarkers is one of the most important areas of research to focus on in future studies of these illnesses.

BRAIN SCAN STUDIES
AND UNDERLYING MECHANISMS

One key area of study, that is just getting started relates to the involvement of distinct regions of the brain in producing distinct symptoms in multisystem illnesses. There have been, as is discussed in Chapter 3 and elsewhere, a number of studies showing changes in positron emission tomography (PET) scans and single-photon emission computed tomography (SPECT) scans of the brains in these multisystem illnesses. The basic proposal, also discussed in Chapter 3 and Chapter 4, is that distinct regions of the brain are involved in producing distinct symptoms. These potential patterns need to be studied in patients, where the precise pattern of symptoms found in specific patients can be compared with their brain scans studied by PET scan, SPECT scan, or NMR techniques.

Does the widespread pain pattern found in FM cases correlate well with the changes in thalamus scans? Does the finding of anxiety behavior correspond to changes in amygdala scans? Do specific region changes correlate with the postexertional malaise symptom characteristic of CFS? Do specific region changes correlate with depressive symptoms in these illnesses? Are particular brain regions, possibly controlling the autonomic nervous system function, show impact correlating with orthostatic intolerance? Each of these possible correlations is suggested in Chapters 3, 5, or 8. They need to be tested, in my judgment.

ANIMAL MODEL STUDIES

There are also a number of important animal model studies that would be very useful. For example, I discussed in Chapter 1 the need for specific animal studies in CFS animal models to confirm the role of nitric oxide and other cycle elements in the etiology of these models. CFS animal model studies might use transgenic mouse deficient in superoxide dismutase activity, enzyme activities that destroy superoxide, to test for the predicted role of superoxide. Superoxide dismutase mimics, low molecular weight compounds that have superoxide dismutase activity, might also be useful in such studies. While a number of supportive animal model studies have provided support for our proposed etiology of MCS, these have not been done in the animal models that have the most compelling similarities to MCS in humans. Such models should be studied to determine whether the predicted roles of the NMDA receptors, of nitric oxide, and of the vanilloid receptor can be confirmed in those systems.

MCS-SPECIFIC STUDIES

Future MCS research is a particularly interesting area to consider. On the one hand, the fit between the NO/ONOO$^-$ cycle and the many diverse and previously puzzling properties of MCS is particularly compelling. In my judgment, it would be extraordinary if the predicted mechanisms involved in MCS were flawed in some fundamental way. However, given the complexity of MCS, there are several potentially important studies that have yet to be performed. For example, the proposed role of the vanilloid receptor as the target for organic solvents in MCS is based on indirect evidence. Certainly, it is appropriate to look at the properties of this receptor from the specific perspective of its potential target role in MCS. It is also desirable to test the effects of complex mixtures of solvents, mixtures of the types that are most often in MCS to determine whether such solvents act synergistically with respect to each other in activating the vanilloid receptor. The role of the vanilloid receptor in MCS should be tested using animal models where its role can be directly tested. The PTSD animal models are strikingly similar to the human disease and may be excellent models to measure roles of NO/ONOO$^-$ cycle elements in causation.

The role of the NMDA receptors in MCS can also be further studied in several ways. For example, the effects of the NMDA antagonist dextromethorphan was inferred from clinical observations, but this effect should be confirmed with a placebo-controlled trial. There are substantial difficulties in doing placebo-controlled trials to study chemical exposure in MCS, difficulties caused in part by the odors that many of these chemicals have. Dextromethorphan studies are not weakened by this issue of odor since the drug is nonvolatile and does not, therefore, carry an odor. I think one of the MCS issues that needs to be tested is the role of NMDA receptors in the peripheral sensitivity mechanisms that often occur in MCS.

CAN WE IDENTIFY A FOCUS OF WHAT DETERMINES THE INITIATION OF THE NO/ONOO⁻ CYCLE?

In Chapter 1, I raised the question about why some become ill but others do not in response to the stressors implicated in initiation of these illnesses. After all, most infections do not lead to cases of CFS and/or FM, and similarly other stressors only produce multisystem illnesses in some but not other individuals. So, why is this? I answered this question *at one level* in Chapter 1, suggesting that variation in genetic background, hormonal balance, the strength of the stressors, the nutritional balance, and possibly the state of the immune system may have substantial roles in determining who becomes ill and who does not. I think that answer has substantial merit, but it only provides an answer at one level—it does not tell us in what way these factors may act. Is there after some critical step, or perhaps more than one step, that determines when the NO/ONOO⁻ cycle is initiated? As was also discussed in Chapter 1, there are known mechanisms for positive feedback loops that are predicted, if they are unimpeded, to produce the cycle, but there also negative feedback loops that may be predicted to impede the generation of the cycle. *What is the switch* that tips the balance in favor of the establishment of the NO/ONOO⁻ cycle?

What I am going to suggest here is a hypothesis, with limited supporting evidence but one that is intriguing nonetheless. Furthermore, the hypothesis should be testable mainly by using animal models. I believe that the critical parameter that may determine whether such a cycle is initiated is prolonged oxidative stress and specifically prolonged superoxide and peroxynitrite elevation. Peroxynitrite may act in two main ways: Firstly by shifting nitric oxide synthase activity toward more superoxide production and less nitric oxide production, and secondly by the effect of prolonged peroxynitrite elevation and oxidative stress on influencing both NF-κB activation and the consequences of NF-κB activation. Let me take these issues one at a time.

As I discussed in Chapter 2, nitric oxide synthases, when deprived of their cofactor tetrahydrobiopterin (BH4), produce substantial amounts of superoxide in place of some of the nitric oxide. This shift toward superoxide production has been reported for all three of the nitric oxide synthases (NOSs), nNOS, eNOS, and iNOS.[1-10] It follows from this that the shift towards superoxide production, in addition to the nitric oxide production, essentially converts the three nitric oxide synthases into peroxynitrite synthases, given the rapid reaction of nitric oxide with superoxide to form peroxynitrite (discussed in Chapter 1). This was concluded by Delgado-Esteban et al.[10] (p. 1148), who stated that "Our results suggest that BH4 deficiency converts neuronal NOS into an efficient peroxynitrite synthase. . . ." The shift of NOS activity towards more superoxide production and less nitric oxide production has been called *uncoupling,* where its intrinsic activity is less tightly coupled to nitric oxide synthesis.

The potential vicious nature of such a shift towards BH4 deficiency can be seen by the fact that peroxynitrite itself is a potent oxidizer of BH4 such that peroxynitrite elevation leads to a deficiency in tetrahydrobiopterin (BH4) levels.[11-14] It can be seen from this that *prolonged elevation of superoxide leading to increased peroxynitrite will lead to BH4 depletion, leading in turn to more peroxynitrite elevation.* This may be a key factor, then, in switching the cell over to the NO/ONOO⁻ cycle.

One point that needs to be made is that, even though the conventional wisdom suggests that most of the superoxide generated in cells comes from the electron transport chain in mitochondria, rather than from nitric oxide synthases or other mechanisms, the generation from NOSs may have an especially important role in the generation of peroxynitrite. This is because those cells and even regions of cells with the most NOS activity have the potential of producing the most superoxide from the NOSs. Because the superoxide and nitric oxide from NOSs will be produced in close proximity to each other due to the concentration of NOS in that location, this will allow much of the superoxide to react with nitric oxide before the superoxide molecules can be destroyed by superoxide dismutases. Thus, the roles of NOSs as potential peroxynitrite synthases may be especially important, even with relatively modest generation of superoxide.

Part of this proposed switch mechanism is diagrammed in Figure 12.1. In that figure, NOS activity is diagrammed as being controlled by a variable switch, indicated by the position of the vertical bar. As that bar moves to the right, it will produce increased uncoupling of NOS activity, leading to increased superoxide (OO•⁻) production and lessened nitric oxide (NO•⁻) production, leading in turn to increased peroxynitrite production. According to the view proposed here, the switch determining whether the NO/ONOO⁻ cycle is initiated is determined by two variable switches: The absolute NOS activity *and* the amount of uncoupling of that activity. It is the combination

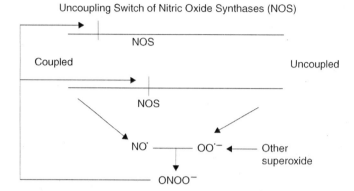

FIGURE 12.1. Uncoupling of nitric oxide synthase (NOS) activity by peroxynitrite-mediated oxidation of tetrahydrobiopterin (BH4). The upright bar of the NOS activity indicates the amount of uncoupling of the NOS activity. Movement to the right indicates increased uncoupling due to BH4 depletion. Peroxynitrite (ONOO⁻) oxidizes BH4, leading to increased uncoupling (increased superoxide production) and lessened coupling of the enzyme to NOS.

of these two that determines whether the cycle is initiated or not and, if it is initiated, how strongly it is initiated.

The switch that turns on the NO/ONOO⁻ cycle may be due to both the intrinsic NOS activity and what has been described as the uncoupling of NOS activity, when the NOS enzyme molecules are deprived of BH4 and therefore synthesize superoxide. This switch, if you will, has the property of a complex dimmer switch. It is quantitatively controlled both by how much intrinsic NOS activity is present and by how much of it is uncoupled due to destruction of BH4. So, it is not a simple on/off switch according to this view, but when it produces prolonged and sufficient peroxynitrite, it flips the NO/ONOO⁻ cycle on.

It can be argued that, instead of a NO/ONOO⁻ cycle, perhaps this cycle should be called the OO⁻/ONOO⁻ cycle, where OO⁻ is the chemical structure for superoxide (oh, oh no cycle?). One of my readers suggested it should be called the "oh no, oh no!" cycle since both superoxide and nitric oxide have essential roles in generating peroxynitrite. In any case, I have no plans to change the name.

The importance of switching nitric oxide synthases away from only nitric oxide production towards greater superoxide production can be seen in the control of the transcription factor NF-κB. NF-κB, as was discussed in

Chapter 1, is a cycle element that is stimulated by peroxynitrite and other oxidants but is inhibited by nitric oxide. Thus, in order to have a shift towards greater NF-κB activity, we need to have a shift towards greater production of or, at least, levels of superoxide. The superoxide will produce a shift toward greater peroxynitrite levels, which stimulate NF-κB, and away from nitric oxide levels, which inhibit NF-κB. How can one test this hypothesis of a central switch mechanism? One way, which will be discussed in Chapter 15, is to use high-level folate supplements to lower this switch towards superoxide production. Such studies to test the effects of high-level folate supplements can be most easily performed in the initiation animal models. I would add that it is possible to provide supplements of tetrahydrobiopterin, as well, to determine their influence on the initiation of these illnesses.

GENETIC STUDIES

One of the most important types of studies that are needed are genetic studies identifying specific genes that have a role in determining with susceptibility to multisystem illnesses. Such studies are still in their early stages, and there are many specific genetic polymorphisms in genes that are expected to interact with the NO/ONOO⁻ cycle and that may have a role, therefore, in determining the chances of initiating these illnesses. The genetic studies that have already been done on these illnesses are already quite important, but I expect that such studies will be progressively much more important in the future.

THERAPY AND PREVENTION

I have always thought that any etiologic mechanism worthy of the name should justify its existence in large part through its ability to predict useful therapeutic approaches. Certainly, the NO/ONOO⁻ cycle predicts quite a number of potential therapies, as you will see in Chapter 15. However, the cycle's complexity makes it difficult if not impossible to find a "magic bullet" that will cure these illnesses. The robust and chronic nature of these illnesses may owe its existence to the complexity of the cycle. Still, a combination of agents that down-regulate different aspects of the cycle may be expected to be more effective than any single agent, and this is an approach that I will take in Chapter 15. It is tragic, in my view, that there have been almost no substantial tests of therapies designed to lower aspects of the NO/ONOO⁻ cycle. I would especially advocate such studies in PTSD because of the essential complete absence of biochemical approaches for the treatment of that multisystem illness. The scientists studying these illnesses and the victims of these illnesses should have common ground in the search for effective therapies—such a search can test, at a practical level, this explanatory model and should help make major improvements in the lives of the patients.

Where there is a high probability that initiating stressors may lead to one or more of these illnesses, prevention can be studied. The stressors leading to PTSD, to Gulf War–syndrome-like illnesses and, in some cases, to MCS responses are often predictable enough to provide useful situations where prevention can be studied. The initiation of FM following certain types of physical trauma may also be predictable enough to provide a useful framework for prevention studies. The prediction here is that agents that help prevent the establishment of the NO/ONOO⁻ cycle will often be effective as preventive agents. A recent study reported the very common of initiation of CFS-like illnesses after symptomatic West Nile virus infection, suggesting another system for testing prevention.

Chapter 13

What About Those Who Say
It Is All in Your Head
or That It All Starts in Your Head?

There are more things in heaven and earth, Horatio, than are dreamt of in your philosophy.

William Shakespeare

There is no question that there are literally many billions of dollars at stake in our understanding of these illnesses—and there are vested interests who would like to prevent insurance coverage for sufferers, prevent disability payments, prevent successful liability suits with regard to chemical exposure and maintain the income stream to the pharmaceutical industry.

Jan van Roijen

TAKE-HOME LESSONS

What has been called psychogenic theory has seven major flaws. It is based on a dualism between the psychological/mental/psychiatric on the one hand and the physical/biological/physiological on the other. This dualism has been rejected by modern science. It is also based on the notions of somatoform disorders and somatization, notions that have serious flaws. When applied to multisystem illnesses, psychogenic advocates have consistently ignored crucial genetic, physiological, and biochemical evidence

Explaining "Unexplained Illnesses"
© 2007 by The Haworth Press, Inc. All rights reserved.
doi:10.1300/5139_13

inconsistent with their views. They also ignore the long history of false psychogenic attribution, claims of psychogenesis for at least nine distinct diseases, which have all been rejected by modern science. The papers of psychogenic advocates substitute emotional terminology for sound argument. They often use flawed logic. They rarely make any clear testable predictions that may be used to distinguish their views from those of physiological explanations, a cardinal sin in science. Despite all of these flaws, their views have had substantial resonance in the medical community, and it is that resonance that produces part of the need for this chapter.

WHY THIS CHAPTER

This chapter is focused on the claims that the multisystem illnesses are not "real" physiological illnesses, that the illnesses are either psychogenic, generated by some usually ill-defined psychological etiology, or that those claiming to suffer from these illnesses are simply malingerers, faking their illnesses. These points of view have been quite commonly embraced either publicly or quietly by many in the medical community. My goal here is to describe why these points of view have become so popular and what flaws I see in these viewpoints.

Why should such a chapter be needed in this book? After all, if I am right about the role of the NO/ONOO⁻ cycle in the etiology of these illnesses, obviously the psychogenic advocates must be wrong so why do we need to consider these issues further? Moreover, there have been quite a number of critiques of their views written earlier,[1-14] so why do we need still another? Both of these are valid questions. My goal here is not to compare the psychogenic point of view[15-24] with my own. I will try to avoid such comparisons in much of this chapter, although I will make a brief overall comparison toward the end of the chapter. It seems to me that the critiques I have seen of these viewpoints are fairly narrowly drawn, although some of them are excellent within the framework in which they were written. However, there is a more comprehensive framework that needs to be considered, which is the focus of this chapter.

SOMATOFORM DISORDERS
AND BELIEF SYSTEMS

Many psychogenic advocates have explained these multisystem illnesses as being due to some kind of aberrant belief system. For example,

Staudenmayer states in his book[20] (p. 21) that "In my view, EI [the term he used for multiple chemical sensitivity (MCS)] is a disorder of belief." Wessely has been quoted* as having stated[7] the following: "I am going to talk not about an illness but about an idea. There is a phenomenon known as myalgic encephalomyelitis or ME. ICD-10 now discourages its use. I will argue that ME is simply a belief, the belief that one has an illness called ME." Typically, the illness belief is claimed to be due not only to the sufferer himself but also to the parents of a child sufferer, medical personnel who "validate" the belief by diagnosing the illness, and the news media and/ or support groups who encourage the illness belief. Often this "belief" is argued to be parallel to that of mass hysteria, where whole groups of people become hysterical due to some type of interaction, where each encourages the hysteria of others.

The parallel between such "belief" and mass hysteria is difficult to maintain given the differences between these multisystem illnesses and mass hysteria. Sirois, in his review of mass hysteria,[25] showed that the best-documented mass hysteria epidemics have several characteristic features that are distinct from those of the occurrence of multisystem illnesses. Most outbreaks of mass hysteria occur in groups of people in close physical proximity to each other such as in a school, village, or factory; in contrast, although there are epidemics of multisystem illnesses such as in sick building syndrome situations or in chronic fatigue syndrome (CFS) epidemics such as the Incline Village epidemic, most cases of multisystem illnesses occur individually, not as epidemics. Most victims of mass hysteria are young, often below age 20 and predominantly below age 40; in contrast, people coming down with multisystem illnesses are often middle aged. Furthermore, most victims of mass hysteria recover within one to 30 days, whereas most multisystem illness victims suffer for years and very often for life. Such recovery has to be viewed as a major distinction between mass hysteria and multisystem illnesses because in CFS, fibromyalgia (FM), and MCS, full recoveries are quite infrequent, and when they do occur, they typically require many months, not days. The only obvious similarity between mass hysteria and multisystem illnesses is that they each show a similar gender distribution, with higher incidence in females than in males. To argue that multisystem illnesses are caused by a belief system based on parallels to mass hysteria is to make at best a very weak argument.

---

*It should be noted that Wessely's recent statements have contained a somewhat a different interpretation of CFS/myalgic encephalomyelitis (ME).

Whether the psychogenic claims are based on claims of a belief system or on some other basis, their understanding of "mechanism," to the extent that one can talk about mechanism, is based on the notion of somatoform disorders, somatization and somatization disorders, and certain related concepts. It is important, therefore, to define these terms and see how they may or may not provide an intellectual base for the notion of psychogenesis of these multisystem illnesses. The following definitions come from Smith[26] (pp. 2-3) and are similar or identical to definitions of the same terms in the scientific literature.

> *Somatoform:* A group of disorders with somatic symptoms that suggest a physical disorder, but for which no organic etiology can be demonstrated. There is presumptive evidence of a psychological basis for the disorder.
> *Somatization:* A process whereby psychological distress is expressed in physical symptoms.
> *Somatization disorder:* A chronic, relapsing psychiatric disorder characterized by at least 13 unexplained medical symptoms from a list of 37 criteria, with at least one such symptom occurring before the age of 30.
> *Somatizers:* Persons who have 6 to 12 unexplained medical symptoms in their lifetimes, with at least one such symptom occurring before age 30.

So, the notion proposed by the psychogenic advocates is that these multisystem illnesses are somatoform disorders and quite possibly somatization disorders and that they are produced by the process of somatization, a process whereby psychological distress produces physical symptoms. In this way, they argue, the appearance of physical symptoms may be a consequence of psychological distress.

There are several problematic issues with both the theory and the practice underlying these definitions and how these may apply to multisystem illnesses. For example, the definition of somatoform demands that no organic etiology can be demonstrated, an almost impossible goal to meet; in practice, what may be argued is that no organic etiology has been demonstrated, a very different thing. This has often led psychogenic advocates to inflate their claims presumably in order to try to meet the requirements of this definition. I have argued in this book and elsewhere that an organic etiology can and has been demonstrated for these multisystem illnesses, so I would contest both of these claims. But the point that should be undisputed is that psychogenic advocates often claim that no such etiology can be demonstrated and that they have not documented. Their failure to imagine an organic etiology does not mean that one cannot exist.

Two of these definitions, for somatizer or for somatization disorder, require that there be unexplained symptoms. These requirements have led to repeated claims of "unexplained symptoms" or "medically unexplained symptoms" in the papers of psychogenic advocates. In most cases they fail to even consider whether the evidence supports this inference. Furthermore, when Dr. Iris Bell or I or others have published explanations for some of these symptoms, our publications have been ignored by those making these claims. One of the more striking examples of the failure to provide any documentation that such symptoms are unexplained is the recent review of Binder and Campbell,[22] whose title starts out with "Medically unexplained symptoms" but makes no attempt whatsoever in this very long review to provide any evidence that these symptoms are unexplained. This is one of many abject failures of psychogenic advocates to pay any attention to the evidence.*

There are three additional problematic features of these definitions:

1. The requirement for unexplained symptoms in the definitions of somatizers and of somatization disorder means that, if today those symptoms are unexplained and tomorrow they are explained, the illness involved immediately switches from one fitting the definition to one not fitting, even though the illness itself has not changed one iota. We are not talking here about switching from an ambiguous status to a nonambiguous one, but rather a switch from one nonambiguous status to another.

2. A second problematic feature is that if a disorder is somatoform, the definition states that "There is presumptive evidence of a psychological basis." So, for some unexplained reason, the default value is that of a psychological etiology even though such etiologies are clearly among the least well-documented ones in medicine. The only rationale for this would be the view that, if we are confused about something, it must be psychological, but that view is clearly wrong. There are many confusing things in medicine.

---

*A key goal for my describing explanations of many of the symptoms of these multisystem illnesses, in Chapter 3 and elsewhere in this book, was to make it as difficult as possible for psychogenic advocates to continue making false claims that these symptoms are unexplained.

3. The third problematic feature of these definitions is that the definition of somatization has little, if any, relationship to the definition of somatization disorder. Somatization is defined in terms of a psychological process leading to the generation of physical symptoms. However, somatization disorder is defined in terms of an arbitrary list of criteria, none of which provide evidence for a psychological as opposed to physiological process. The consequence of this is that an illness may meet the definition of being a somatization disorder without involving the process of somatization. However, the contrary is widely assumed in the literature: psychogenic advocates and others widely assume that, if an illness meets the definition for somatization disorder, then the process of somatization must be involved.

The features of these definitions mean that the foundation upon which psychogenesis is built has substantial flaws. Each of the problematic features of these definitions creates a conceptual or practical problem for the whole concept of psychogenesis.

Janca[27] recently reviewed papers expressing reservations about the basic concepts of somatization and of somatoform disorder. He summarizes the field as follows (p. 65): "If one were to find a common denominator of the papers covered in this review, it is a general agreement amongst the authors that the current concepts of somatization and somatoform disorders have serious theoretical and practical limitations in both research and clinical settings." He further suggests that the time has come to seriously rethink these concepts so as to "find better nosological solutions for the forthcoming revisions of classification systems in psychiatry and medicine." Other criticisms of the concept of somatization and the way it has been used in practice have been published by Epstein et al.[28]

Per Dalen, MD, PhD, and professor of psychiatry, stated[8] in reference to these multisystem illnesses (p. xiii): "For some years now I have been convinced that the concept of somatization is being exploited for reasons that are only partly transparent. Scientifically there is no basis for the remarkable expansion of this field. The lives of large numbers of patients are touched and often made more difficult by what is going on. Psychiatry is apparently being abused, and it is of course very important to find out more about the background in order to do something about it."

The flaws in the concepts of somatoform disorders, somatization, and somatization disorders necessarily produce flaws in the concept of psychogenesis because psychogenesis is based on these concepts.

MALINGERING

Malingering is not an example of psychogenesis but is considered here because it is an interpretation of these multisystem illnesses that also suggests they are not true physiological illnesses. Malingering is usually described as faking illness for secondary gain. Examples are where an individual may pretend to be ill to avoid some unpleasant or dangerous task, such as avoiding military service. DSM-IV[29] (p. 457) states that "obvious goals such as financial compensation, avoidance of duty, evasion of criminal prosecution or obtaining of drugs are apparent in malingering." There have been many claims in the literature suggesting that people claiming to have one or more of these multisystem illnesses are malingerers.[30-33] However, it is difficult to find convincing evidence of this.

One of the more thoughtful studies of possible malingering is the study of Mittenberg et al.[31] in which they attempted to assess "probable rates of malingering" among apparent cases of "fibromyalgia or chronic fatigue" as well as in a variety of other disorders. They did this by surveying 144 experienced neuropsychologists, using diagnostic impressions of nine different criteria to assess "probable malingering." They came to the inclusion that approximately 38 percent of "fibromyalgia/chronic fatigue" patients are probable malingerers.[31] It is instructive to look at some of these criteria to see what flaws may be apparent in applying them to multisystem illnesses:

1. *Severity of cognitive impairment inconsistent with condition.* Given the great variation in symptoms in these illnesses, how does one assess this inconsistency? The answer to that is not clear. In the Epstein et al.[28] review, they state that (p. 217) "For most illnesses, somatic experience is highly variable. The correlation between symptoms and observed pathological changes is poor in many conditions including peptic ulcer, upper respiratory tract symptoms and back pain."
2. *Pattern of cognitive test performance inconsistent with condition.* Same concerns as for item 1.
3. *Scores below empirical cutoffs on forced choice tests.* How does one determine empirical cutoffs when the diagnosis itself is at issue?
4. *Discrepancies among records, self-report and observed behavior.* How reliable are the medical records involved? It is not unusual in medicine for self-reported symptoms to differ from those inferred from behavior; does this necessarily mean that malingering is occurring?

5. *Implausible self-reported symptoms in interview.* Given how variable the symptoms are in these multisystem illnesses, how can a neuropsychologist judge such implausibility? Symptoms of MCS appeared to be implausible until now, when we finally have an explanation for each of its puzzling symptoms.

6. *Implausible changes in test scores across repeated examinations.* Given the repeated reports of high variability in severity of symptoms over time with these multisystem illnesses, what does implausibility mean here?

If you look at these assessments, it is apparent that each of these is, at best, a guess. Furthermore, the features of these illnesses that make them differ from many other diseases, high-level variability from one patient to another, diversity of symptoms found in individual patients, as well as their previously unexplained nature, may well lead to elevated levels of estimates of "probable malingering." The basic problem is that, in the absence of a specific biomarker that provides an objectively measurable diagnostic criterion, all we have is guesses, and even "informed guesses" of experienced neuropsychologists have no objectively measurable validity with these illnesses.

There are two other issues that need to be considered with regard to the notion of malingering. Because malingerers presumably fake illness because of secondary gain, is there any plausible secondary gain in the cases of these multisystem illnesses? Since people diagnosed with these illnesses are typically impacted by the difficulty in maintaining employment, by their inability to perform daily tasks, and by their inability to maintain anything resembling a normal social life, it is hard to see how they could have any secondary gain that would lead them to fake such illness. We typically gain status and take pleasure in things that require either cognitive activity or physical activity or both, and both of these are usually impacted in these individuals. We often see marriages disintegrate, friendships deteriorate, poverty descend, and self-empowerment disappear. It is not unusual for suicides to result. Where, then, is the secondary gain? The only possible objective case for secondary gain that may be apparent is in the small minority of cases where sufferers try to obtain disability support or compensation for chemical exposure. In these cases, which are typically a small minority of such cases overall, the sufferers face a long and arduous process with no guarantee of success. They also face a Catch-22 situation—their seeking such support provides antagonists with the only evidence that there may be such secondary gain. Psychologists sometimes argue that there may be secondary gain in these patients from their ability to call attention to themselves. Here the problem comes in when psychologists or psychiatrists convert a theoretical possibility into a probability and then that into certainty in the absence of any objective data supporting such conversions. As we will see in the following text, it has not been unusual in instances such as this for some psychologists and psychiatrists to repeatedly overinterpret the available information.

The last issue that needs to be raised is that of objectively measurable aberrations in these illnesses. It should be clear from the various studies of such things as positron emission tomography (PET) scan or single-photon emission computed tomography (SPECT) scan abnormalities, oxidative stress, nitric oxide increases, mitochondrial/energy metabolism dysfunction, and others I have discussed elsewhere that there are no apparent mechanisms by which these abnormalities can be generated by malingering. Certainly, the advocates of a malingering interpretation of these illnesses make no such claims. Rather, they ignore all of this data, as do the psychogenic advocates. So, it should be clear that most of these patients cannot be malingerers, because as a group they show multiple objectively measurable defects.

Still, these types of measurements could be used to independently assess the "probable malingerers" that Mitterberg et al.[31] claim to have identified. If the 38 percent of these FM/CFS individuals are truly malingerers, they should have no statistically significant differences from normal controls in their markers of oxidative stress, nitric oxide, etc. Of course, tests like these have not been performed.

Malingering does not explain the majority of individuals with these multisystem illnesses, and it is doubtful that it explains even the minority subset previously described as being "probable malingerers." I will not give much further consideration to the issue of malingering in the rest of the chapter, but will focus, rather, on the issue of psychogenesis.

WHY DO THESE VIEWS HAVE SO MUCH RESONANCE WITHIN THE MEDICAL COMMUNITY?

There are two reasons why these psychogenic views have so much resonance in the medical community. The first of these is that the psychogenic views are very close to what medical students are taught in medical school. For example, in a chapter in *The Cambridge Illustrated History of Medicine*, Porter[34] (p. 111) describes the idea of the culture of sickness stating that "Being ill becomes a way of life accorded social sanction and medical encouragement." He goes on to describe the views of Talcott Parsons, an

American sociologist who formulated the idea of the sick role. In it, an individual might be allowed to retire under the guise of being ill, temporarily relieved of social responsibilities. Porter's key paragraph (p. 111) is as follows:

> The existential side of playing sick is psychosomatic illness, whose intriguing history has been traced by Edward Shorter. He focused on what he calls "somatizers"—that is, people suffering from "pain and fatigue that have no physical cause." These are patients frustrating to no-nonsense physicians such as the early-twentieth century Kentucky doctor who thought a 'good spanking, sometimes even a good "cussing" was the surest way with such evident hypochondriacs.' Most of those suffering in the past two centuries from conditions variously called "nervous spine," "neurasthenia," "fits," and nowadays myalgic encephalomyelitis, or ME (also called "yuppie flu" or chronic fatigue syndrome) and perhaps repetitive strain injury (RSI) have nothing intrinsically organically wrong with them, argued Shorter, but have been consciously or unconsciously seeking solace, attention, or social excuses. Such somatizers have produced a fascinating succession of phantom diseases, Shorter suggested, the "unconscious", selecting convenient suits of somatoform manifestations from a wider "symptom pool."

Another example that is relevant to what physicians are taught in medical school is from the forward by Marmor in the textbook *Clinical Psychiatry for the Primary Physician*[35] (p. vii), who wrote as follows: "It is well known that anywhere from 50 to 75 percent of all persons who consult physicians for physical symptomatology have complicating or contributing mental or emotional problems. Thus, it is the primary physician who constitutes the first line of defense, so to speak, in the mental health care of most people." Clearly, if you are a physician and you have a patient consulting you for an illness for which the standard clinical tests are in the normal range, and the patient is ill based primarily on what are described as self-reported symptoms, and you have been taught that over half of your patient visits are likely to be primarily for mental or emotional reasons, you are likely to think that the patient is there for those reasons.

It can be seen from the first of these quotations that the sickness role is taught in the medical curriculum, and this source specifically includes chronic fatigue syndrome and a variety of related "phantom diseases." You can see from the second quotation that, given the claimed frequency of contributing emotional/mental problems among patients, there will be a strong tendency to interpret puzzling illnesses as being emotional/mental, whatever their true etiology may be. Whatever the flaws may be in views of the psychogenic interpretation of multisystem illnesses, it should not be surprising that the psychogenic interpretation finds receptivity in the minds of physicians and other medical personnel—it is quite similar to views taught to them in medical school.

A second source of such receptivity is likely to come from the needs of physicians to feel empowered in their ability to treat their patients. No physician wants to feel completely helpless in his or her ability to understand and treat any "real" physiological illness. The reactions of physicians to the challenge of patients for whom they can do little are demonstrated by a statement published by Epstein et al:[28]

> Quality of care may relate in part to physicians' difficulty tolerating uncertainty and their need to feel effective. In response to patients who can offer the physician neither certainty nor efficacy, physicians use blaming language ("amplifying," "supratentorial," "difficult") and attempt to "withdraw attention from the patient" through referral or avoidance. (p. 218)

One of the aspects that exacerbates the division between physician and the patient suffering from these multisystem illnesses is that, if a physician interprets the illness as being primarily or entirely psychiatric and refers the patient to a psychiatrist, resistance by the patient is viewed as lack of cooperation in treatment. And, as stated in Stoudemire's textbook[36] (p. 26), "Patients who do not cooperate with their treatment are also viewed negatively by the medical profession. Negative labels, such as 'crock, troll, turkey, gomer,' are often invoked to characterize such patients who do not fit into the traditional sick role model. Once patients get labeled in this manner, physicians often feel less obligated to follow through on the rest of their own responsibilities and obligations of taking care of the patient."

So, both the training of physicians in medical schools and their human weaknesses as clinicians cause them to be receptive to the psychogenic views of multisystem illnesses despite flaws in these views.*

---

*My goal here is not to excuse this approach of many physicians. Nor is it to either agree or disagree with the 50 to 75 percent figure of emotional/mental reasons for consulting physicians given by Marmor, although I think these figures may be high. It is, rather, to develop an understanding in both patient and physician on the origin of the clear resonance that psychogenic views have had in the medical community, despite the many scientific flaws that these views have.

DUALISM: THE ACHILLES' HEEL
OF PSYCHOGENESIS

The basic tenet of psychogenesis is that these illnesses all start in the psychological/psychiatric/mental sphere and that none of the basic etiology of these illnesses involves real physiological mechanisms. As stated by Staudenmayer[20] (p. 20), "The core presupposition of psychogenic theory is that psychological factors are necessary and sufficient to account for the clinical presentations of EI patients. Psychogenic theory emphasizes belief, somatization, psychophysiologic stress and anxiety responses, and psychogenic etiology." What the psychogenic advocates have done is to draw a line in the sand between the psychological/psychiatric/mental on the one hand and the physical/biological/physiological on the other, stating that all of the initial causality and perhaps all of the complete causality is on the psychological side of the line. In other words, their entire case is based on a dualism between the psychological/psychiatric/mental on the one hand and the physical/biological/physiological on the other. However, this proposed dualism, which dates from Descartes, does not exist.

This dualism has been firmly rejected by the American Psychiatric Association in DSM-IV[29] (p. xxi), often described as the psychiatrists' bible— "the term mental disorder unfortunately implies a distinction between 'mental' disorders and 'physical' disorders that is a reductionist anachronism of mind/body dualism. A compelling literature documents that there is much 'physical' in 'mental' disorders and much 'mental' in 'physical' disorders." It should be noted that the psychiatrists may be viewed as having a vested interest in preserving this dualism, so their rejection of it should lead us to admire their intellectual honesty. Their position also assures us of the compelling nature of the evidence leading to this rejection.

The connection between this dualism with CFS and related illnesses and the distortions it engenders for our understanding of them was recently explored by Deary,[37] who also suggests alternative interpretations of these illnesses, not dependent on this dualism.

The nonexistent dualism was also an element in a paper by Mayou et al.[38] recommending what they called the "radical option" of dropping all subcategories currently listed under somatoform disorders in DSM-IV. The fact that "the (somatoform) category is inherently dualistic" was only one of eight reasons behind this recommendation to drop the entire category[38] (p. 849). It should be noted that one of the authors of this paper is Michael Sharpe, a British psychiatrist who has often been identified as a psychogenesis advocate. I believe, therefore, that Sharpe showed great intellectual courage in taking this important step.

The psychogenic advocate Gots argues for this dualism in his paper[15] titled "Multiple chemical sensitivities: distinguishing between psychogenic and toxicodynamic." This leads him to some stunning leaps of logic such as the following (p. S10): "Stimulation of a neurotransmitter or release of a hormone occurs in response to stimulus. Evidence of response to stress or phobia, such as EEG changes or elevated cortisol levels, helps to describe part of the organic interface between stimulus and response and supplements our knowledge of how the mind produces symptoms. *These responses, however, are not indicative of organic dysfunction and do not eliminate the role of the mind in the phobic or stress response*" (italics added). So, Gots would have us believe that, because these are produced in response to psychological stress, cortisol or EEG changes are of no organic consequence, incapable producing organic dysfunction. Taken to its logical conclusion, this same reasoning would have us believe that, if a person responds to psychological stress by committing suicide, he or she is not "organically" dead. The reason for Gots's commitment to this discarded dualism becomes clear in another part of his paper.[15] He argues (p. S9) that "Manufacturers cannot be held responsible for responses that depend on psychological processes."

Binder and Campbell take such flaws in logic one step further in their 2004 review.[22] In discussing the issue of some neuroendocrine abnormalities in FM, they state that (p. 374): "It is believed by some investigators that there are neuroendocrine abnormalities associated with fibromyalgia and that the illness is caused by abnormal sensory processing. *However emotional problems also are associated with neuroendocrine disorders. We know of no evidence of neuroendocrine abnormalities specific to that condition.* There was evidence of reduced cerebral blood flow in the thalamus and pontine tegmentum in patients with fibromyalgia, *but similar findings are nonspecific and occur in psychiatric patients*" (italics added and references deleted). Binder and Campbell would have us believe that such real physiological changes in FM are of no consequence because they also occur elsewhere in patients with "emotional" or "psychiatric" disorders. The implication is that because a physiological correlate occurs in a psychiatric or emotional condition, it is forever discounted even when it occurs in another, possibly unrelated, illness. They use a similar leap of logic in describing a CFS study as follows (p. 375): "A fluorine (sic)-deoxyglucose positron emission tomography (PET) study suggested that hypometabolism of the brain stem was found only in CFS and not in depression, *but a study using the same technique found no differences between a group with CFS and a group with somatization disorder*" (references removed and italics added). It appears that Binder and Campbell wish to not only discount real objectively measurable physical correlates in psychiatric/emotional disorders but to discount those same correlates when they are found elsewhere because of some sort of guilt by association. Let me state, for the record, that objectively measurable physiological correlates of illness are biologically and medically significant whether they are specific or nonspecific. Certainly, a large number of standard clinical tests measure correlates whose changes are not completely specific but are nevertheless medically significant. If such changed correlates are found in psychiatric/emotional illnesses, they provide still further evidence, should that be needed, that the dualism was correctly discarded.

Another flaw in logic occurred in the letter published by Black on the apparent effectiveness of the drug paroxetine in the treatment of MCS.[39] Paroxetine, as you may recall from Chapter 6, is an inhibitor of nitric oxide synthase activity as well as being a serotonin reuptake inhibitor and is a drug that has been used to treat certain psychiatric disorders. Black reports that this drug was effective in the treatment of an MCS patient and concludes that (p. 1436) "This case joins two others in showing *that some patients diagnosed with multiple chemical sensitivity have an underlying psychiatric disorder that, when identified, responds to medication therapy*" (references deleted and italics added). Black infers that, because paroxetine has been effective in the treatment of some psychiatric disorders, it must be acting to correct a psychiatric flaw in these cases. Clearly, that is illogical and the flaw in logic appears to be based on his being stuck with this dualistic frame of thought. The "logic" used is the same as if I were to propose: Aspirin cures headaches. Aspirin decreases blood clotting. Therefore, headaches cause blood clotting. If I were to write a letter to the editor of a scientific journal making that argument, I doubt that you can find an editor who would hesitate more than a millisecond or so before pushing the reject button. But Black makes the same error in logic and it gets published.

In summary, the fact that what has been called psychogenic theory is based on a rejected dualism is sufficient reason to reject such theory. There are additional substantial reasons.

LONG HISTORY OF FALSE PSYCHOGENIC ATTRIBUTION IN MEDICINE

There is a whole series of diseases that has been attributed to a psychogenic etiology and in each such disease, that attribution has been rejected by modern medical science. The reasoning and errors that led to these false attributions are interesting and one would think that the current psychogenic advocates should acknowledge this history and show that they are not simply repeating these errors today. What they have done, however, is to ignore the existence of this history, leading us to wonder why?

I wish to briefly discuss several examples of such false attribution. Aring published a paper titled "Observations on multiple sclerosis and conversion hysteria," positing what is now called a psychogenic etiology for multiple sclerosis (MS), with MS largely generated by hysteria.[40] In it he quotes from Wilson (p. 666) as follows: ". . . symptoms are still chiefly if not solely subjective where a superficial though perhaps natural diagnosis of hysteria is apt to be made. . . . Examination discloses no single unequivocal sign of 'organic' nervous disease. . . ." Later, Aring states that (p. 666) "The neurological literature abounds with references to the association of multiple sclerosis and hysteria." Still later, he describes the work of Langworthy and others as follows (p. 667): "In their studies they noted the basic hysterical personality structure of certain patients with multiple sclerosis long before they developed signs of the neurological disease." So, here we have MS, a neurological disease now known to be caused by demyelination of neurons and subsequent neuronal dysfunction, ascribed to "hysteria" in terms very similar to those used currently to describe the multisystem illnesses by psychogenic advocates.

Parkinson's disease was confidently described as developing in people with histories of an insecure childhood who exhibited poor adjustment to previous stresses.[41] It was also described elsewhere[42] (p. 13) as follows: "Parkinsonism, postencephalitic as well as senile, is a syndrome characteristic of a specific personality type. The Parkinsonian personality is characterized by urge toward action, expressed through motor activity and through industriousness; striving for independence, authority, and success within a rigid, usually moralistic behavior pattern. The following factors appear to be responsible for this personality structure. . . ."

Psychogenic type interpretations have been touted for lupus[43] and a number of other diseases. Interstitial cystitis was described in a major medical textbook[44] as being the result of emotional disturbance—a pathway for the discharge of unconscious hatred. Migraine headache is another disease ascribed to psychogenesis, with the migraine personality being described as perfectionistic and inflexible, characterized by tension, dissatisfaction, and resentment.[45] As the pathophysiology of migraine has become better understood, the role of psychological factors has been steadily downgraded.

Dorfman reviewed in his book[46] a large number of proposed psychogenic roles in human disease. Among the diseases he discusses are rheumatoid arthritis, asthma, peptic (gastric) ulcers, and ulcerative colitis. All of these are now known to have etiologies dominated by identified physiological processes, although in some cases important aspects of the physiology are still unknown. It is instructive to read some the passages in Dorfman[46] to see how pervasive this psychogenic misattribution was.

Dorfman states (p. 73) that "The role of chronic repressed hostility and resentment (in rheumatoid arthritis) is considered to be significant. Like the hypertensive, the patient with rheumatoid arthritis has conditioned himself and learned to control aggressive and hostile impulses. In reviewing the individual's history, it is frequently noted that the parents were very restrictive; punishment was often provided by the curtailment of physical freedom. Alexander noted that patients with rheumatoid arthritis tried to control their environment with an 'iron hand' (a symbolic and dramatic portrayal of the physical deformities often seen in advanced stages of disease). Alexander noted that females were tomboys while in their adolescence, with an inordinate and exaggerated need for physical exercise. He finds that the onset of the disease is often precipitated by curtailment of physical activity. . . ."

Dorman argues that asthma has important psychogenic aspect to its etiology as follows (p. 77):

> French and Alexander regarded asthma as a substitute for crying; an asthmatic attack was equated with the frustrated cry of an infant. Clinically, some patients learned to avert an asthmatic episode by crying. At times under psychotherapy, when patients began to express emotions which were formerly repressed, the asthma improved. The central conflict in bronchial asthma is said to lie in the relationship with the mother; attacks are frequently precipitated by pending or actual separation. Acute exacerbations are thus frequently precipitated by leaving home, engagement, marriage, etc., when the patient is too dependent to make the transition to a more independent existence. Bastiaans and Groen (a psychoanalyst and an internist) attempted to integrate the allergic and the psychogenic aspects of the etiology of asthma. They viewed the illness as a three-pronged affair: a) a constitutional tendency to allergy; b) a type of childhood experience in which the patient's mother or parent surrogate, exposed him to a 'loving tyranny' and c) an acute conflict-producing situation in which the patient felt compelled to submit helplessly to an authoritative figure towards whom he held mixed feelings of hostility and dependency. The authors believe that when oppressive feelings become linked with certain provocative events, a process of conditioning is established so that the patient reacts to hair trigger stimuli and bronchoplasm.

In peptic (gastric) ulcer, Dorfman (p. 23, 24) noted that psychogenic factors alone cannot cause the disease but states that "Somatic, constitutional and socio-cultural factors all play significant roles. In exploring the psychogenic factors, it is interesting to note that milk remains the one item which is not only innocuous but quite essential in the diet of the ulcer patient. Psychoanalytic considerations can aid in interpreting this fact since 'food is equated with love,' and the milk may be reminiscent of the gratification provided by this product in infancy. Even those who were not breast-fed as infants were given milk which was bottled or at least distributed by their mothers or mother-substitutes." Dorfman later states "Most of those with peptic ulceration will balk at the mention of possible psychiatric referral for consultation or treatment. The roots for this reluctance may very well be related to the persistent need for their façade 'to be independent'; it may also be a subtle derivative of adolescent rebellion. At any rate, these patients often resent any implication that would place them in the 'dependent position' of possibly requiring psychiatric help." These and other statements of the claimed partial psychogenesis of gastric ulcers produced considerable difficulty to the attempt to get acceptance of the view that these ulcers were caused by a bacterial infection of the bacterium *Helicobacter pylori*. Even after there was very clear evidence for an infectious etiology for gastric ulcers and a simple, effective antibiotic treatment was available, it still took about 10 years for the medical community to widely accept this new view.* Strong statements on psychogenesis can have powerful destructive influences and the gastric ulcer example is a clear-cut example of that.

You cannot fault people for looking at a variety of explanatory models to try to find explanations for the etiology of illnesses. But you can fault them for overinterpreting their data and overstating what is supported by those data. You can also fault them for uncritically quoting unsupported and poorly supported opinion. In the current time, you can fault them for setting up a false dichotomy between psychogenic versus physiological attribution, a dichotomy based on a false dualism, as I state elsewhere in this chapter. Psychological factors can influence the course of physical illness, but it is important not to overinterpret or misinterpret any evidence presumably supporting such a role. You will see later in this chapter that the current psy-

---

*The 2005 Nobel Prize in physiology and medicine was given to two Australian physicians who demonstrated the infectious etiology of gastric ulcers. This may be viewed as surprising, given that over 100 other diseases had each been previously demonstrated to have an infectious etiology, leading one to ask why such a demonstration for gastric ulcers was viewed by the Nobel committee as having such significance. It seems clear that the many confidently made false claims of a primarily psychogenic etiology of gastric ulcers led the Nobel committee to view this demonstration with special medical significance.

chogenic advocates regarding multisystem illnesses make other, even more serious errors than those considered in this section, so that rather than learning from the errors of the past, they seem to be intent on exceeding them.

There are other important lessons that should, in my judgment, be derived from the history of false psychogenic attribution. Perhaps this can be seen most clearly in both MS and lupus. Both of these show considerable variation in symptoms from one case to another, providing psychogenic advocates some cover for their speculations about these diseases. Both typically showed no obvious abnormalities in many standard clinical tests, again paralleling the observations of the multisystem illnesses. Like many other chronic diseases, both were associated with at least occasional psychiatric symptoms. It was only after considerable study was done to identify specific biomarkers for each of these diseases that the psychogenic speculation was finally laid to rest. In MS, this involved the demonstration of extensive demyelination in regions of the brain and spinal cord, as being characteristic and demonstrable biomarker for that disease. In lupus, it was the demonstration of antinuclear antibodies (ANA) that provided the specific biomarker and evidence for its autoimmune etiology. What we obviously need in the case of CFS, MCS, and FM is a dedicated search for such biomarkers, and it is for that reason that I have indicated, elsewhere in this book, where I think those searches should be focused.

Those who ignore the lessons of history are doomed to repeat them.

George Santayana

GENETICS: THE ULTIMATE PROOF
OF A BIOLOGICAL ROLE IN CAUSATION

Genes act by determining the structure, amounts, and biological distribution of proteins in the body. They determine much of the chemistry and, therefore, the biology of the body. It follows that, if genes influence any property of the organism, they do this through some sort of biological mechanism. It follows from this that, if genes have roles in influencing the incidence and prevalence of multisystem illnesses, they have a causal role through their influence on biology. This is almost a trivial point, but one that has devastating implications for either the psychogenic school or the related malingering school. Genes may, of course, influence psychology as well as biology, but when they do, they do so via the biology. I have cited quite a number of studies of genetic roles of these multisystem illnesses, in Chapter 1, Chapter 5, and Chapter 7, several of which provide support for several aspects of the NO/ONOO⁻ cycle mechanism. What the psychogenic advocates state is that it all starts with psychology not biology. It follows that any genetic roles, and such roles are by definition causal roles, show that the psychogenic advocates are wrong. Similarly, in the absence of data that the genes involved influence the tendency to become a malingerer, genetic data are inconsistent with a malingering interpretation as well.

So, how do the psychogenic or malingering advocates deal with the genetic studies of these multisystem illnesses? They ignore their existence. With one exception, which I will discuss in the following text, they universally ignore the genetic studies of these illnesses. Evidently, the psychogenic/malingering advocates feel that failing to cite such studies is the equivalent of their not existing at all—out of sight, out of mind.

I have tried in most of this chapter to avoid comparing the psychogenic interpretation of these illnesses with my own. However, with the genetic data, the comparison is so compelling, it should not be avoided. As you have seen in Chapter 5, two of the genes implicated in determining the incidence of CFS may act by regulating nitric oxide levels and some others may act through superoxide. Genes give important information about mechanism. In many situations they provide the most profound such clues because they provide evidence for important causal roles in real live people.

I would like to talk about two related and important genetic studies on MCS, but before doing so, I would like to provide some background information. Cases of MCS, as I discussed in Chapter 7, are often preceded by and presumably initiated by chemical exposure incidents, with organophosphorus/carbamate pesticides and neurotoxins forming one class of such chemicals and volatile organic solvents forming a second such class. The two additional pesticide classes that I discussed in Chapter 7 are not relevant to this discussion. So, we have *prima facie* evidence for organophosphorus compounds and organic solvents acting as short-term stressors, initiating these illnesses. The psychogenic advocates universally ignore the substantial literature implicating these chemicals in MCS initiation.

Haley et al.[47] published an important genetic study of the Gulf War syndrome sufferers, showing that a particular form of the *PON1* gene occurs in substantially higher frequencies among these sufferers than among unaffected controls. The *PON1* gene encodes a protein that metabolizes organophosphorus neurotoxins including sarin gas, which Gulf War military personnel were presumably exposed to. The particular form of the *PON1* gene associated with Gulf War syndrome is the form that causes a lessened ability to metabolize sarin gas. The role of the *PON1* gene in determining sensitivity to organophosphorus pesticides and other toxins has been reviewed recently.[48] So, the probable interpretation here should be obvious—lowered ability to metabolize these toxins leads to much higher accumulation in the body and consequent higher neurotoxicity leading to increased initiation of MCS and related illnesses. There are two possible criticisms of this inference. One is that it is possible that the *PON1* gene has some different physiological role in the initiation of MCS. That is possible, but the connection between the activity of the protein it produces and that of organophosphorus toxin metabolism makes that seem unlikely. The second possible criticism concerns whether this study is reproducible, and that concern has been allayed by a recent study from Toronto.

The Toronto study[49] reported that a similar *PON1* genetic role was found with a group of civilian MCS sufferers. This provides evidence for the reproducibility of the *PON1* gene role and expands its role to civilian MCS sufferers who may have been exposed to organophosphorus pesticides. The Toronto study also implicated five other genes, each involved in producing proteins active in metabolizing compounds previously found to initiate MCS—organic solvents or organophophorus compounds. This study provides strong further conformation that these compounds act as toxins in initiating MCS and that their chemical form is, therefore, very important in determining their toxicity. This is an important study, and in my judgement, it completely blows any notion of psychogenesis of MCS out of the water. The studies of these additional genes have not yet been confirmed by other laboratories, but I am told that a German group has some similar, as yet unpublished, results.

Another interesting genetic study on MCS was published by Binkley et al.[50] a group that makes clear their interest in and support for some sort of psychogenic mechanism for MCS. They use the term idiopathic environmental intolerance (IEI) for MCS, a term favored by the psychogenic school. Binkley et al.[50] report that people with MCS/IEI have a statistically significant higher frequency of a form of the CCK-B gene as compared with normals, a form that produces higher activity of the CCK-B receptor. This same form is associated with higher incidences of panic disorder. They state that (p. 889) "The association of specific CCK-B receptor alleles in patients with both IEI and panic disorder suggests they may share an underlying neurogenetic basis." Let me state that I agree with their inference. Both the increased MCS and panic disorder may be caused by the well-documented activity of the CCK-B receptors in stimulating the NMDA receptors, as discussed in Chapter 7 and elsewhere.[51] The irony is that their study helps refute the term they prefer, idiopathic environmental intolerance, because idiopathic means of unknown causation, and their study provides support for the view that part of the cause can be excessive CCK-B activity. Because the CCK-B receptor can, in turn, stimulate NMDA activity, it provides support for the NO/ONOO⁻ cycle and neural sensitization mechanisms for MCS.

These and other studies reporting substantial genetic roles in the etiology of multisystem illness all provide critical evidence for biological as opposed to psychogenic causation. They, therefore, provide still another Achilles' heel for the notion of psychogenesis. Like other such evidence, these studies have been consistently ignored by psychogenic advocates.

IS PTSD A PSYCHOGENIC ILLNESS?

Of the four multisystem illnesses, the one where one can make the strongest argument for its being psychogenic is obviously post-traumatic stress disorder (PTSD). After all, most cases of PTSD are initiated by severe psychological stress and the disease has been long classified as being psychiatric because of its most characteristic symptoms. In a commonsense way, there should be no question that PTSD is psychogenic. However, if you take the position of the psychogenic advocates, that "that psychological factors *are necessary and sufficient* to account for the clinical presentations" of psychogenic illnesses[20] (p. 20), then PTSD is clearly not psychogenic. Their position still runs afoul of being dependent on the rejected dualism. It still runs afoul of the reported genetic role in PTSD and the evidence for real, biological changes that are involved in the pathophysiology of the disease.

PTSD may be the best example of the four multisystem illnesses of an illness that is truly biopsychosocial, in the sense that we not only have powerful evidence for a psychological role but also substantial evidence for social and biological roles as well. There is good, published evidence for social factors; for example, rape victims with good social support succumb to PTSD much less frequently than do those without such support. Then there are all of the biological factors that, I argued in Chapter 9, can be understood in terms of a NO/ONOO⁻ cycle involvement in the etiology. PTSD may be biopsychosocial not in the ill-defined way that term has been used to describe CFS but rather in a well-defined way in which biological, psychological, and social factors each have specifically described and important roles.

OBJECTIVELY MEASURABLE CORRELATES
AND TESTABLE PREDICTIONS?

There are, as we have seen elsewhere in this book, a large number of objectively measurable correlates of the multisystem illnesses. While these show considerable variation from one individual to another, they show, at least in aggregate, that there are real physiological changes that have occurred in those suffering from multisystem illnesses. In the early psychogenic literature, advocates usually argued that there were flaws in at least some of this data. But as the data have become more and more convincing, what they have taken to doing is ignoring it, in the apparent hope that it might go away. Clearly, the question that needs to be raised of these psychogenic advocates is what aberrant correlates are consistent with their hypothesis and what mechanisms are known that show such consistency.

One of the frustrations one faces in reading the psychogenic literature is the complete lack of clearly stated testable predictions in these papers. Scientific hypotheses must have testable predictions, things that when tested can potentially lead to the falsification, with such predictions differing from those of alternative hypotheses. It is this testability that distinguishes a scientific hypothesis from mythology. Staudenmayer is well aware of this, using what he claims is the lack of such predictions to criticize those advocating physiological explanations for MCS.[20] Yet, he himself and other psychogenic advocates have carefully avoided making such predictions. I have scoured his book for any statements that might serve as surrogates for such predictions and have come up with one, a statement that I quoted earlier in this chapter[20] (p. 20): "The core presupposition of psychogenic theory is that psychological factors *are necessary and sufficient* to account for the clinical presentations of EI patients. Psychogenic theory emphasizes belief, somatization, psychophysiologic stress and anxiety responses, and psychogenic etiology" (italics added). So, if psychological factors are necessary and sufficient, then it follows that the genetic evidence discussed in the preceding section are sufficient to reject psychogenic theory, as is its dependency on dualistic reasoning.

But what about other factors, such as the role of objectively measurable physiological correlates? Are they consistent with predictions of psychogenic theory? Here, the obfuscation of the psychogenic advocates makes it difficult to clearly answer these questions. I would argue that they have provided no mechanisms whereby psychogenesis can generate mitochondrial dysfunction or oxidative stress or nitric oxide increases or any of a large number of other objectively measurable physiological correlates, and it is clearly their responsibility to do so or to concede that their hypothesis is unsupportable. What is clear from Staudenmayer's statement is that therapies that work based on clear physiological mechanisms are inconsistent with the psychogenic theory. Therapies that work based on improving mitochondrial function, based on lowering nitric oxide levels or based on lowering NMDA activity, are inconsistent with their hypothesis, and thus the trial data that are available for each of these should lead to rejection of their views.

I would like to convey to you a personal experience that I had in trying to get some psychogenic advocates to come to terms with the issue of whether the objectively measurable physiological correlates in CFS are consistent with their views. Three psychiatrists, Stanley, Peters, and Salmon (S, P, & S) wrote an editorial in the *British Journal of General Practice*[52] arguing that chronic fatigue syndrome/myalgic encephalomyelitis is a "social epidemic," where what they described as "persistent unexplained physical symptoms" are generated by psychogenic mechanisms. I responded in a letter to the editor[53] pointing out that there were seven distinct objectively measurable physiological correlates of CFS that had each been reported by more than one research group and that they must "either show that each of these studies from multiple research groups are invalid or that they are consistent with their interpretation." The seven that I listed were immune (NK cell) dysfunction, elevated levels of inflammatory cytokines, elevated levels of neopterin, elevated levels of oxidative damage, orthostatic intolerance, elevated levels of the 37 kDa RNase L, energy metabolism/mitochondrial dysfunction, and neuroendocrine dysfunction. Obviously, what I was trying to do was to determine how they interpreted these physiological correlates and what evidence supported their interpretation.

The response that I got[54] was the following:

"It is a naïve form of reductionism to make the assumption that a correlation of physiology with illness behavior necessarily indicates that the former caused the latter." That is certainly true, although nowhere did I make the stated assumption. Both illness behavior and the correlates could have a common cause or the correlates could cause the illness behavior. Having raised this "naïve form of reductionism," S, P, & S completely failed to clarify what sort of connection there might be between the correlates and the illness behavior that might be consistent with their hypothesis. They then raise a second claim stating "Indeed, were Professor Pall's view to be adopted, then many of the distressing phenomena with physiological correlates that doctors do not currently regard as diseases would have to be so designated." I did not express a view, but rather raised a question; so, it is not clear how S, P, & S could construe my view, let alone infer, that it said anything about the disease status of these illnesses. They go on to conclude that "There is, therefore, no need for us to question the validity of the physiological findings: if they are correlates or secondary consequences, this is entirely consistent with the social origins of persistent unexplained physical symptoms." So, here we have S, P, & S making a sweeping conclusion about all seven of these correlates based on no evidence whatsoever. S, P, & S and indeed many psychogenic advocates live in a different universe where sweeping scientific conclusions can be made without any reference to evidence whatsoever. Amazing!

Some scientists, facing the difficulty (I would strongly argue impossibility) of providing evidence in support of a psychogenic view of the multisystem illnesses, have taken the tack of claiming they are biopsychosocial (BPS) illnesses. This raises another question. If they are unwilling or unable to make any clear-cut predictions of a psychogenic model, how can they possibly make any testable predictions of an ill-defined BPS model? Until we have some well-defined, testable predictions of the BPS model that distinguish it from any physiological etiology, it cannot be considered a scientific hypothesis and should not, therefore, be considered further.

WHAT ELSE IS IN THEIR PAPERS?

To provide you with a feeling for what is in their papers, I have reprinted two abstracts and then will discuss a third paper in this area. The first by T.W. Bohr, argues that FM is caused by psychogenesis.[55]

Fibromyalgia Syndrome and Myofascial Pain Syndrome: Do They Exist?

It is in the healing business that the temptations of junk science are the strongest and the controls against it the weakest. Despite their subjective nature, these syndromes (particularly MPS) have little reliability and validity, and advocates paint them as "objective." Despite a legacy of poor-quality science, enthusiasts continue to cite small, methodologically flawed studies purporting to show biologic variables for these syndromes. Despite a wealth of traditional pain research, disciples continue to ignore the placebo effect, demonstrating a therapeutic hubris despite studies showing a dismal natural history for FS. In reviewing the literature on MPS and FS, F.M.R. Walshe's sage words come to mind that the advocates of these syndromes are "better armed with technique than with judgment." A sympathetic observer might claim that labeling patients with monikers of nondiseases such as FS and MPS may not be such a bad thing. After all, there is still a stigma for psychiatric disease in our society, and even telling a sufferer that this plays only a partial role may put that patient on the defensive. Labeling may have iatrogenic consequences, however, particularly in the setting of the work place. Furthermore, review of a typical support group newsletter gives ipso facto proof of this noxious potential. The author of a flyer stuffed inside the newsletter complains that getting social security and disability benefits for "the invisible disability" can be "an uphill battle. But don't loose [*sic*] hope." Apparently the "seriousness of the condition" is not appreciated by the medical community at large, and "clinician bias may well be the largest threat," according to Boston epidemiologist Dr. John Mason. Sufferers are urged to trek to their local medical library and pull four particular articles claiming FS patients have more "stress," "daily hassles," and difficulty working compared with arthritis patients. If articles can't be located, patients are told to ask their lawyers for help. Although "Chronic Fatigue Syndrome" and FS are not considered by everyone to be the same malady, the "National Institute of Health [*sic*] has lumped these two conditions together. This could work in your favor." (A U.S. political advocacy packet is available for $8, but a list of U.S. senators with Washington, DC addresses is freely provided.) These persons see themselves as victims worthy of a star appearance on the Oprah Winfrey show. A sense of bitterness emerges; one literally bed-bound Texas homemaker writes in *Parents* magazine that "Some doctors may give up and tell you that you are a hypochondriac."

Despite the training that scientists receive to avoid emotion laden and obviously biased nomenclature, this abstract is full of such nomenclature. We see "temptations of junk science," "enthusiasts," "methodologically flawed studies," "therapeutic hubris," "dismal natural history," "sage words," "nondiseases," to mention only some. You also see that Bohr goes on to scoff at the poor people who suffer from these illnesses and are trying to make sense out of their state of ill health despite the cognitive dysfunction that commonly accompanies these conditions. You see him citing a statement from F.M.R. Walshe not for some experimental result that may support Bohr's conclusions but because Walshe's opinion provides him with support. This is extraordinarily common in the papers of these psychogenic school advocates; they cite others mainly for their unsupported or poorly supported opinions rather than for some important piece of data that may provide objective evidence. When you couple this to the widespread ignoring of evidence that provides prima facie evidence against their point of view, psychogenic advocates leave the tenets of science far behind.

The second abstract is by Herman Staudenmayer.[56]

Clinical Consequences of the EI/MCS "Diagnosis": Two Paths

There are two distinct paths down which patients "diagnosed" with environmental illness/multiple chemical sensitivities (EI/MCS) can travel. Along the first path, beliefs about low-level, multiple chemical sensitivities as the cause of physical and psychological symptoms are instilled and reinforced by a host of factors including toxicogenic speculation, iatrogenic influence mediated by unsubstantiated diagnostic and treatment practices, patient support/advocacy networks, and social contagion. Intrapsychic factors also reinforce this path through the motivational mechanism of factitious malingering, or unconscious primary and secondary gain, mediated through psychological defenses, particularly projection of cause of illness onto the physical environment. The second path involves restructuring distorted beliefs about chemical sensitivities. Explanations of the placebo effect, the physiology of the stress response, and the symptoms of anxiety and panic facilitate the direction of EI/MCS patients onto this path. A decision model is presented to discriminate among toxicogenic and psychogenic explanations of the EI/MCS phenomenon, based on appraisal of reaction and physiologic and cognitive responses during provocation chamber challenges under double-blind, placebo-controlled conditions. These studies have been helpful therapeutically for some patients in selecting the path that leads to wellness. This paper suggests how various therapeutic techniques can be employed with difficult patients. Often, supportive psychotherapy establishes a therapeutic alliance which facilitates cognitive therapy to restructure distorted beliefs. In the process of finding alternative explanations to chemical sensitivities, the etiology of symptoms is related to stressful life events, including childhood experiences which may have disrupted normal personality development and coping capacity. Furthermore, biological and physiological sequelae stemming from early, chronic trauma have been identified which could explain many of the multisystem complaints. The incidence of childhood abuse reported by EI/MCS patients is strikingly high, and it is recollection of trauma that many EI/MCS patients avoid by displacing the psychologic and physiologic adults sequelae onto the physical environment. The reenactment of these experiences may be necessary in the therapy of some affected individuals. Despite the significant therapeutic effort expanded, some patients who are imprisoned by a closed belief system about the harmful effects of chemical sensitivities are resigned to travel down the path which ultimately leads to despair and depression, social isolation, and even death.

Here you also see several emotion-laden phrases and recognition of psychological but not much better documented physiological stressors in the initiation of MCS. You also see something that was missing in the Bohr abstract. Bohr satisfied himself with criticizing those supporting a physiological explanation for FM, whereas Staudenmayer *states as facts* what are at best suppositions supporting a psychogenic view of MCS (or what he calls EI). He states *as a matter of fact* that "beliefs about low-level, multiple chemical sensitivities as the cause of physical and psychological symptoms are instilled and reinforced by a host of factors including toxicogenic speculation, iatrogenic influence mediated by unsubstantiated diagnostic and treatment practices, patient support/advocacy networks, and social contagion. Intrapsychic factors also reinforce this path through the motivational mechanism of factitious malingering, or unconscious primary and secondary gain, mediated through psychological defenses, particularly projection of cause of illness onto the physical environment. The second path involves restructuring distorted beliefs about chemical sensitivities." These positions are, at best, poorly documented suppositions, supported by little or no empirical evidence. You do not see in either of these abstracts any indication whatsoever that there is empirical support for their views. Given the fact that Bohr, Staudenmayer, and other psychogenic advocates regularly ignore all evidence for physiological mechanisms causing these illnesses, it can be argued that they are posing a myth rather than a scientific hypothesis.

Is there an answer to the question raised by Staudenmayer on p. 15 of his book[20] "Is there any plausible rationale for a biological, toxicogenic, chemical-receptor mechanism that can honestly claim to account for the bizarre, hysterical, and sometimes frank delusional presentations of many severely affected EI patients"? My answer is provided in Chapter 7. It may be argued that the delusions are more characteristic of the psychogenic advocates than of the sufferers of these illnesses.

I would like to consider one other quite recent paper of some psychogenic advocates, this one published on FM by Hazemaijer and Rasker.[57] This paper, in a conclusion section of their abstract, states "For prevention and treatment of fibromyalgia, doctors as well as politicians and media have to start by fundamentally changing the therapeutic domain. In such a renewed setting, fibromyalgia cannot become manifest in an individual and thus fibromyalgia syndrome can no longer exist. A firm public message that symptoms can be psychological in origin to prevent their spread, as Wessely recently stated in the comparable case of mass psychogenic illness, is only part of the answer." Elsewhere they state "Fibromyalgia is 'not an entity that can be described and explained; it is rather a subjective experience comprising pain and fatigue': 'puzzling syndrome'. But at the same time these invisible experiences have a visible (form of) appearance: the fibromyalgia syndrome. *From a positivistic point of view, fibromyalgia cannot even exist because we cannot demonstrate it objectively*" (references removed and italics added). The italicized statement is interesting because it clearly demonstrates fundamental flaws. Firstly because they cannot "demonstrate" FM while others have. For example, others report important and objectively measurable changes that "demonstrate" FM, in such things as brain scan responses to what in normal people are modest stimuli; similarly, others show changes in spinal cord processing of modestly painful stimuli, excessive NMDA activity, increased oxidative stress, mitochondrial/energy metabolism dysfunction, and increased nitric oxide levels. Even if you discount these data, and you cannot do so without critiquing them, something Hazemaijer and Rasker fail to do, there is still a flaw in the argument. Just because something has not been demonstrated, it does not mean that it cannot be demonstrated. And something that has not been demonstrated may still exist from a positivistic or other point of view. Hazemaijer and Rasker would have you believe that the backside of the moon did not exist until we sent a satellite around to look at it.

One cannot find any clearly stated testable predictions that may be used to test their hypothesis in the Hazemaijer and Rasker paper,[57] with one possible exception. They stated, as I quoted earlier, that "In such a renewed setting, fibromyalgia cannot become manifest in an individual." In other words, FM cannot exist where what they call the "therapeutic domain" encouraging it, does not exist. There are, in fact, epidemiological data that I would argue refute that prediction and show, therefore, that Hazemaijer and Rasker's hypothesis should be rejected. The prevalence of FM in both Bangladesh[58] and Mexico[59] are reported to be similar to those in the United States and western Europe, and neither Bangladesh nor Mexico can be argued to have a therapeutic domain that would encourage FM. The Bangladeshi study is quite recent, but the Mexican study predated the Hazemaijer and Rasker paper, and like other evidence that contradicts their hypothesis, they fail to cite it or discuss it. There are other studies that refute their prediction. A Turkish study of FM in women reported similar prevalence to those found in the United States and other Western countries.[60] A careful study by White and Thompsom of the prevalence of FM in the North American Amish community found substantially higher incidence of FM among the Amish[61] than in the United States and Canada generally. It is difficult to find a community in North America more isolated from what Hazemaijer and Rasker call the therapeutic domain than the Amish. All of the available evidence appears to show that the prediction of Hazemaijer and Rasker is not fulfilled.

Other things that Hazemaijer and Rasker[57] ignore include the substantial literature on the role of short term stressors including physical trauma and infection in the initiation of cases of FM, they ignore the evidence for a genetic role in FM, they ignore the many reports of objectively measurable physiological correlates of FM, and they ignore its comorbidity with well-accepted diseases such as migraine, lupus, and rheumatoid arthritis.

The papers of psychogenic advocates correctly note that a substantial fraction of people diagnosed with these illnesses have some psychiatric symptoms. What they fail to point out is that most, perhaps all, serious chronic illnesses show similar patterns. The fact that substantial numbers of people with cancer, MS, or rheumatoid arthritis have psychiatric symptoms does not mean that any of these are psychogenic. This criticism is important and should at least be responded to rather than simply ignored.

One of the great puzzles about the psychogenic literature regarding these multisystem illnesses is how do so many bad papers get published? How do so many papers dominated by emotion-laden phrases, by transparent falsehoods, by logical flaws, by overstated claims, and by unsupported or poorly supported opinion get published in what appear to be respectable, peer-reviewed journals? These papers consistently ignore massive amounts of contrary data and opinion and cannot, therefore, lay claim to objective assessment of the literature. Most of us find the peer-review system is generally pretty effective in keeping us scientists honest, but that function is nowhere evident with the psychogenic literature. This is by far the largest failure of the peer-review system that I am aware of, a system that in my experience usually works pretty well despite the defects associated with almost any human endeavor. I am almost tempted to call this failure inexplicable.

I cannot help speculate on the origin of this failure of peer review and, indeed, the abject failure of the psychogenic advocates to uphold even the minimum of scientific standards. I cannot help wondering whether it is based on the fact that most victims of these illnesses are women. There is a long history of sex discrimination in medicine, and while I would like to think we are more enlightened in the twenty-first century, this pattern suggests that perhaps we are not.

The Latest Staudemayer et al. Papers on MCS

Staudemayer and three coauthors published two back-to-back papers on MCS in a new journal of very limited circulation,[23,24] representing their latest views on MCS mechanisms. Because these were recently published, it was of interest to see if there were any new developments in their psychogenic views and how they dealt with all of the new evidence and theory regarding the physiological mechanisms involved in MCS. Both papers were based on a much earlier paper by Hill[62] on the possible roles of physical, chemical, and other hazards in the environment and possible consequent illness. Hill suggests nine distinct criteria that should be looked at in assessing a possible causal role of environmental factors in initiating illness but suggests that these should not be used in a dogmatic fashion. For example, Hill states in his discussion of his first criterion[62] (p. 296), strength of association, that "in thus putting emphasis upon the strength of an association we must, nevertheless, look at the obverse of the coin. We must not be too ready to dismiss a cause-and-effect hypothesis merely on the grounds that the observed association appears to be slight. There are many occasions in medicine when this is in truth so." Later in his paper (p. 299), Hill states that "None of my nine viewpoints can bring indisputable evidence for or against the cause-and-effect hypothesis and none can be required as a *sine qua non*. What they can do, with greater or lesser strength, is to help us make up our minds on the fundamental question—is there any other way of explaining the set of facts before us, is there any other answer equally, or more, likely than cause and effect?"

The literature implicates a large range of chemicals in the initiation of MCS, as well in triggering symptoms of MCS, making both quantitative and specificity relationships much more difficult to document, but with that caveat, Hill's criteria are very useful criteria for the analysis of MCS. Staudenmayer et al.[23,24] have used the term idiopathic environmental intolerance (IEI) instead of MCS, an unfortunate term because it prejudges the issue of whether this illness is truly idiopathic, that is without known cause or causes. I will spend all of my discussion on the first of the two papers,[23] the one considering the support for what the authors call "toxicogenic theory," going through each of the nine Hill criteria[62] one at a time.

The first Hill criterion, strength of association, raises the question of how strong the association is between initiation of cases of MCS and chemical exposure. Have people who have been exposed to higher amounts of the chemicals implicated in MCS developed more cases of the illness? There are three obvious examples providing support for this strength of association. One is the reported increase in sick building syndrome situations following the decrease in air flow in buildings as an energy conservation measure. The second is the parallel between the production of synthetic organic chemicals and the increased scientific literature on MCS. The third is genetic evidence on susceptibility. I will discuss each of these in sequence.

During the 1970s, there were changes in air flow standards that preceded a very substantial increase in sick building syndrome situations. Ashford and Miller[63] described the drop in air flow standards in the Unites States, which came into effect in 1973, such that air flow required in both older buildings and in newly constructed "tight" buildings could be substantially decreased. Ashford and Miller[63] state (p. 16) that "Remarkably, these sources present in indoor air are the same ones individuals with multiple chemical sensitivities identify as provoking their vague and seemingly inexplicable symptoms. With their homes and workplaces already filled with synthetic materials that off-gas, gas furnaces, cigarette smoke, and other sources of pollutants, Americans sealed their buildings for energy efficiency. Not surprisingly, indoor air pollution levels rose dramatically, and so did health complaints." By the mid to late 1980s, the U.S. Environmental Protection Agency was reporting that sick building syndrome situations constituted about 50 percent of the environmental complaints called to their attention. So, one sees an apparent association between indoor air pollution and MCS cases associated with sick building syndrome. There is a broader association between synthetic organic chemical production in the United States, which increased approximately 15-fold between 1945 and 1980 (p. 18 of Reference 63) and the increased awareness of MCS. Because we do not have good epidemiological data on the prevalence of MCS during the early phases of this epidemic, we are forced to rely on indirect estimates of the interest in this illness. A good example of such indirect estimates is the data shown in Table 13.1, which is based on the MCS database developed by Albert Donnay.[64] It can be seen that the increase in MCS papers in this database parallels the dramatic rise in organic chemical synthesis and in appar-

TABLE 13.1. Numbers of papers published on MCS in different time periods.

Years involved	Number of MCS papers	MCS papers per year
1945-1965	15	0.71
1976-1985	50	5.0
1986-1995	303	30.3
1996-1999	227	56.75

Total scientific papers up to 1999: 595.

ent exposure to indoor chemicals. This database[64] also documents that most of the papers that express views on a physiological basis of MCS versus a psychogenic basis favor a physiological interpretation.

The third obvious argument for strength of association is based on the evidence that people who are less able to metabolize initiating chemicals are at greater risk of developing MCS and related illnesses. The first critical study that I have already discussed is that of Haley and coworkers, showing that Gulf War syndrome was more common in individuals carrying a *PON1* gene polymorphism producing lessened ability to metabolize organophosphorus neurotoxins including pesticides and sarin gas.[47] This provided clear-cut evidence for an association. The more recent and very important Toronto study by McKeown-Eyssen et al.[49] was published after these two Staudenmayer et al. papers, and so we cannot expect them to cite that paper, but we can expect them to cite and discuss the Haley study and others relating to the two earlier factors supporting strength of association. So, what do Staudemayer et al. have to say about any of this evidence supporting strength of association between chemical exposure and MCS? Nothing. They do not cite the relevant studies in this context nor do they discuss any of these three types of evidence supporting a strength of association. Later, in what they describe as their "evidence-based review," they conclude[23] (p. 244) that "toxicogenic theory fails to meet any of the Hill criteria." From the consideration of this first criterion, it appears that the failure is not of toxicogenic theory but rather of Staudenmayer et al.[23] to objectively assess the available evidence. The point here is not that this evidence is immune from criticism. In a system as complex as MCS, it is rare that any evidence is immune from criticism. In the case of MCS, because there is not sufficient epidemiological evidence on the prevalence of this illness in earlier years, we are forced to use the amount of MCS scientific literature as a surrogate suggesting increased prevalence over time. An "evidence-based review," as claimed by Staudenmayer et al. (p. 244), should be based on an objective assessment of the available evidence.

The second Hill criterion is consistency. Hill[62] (p. 296) asks "Has it been repeatedly observed by different persons, in different places, circumstances and times?" Similar observations have been made about MCS in papers written in the United States, in Canada, in at least nine European countries, in Japan, and in Australia, with some of these descriptions going back 40 years or more, providing substantial support for consistency. Miller[65] (p. 445) commented on the similarity of reports from different countries, stating "numerous investigators from different geographic regions have published strikingly similar descriptions of individuals who report disabling illnesses after exposure to recognized environmental contaminants." Staudenmayer et al.[23] (p. 238) completely ignore all of this literature, concluding that "Research presented in support of toxicogenic theory has thus failed two fundamental components of consistency. . . ."

The third Hill criterion is specificity. Clearly, the chemicals implicated in the initiation of cases of MCS are of several types, as I have discussed in Chapter 7, and are relatively diverse, including organic solvents and three classes of pesticides. So, we have some specificity here, but not a high level of specificity. I have argued that these are all specific, in that they can all lead to increased NMDA activity. Hill states that[62] (p. 297) "We must not, however, over-emphasize the importance of the (specificity) characteristic." Hill talks about milk- or waterborne infections as being very diverse, therefore lacking high level specificity. He concludes (p. 297) "In short, if specificity exists, we may be able to draw conclusions without hesitation; if it is not apparent, we are not thereby necessarily left sitting irresolutely on the fence." You may be able to guess the position of Staudenmayer et al. on specificity. They fail to cite any of the relevant literature while providing a long (one full page) discussion that is largely irrelevant to the issue of causal specificity, the issue raised by Hill.

Temporality is Hill's fourth criterion. Hill asks the question with respect to possible dietary role in illness (p. 297) "Does a particular diet lead to disease or do the early stages of disease lead to those peculiar dietary habits?" So, the key issue in the temporality criterion is as follows: Does exposure to the particular stressor being considered precede or follow the initiation of illness? In the case of MCS, the issue is whether exposure to any putative chemical initiator of MCS preceded the onset of illness. Ashford and Miller in both their 1991 first edition and in the 1998 second edition[63] reviewed evidence that supported their conclusion that chemical sensitivity is first initiated by a single high-level chemical exposure or multiple lower-level exposures followed by the chronic phase of illness during which chemicals trigger the production of symptoms. Cullen's early studies reported many examples of previous chemical exposure leading to development of MCS, even requiring evidence of such previous chemical exposure for diagnosis of that illness.[66] There are many other publications reporting MCS initiation following previous pesticide exposure or specific organic solvent exposures or sick building situations involving either remodeling associated with outgassing of organic solvents or with mold infestations.[67-89] Miller[90] reviewed 23 distinct studies or groups of people reporting new-onset chemical intolerance following well-defined chemical exposure events, described in References 59 and 64, including 12 additional papers not cited here. I find that two of the publications are particularly compelling. One of these is the Miller and Mitzel paper,[68] reporting on two series of MCS patients, those cases preceded by organophosphorus pesticide exposures and those preceded by sick building syndrome, the latter involving building remodeling and consequent increased exposure to outgassed organic solvents. Another interesting publication is the volume edited by Alison Johnson,[86] where a series of MCS sufferers described their own experiences. Of the 57 MCS cases described in their own words, 52 of these had their chemical sensitivity initiated by an identified, specific previous chemical exposures. The chemical exposures for these 52 were quite similar to those described in the previous MCS literature, often involving pesticide exposure or sick building syndrome situations including those involving new carpeting, new paint, and other building renovations. Other exposures included the various chemicals to which Gulf War syndrome veterans were exposed, a variety of solvents including formaldehyde, trichloroethylene, cleaning solvents, or other organic solvents, gas leaks, diesel fuel and burning fuel fumes, or other unidentified odiferous chemicals. Fully 52 out of 57 (91 percent) of the MCS sufferers dated their initial sensitivity to a specific chemical exposure. Part of the reason I find the Johnson volume so compelling is that these cases are described in the words of the victims, so they are not filtered through the possibly biased views of any scientist, and yet the reader can easily see the patterns of initiation and the similarities those patterns have to previously published studies. Recent studies in Spain[85] and in Japan[87,89] report similar patterns of chemicals involved in the initiation of MCS cases, as have been reported in many earlier studies.

The reported role of chemicals in both the initiation of cases of MCS and in producing sensitivity symptoms was well known to Gots[15] (p. S11) who argued "There is no known mechanism whereby low levels of chemicals can interact adversely with numerous organ systems. Even theories of advanced clinicians arguing for an intense organic etiology fail to do this [sic]." Of course, you have seen in Chapter 7 and elsewhere how such diverse chemicals may produce this pattern of symptoms. Since Gots was aware of the literature on chemical exposure preceding apparent onset of MCS, however much he wants to dismiss its significance, how can Staudenmayer et al. seven years later after many additional papers have been published on it, after several reviews have discussed it in substantial detail, be apparently completely unaware of its existence in their "evidence-based review"?

Needless to say, Staudenmayer et al.[23] fail to discuss or cite any of the relevant literature, focusing instead on a series of irrelevant psychological issues, having nothing to do with the question of whether chemical exposure precedes chemical sensitivity in MCS. I have cited 24 distinct studies providing evidence for temporality in MCS, and Miller[90] cites 12 additional studies many of which were cited and discussed in earlier studies. Of these, 30 predated the Staudenmayer et al., submission and consequently could have been cited and discussed by them. None were. They fail to even discuss the important Miller and Mitzel paper,[68] which was itself cited by others 62 times before the submission of the Staudenmayer et al. paper, according to the Web of Science database. Their failure to cite and discuss this paper was despite the fact that its title alone clearly implies its relevance to this Hill criterion. It appears that Staudenmayer et al.[23] have invented a new type of scientific paper—an "evidence-based review" (p. 244) devoid of evidence.

The next criterion of Hill is that of biological gradient; is there a measurable dose–response relationship between the putative causal agent and the illness response? This is a criterion that is often difficult to fulfill even in otherwise convincing cases of environmental causality, because, as Hill states (p. 298) "Often the difficulty is to secure some satisfactory quantitative measure of the environment which will permit us to explore this dose-response." This difficulty is made more challenging in the case of MCS because of the diversity of chemicals implicated in initiating it and because of the possible synergism among those chemicals. Here again, I would argue that the best evidence for some sort of dose–response curve relationship is the genetic evidence, where decreased metabolism of organophosphorus compounds presumably involved leads to increased incidence of MCS. The complex genetics found by the Toronto group[49] provides an explanation for the diverse responses in different individuals to chemical exposure.

The sixth Hill criterion is that of plausibility; is there a biologically plausible mechanism for MCS and specifically for the initiation of MCS cases by previous chemical exposure? You have already seen such a detailed, biologically plausible mechanism discussed in Chapter 7 a mechanism that explains each of the most puzzling features of MCS. This includes the role of four distinct classes of chemicals in MCS, its chronic nature, and the exquisite chemical sensitivity found in MCS. I would argue that my 2002 *FASEB Journal* paper on MCS,[51] which predated the submission of the Staudenmayer et al. review,[23] provides the most convincing evidence supporting a specific and detailed plausible mechanism for MCS. This paper was published in a journal with the highest citation impact factor of any journal that has published an MCS paper. My paper,[51] consequently, is difficult to ignore, based on the prestige of the publishing journal. Needless to say, Staudenmayer et al. have done exactly that.

The seventh Hill criterion[62] (p. 298) is that of coherence, that the interpretation should not "conflict with the generally known facts of the natural history and biology of the disease." Hill gives an example fulfilling this criterion, of the increase of cigarette smoking paralleling the subsequent rise in lung cancer. The increase in awareness of MCS and of scientific scrutiny of this illness closely parallel the rise in synthetic organic chemical production, the specific rise in the use of the three classes of pesticides implicated in MCS, and the decrease in indoor air flow, as I have already noted. Thus, there appears to be a substantial similarity between the evidence available in MCS and the evidence Hill suggests provides excellent support for fulfillment of his seventh criterion, although in MCS the lack of earlier epidemiologic studies forces us to use the increase in publication activity on MCS as a surrogate for increased prevalence of the illness. None of this is discussed by Staudenmayer et al. They do discuss the genetic evidence for a role of the CCK-B receptor,[50] but only in the context that this receptor has a role in panic disorder, not in the context of its role in stimulating NMDA activity and the apparent role of such NMDA activity in the physiology of MCS. So again, we have apparent bias dominating this "evidence-based review."

The eighth criterion is that of experimental intervention. The best published evidence for such intervention is with animal models, where I have cited such model studies as implicating excessive NMDA activity, nitric oxide, and, in one case, excessive cholinergic activity. Much of this was discussed in both Chapter 1 and Chapter 7, as well as in Reference 51. An example of experimental intervention in humans was reported in the extensive study of chemical sensitivity responses among employees of the prestigious Brigham and Women's Hospital[88] when that hospital was suffering from substantial levels of internal pollutants due in part to insufficient air flow. The authors of that study reported a substantial decrease in subsequent sensitivity induction following major improvements to the ventilation systems. In this highly studied situation, an experimental intervention apparently led to a decrease in initiation of new chemical sensitivity cases.

The ninth Hill criterion is that of analogy; are there analogies to other diseases or disorders? Staudenmayer et al.[23] (p. 243) state that "Proponents of toxicogenic theory contend that IEI is not analogous to any known toxic syndrome. Therefore, it is uncontested that the criterion of analogy does not apply to toxicogenic theory." Both of these sentences are clearly untrue. Meggs and others have discussed the analogy between MCS and RADS, and RUDS and skin hypersensitivity, as was discussed in Chapter 7.

Indeed, as was also discussed in that chapter as well as by Meggs, there is a compelling analogy between MCS and asthma. Another analogy is that of migraine, where migraine susceptibility is reported to be initiated by the same chemical exposures involved in initiation of MCS and where chemicals are reported to trigger migraine attacks.[65,76,91] I discussed the comorbidity of migraines with this whole group of illnesses in Chapter 2. The role of neurogenic inflammation, excessive nitric oxide and central sensitization in migraines[91-93] suggests that this analogy may involve profound similarities of etiology. The other analogy that has been raised in the "toxicogenic" literature is that of hyperalgesia and allodynia, where a painful trauma leads to chronic sensitivity to very mild touch, stimuli that were previously either only mildly painful or not painful at all. Perhaps none of the four authors of the Staudenmayer et al. paper ever stubbed his or her toe and found that it led to excruciating pain responses to previously mild stimuli. As I have noted elsewhere in this book, it appears that the mechanisms of hyperalgesia (and presumably allodynia) appear to be strikingly similar to those involved in MCS.

Again, it is not my view that the types of evidence providing support for these nine criteria are immune from criticism. As Hill observed, it is exactly because such criticisms are commonly found in evidence relating to possible environmental illness that it makes sense to consider nine criteria rather than just one or a few. I would argue that of the nine, the strongest evidence supporting what Staudenmayer et al. refer to as "toxigenic mechanisms" are found in five: strength of association (#1), consistency (#2), temporality (#4), plausibility (#6), and analogy (#9). I also consider the animal data for #8, experimental, to be very substantial, but because Hill himself does not discuss animal model data, it is not clear whether or not he would agree with this assessment.

Ashford and Miller, on pp 273-275 of their book,[62] discussed all nine of Hill's criteria, finding evidence for the fulfilling of at least six of them for MCS. Staudenmayer et al.[23] do not acknowledge this or try to refute any of Ashford and Miller's earlier arguments. The complete inability Staudenmayer et al. to find any evidence for "toxicogenic mechanisms" that fulfill any of Hill's nine criteria speaks to the unusual bias in their "evidence-based review." I have, in the past, tried to avoid reading the papers of these psychogenic advocates because I find such reading to be intellectually degrading and emotionally draining. This was certainly my response to this Staudenmayer et al. paper. When I see the shoddiness of the work, I react with anger and with sorrow. Anger and sorrow for the victims of these illnesses, who deserve so much better, and for the scientific community whose disciplines and whose standards are degraded by this work.

A COMPARISON OF THE NO/ONOO⁻ CYCLE WITH PSYCHOGENESIS AND MALINGERING IN MULTISYSTEM ILLNESSES

I have been trying, as you may have noticed, to avoid repeatedly comparing the NO/ONOO⁻ cycle mechanism of these multisystem illnesses with the either "psychogenic theory" or malingering. Now, however, in Table 13.2, I have made such a series of comparisons. Not surprisingly, both psychogenic theory and malingering come off very poorly in such a head-to-head comparison. This is a direct consequence of both the available evidence and theory.

How Do Psychiatrists and Psychologists View Psychogenesis of Multisystem Illnesses?

Psychiatrists and psychologists have been advocates of psychogenesis of multisystem illnesses and are also critics of these views.[3,8,10] The book by Taylor, Friedberg, and Jason,[94] two psychologists and one psychiatrist, makes it clear that they view CFS, FM, and MCS as true physiological illnesses. The American Psychiatric Association in DSM-IV[29] does not claim any of these three illnesses as being psychiatric, although PTSD is classified as psychiatric. DSM-IV does claim somatoform disorders and somatization disorders, although, as I discussed earlier, those positions have come under very substantial attack by many psychiatrists.

Psychiatry and psychology has moved consistently over the past 30 years toward becoming more scientific in their approach, developing testable theories and testing them empirically, focusing on therapies that can be empirically tested, and becoming more integrated with other medical and scientific disciplines including the neurosciences. They have done so despite the staggering complexities that are at the center of their disciplines and the consequent difficulties in doing so. While some have argued that they have not moved quickly enough or vigorously enough, there is no question of the direction in which these disciplines are headed.

My own critique of psychogenesis of multisystem illnesses should not be construed in any way as a critique of psychiatry and psychology. I am greatly impressed by the wisdom needed to deal effectively with these incredibly complex areas that are so important to our understanding of the human condition. It is, rather a critique of those who either lack the needed wisdom or have sold their integrity, leading them to make many unsupported and poorly supported claims.

TABLE 13.2. Comparison of "psychogenic theory," malingering, and the NO/ONOO⁻ cycle.

	₁NO/ONOO⁻ cycle	Psychogenic theory, including somatoform and belief systems	₂Malingering
Provides explanations for roles of short term stressors	Yes, explained in terms of nitric oxide/peroxynitrite increases.	No, only psychological stressors recognized.	No.
Explanation of symptoms and signs	Yes, detailed explanations of both common and unique symptoms and signs.	No, proclaimed as "unexplained."	No, proclaimed as "unexplained."
Dependent on mental/physical dualism	No, explicitly rejects such dualism.	Yes.	??
Explanation for chronic nature	Yes, explained in terms of the NO/ONOO⁻ cycle.	No. Parallel with mass hysteria is weak and mass hysteria victims usually recover quickly.	No. Because many of these people obvious suffer greatly from their illnesses, this is difficult to explain by secondary rewards.
Makes verified and verifiable predictions	Yes, with extensive verification to date; others need to be tested.	No. To the extent that predictions can be inferred, they are not verified	No. Predictions of lack of physiological change are not verified.
Supported by genetic studies	Yes, especially in the case of CFS and MCS.	No. Genetic literature ignored; genetics demonstrates biological causation	No. Genetic literature ignored; genetics demonstrates biological causation.
Supported by other physiological observations	Yes, extensively.	No, physiological literature largely ignored. Based mainly on unsupported opinion.	No, physiological literature largely ignored. Based mainly on unsupported opinion.
Supported by animal model data	Yes.	No, animal model data is ignored.	No, animal model data is ignored.
Provides explanation for overlaps among multi-system illnesses	Yes, based on common mechanism.	Yes, based on common "mechanism."	No.
Provides explanations for comorbidity with well-accepted diseases	Yes, such diseases as lupus, asthma, rheumatoid arthritis, and migraine share a common biochemistry and physiology.	No. The studies of such comorbidity are universally ignored.	No. The studies of such comorbidity are universally ignored.

I have been contacted by quite a number of psychiatrists and psychologists who have expressed interest in my work and I would warmly welcome more contacts with these important disciplines.

The Damage Created

It is difficult to encompass the damage created by the psychogenic advocates. They have made it difficult to obtain research funding on the physiological basis of these multisystem illnesses. This difficulty has been particularly profound for MCS, where, not coincidentally, the fear of massive liability has created major vested interests among industries that have a legitimate fear of law suits that may parallel the liability of the cigarette companies. What is not legitimate is to use their economic and political influence to stifle the scientific and health needs. And what is not legitimate is to continue the fiction that MCS is unrelated to chemical exposure, such that millions of additional people inevitably become chemically sensitive due to what should be avoidable chemical exposures. Responsibility for these millions of additional new cases of MCS should be placed squarely on the door of the psychogenic advocates and their financial supporters.

The strange position of many psychogenic advocates in arguing that these illnesses are unexplained while simultaneously arguing against conducting research into their causes has been commented on by Martin Walker in his book *Skewed*.[9] Walker states that (p. 64) "Arguments that the cause of CFS, MCS, ME or GWS is psychological serve a significant purpose: in addition to simply labeling sufferers as being mentally unwell and creating a market for pharmaceuticals, they also dull the determination to inquire into other causes. This is one way in which we can identify individuals and groups involved in defending the status quo; like no other physicians or medical scientists in history, these people all argue that it is counter-productive to look for any biological cause of these illnesses and that detailed clinical investigations are not appropriate."

Those who fear illegitimate claims of liability, whether they are insurance companies concerned about disability claims or claims for health benefits or companies using or producing synthetic chemicals, such companies have an obvious route to minimize such claims. They should be using their influence with the media, with political organizations, and with scientists to push for research leading to the development of specific biomarkers of these illnesses such that any illegitimate claims can be falsified. Their failure to do this is sufficient evidence to infer that these powerful and very canny organizations have a different goal entirely: it is to deny legitimate claims and therefore deny any culpability on their part. To the extent that psychogenic advocates act to encourage such behavior, they have a lot to answer for; to the extent that they make it difficult to develop truly effective therapies for these illnesses, they have still more. And, of course, they provide cover for the neglect of the medical care community. In the case of MCS, they also allow the continued unsafe use of synthetic chemicals, such that many additional and completely preventable cases of MCS will occur.

Let me state that I do not think that all psychogenic advocates have simply sold their integrity to vested interests, although I do believe that many of them have done so. What they need to do in order to reestablish confidence in their integrity is to start following the tenets of science. As I have stated, I believe that this will inevitably lead them to abandon their psychogenic views.

The lack of funding for research on these illnesses can be assessed by doing two types of comparisons. The first is the tiny amount of funding available through publicly funded foundations when compared with other illnesses of similar prevalence or similar overall health impact. Funding for research on multisystem illnesses is tiny compared with that available for diabetes, let alone others of lower prevalence such as MS or Parkinson's disease. I am not arguing that these other diseases are overfunded but rather that the neglect of funding for multisystem illnesses can only be rationalized as being due to the obfuscation that the psychogenic advocates have generated. When you look at funding through the NIH for research on these illnesses, it has been similarly disgraceful. NIEHS has never put out an RFA (request for applications, for which a pot of money has been set aside) aimed at MCS research. It has never put out an RFA aimed at developing specific biomarkers for these illnesses despite the obvious need for such biomarkers. What we see is neglect generating more neglect, with much of the original neglect being due to the smoke screen put out by psychogenic advocates.

While the most severe long-term damage created by psychogenic advocates has been to the research prospects for these illnesses, the most severe shorter-term impact has clearly been to the sufferers of these illnesses and their families. Family ties have been torn asunder by claims that sufferers are simply malingering or that they simply have a mistaken "belief system." Where families have supported their family member, believing that they are truly ill based in part of their intimate knowledge of the individual, they have often been accused of encouraging illness behavior. Based on such claims, children sufferers have been legally removed from the home in the United Kingdom. Mothers have been blamed in the past for the illness behavior of their asthmatic or autistic children, and we see the same sort of accusations occurring today with multisystem illnesses. Have we really progressed so little from the ignorance of the dark ages? Let me state for the record that there is no excuse for making overreaching psychogenic claims, producing such damage, in the absence of near certainty that the advocates are right. They cannot claim near certainty when they regularly ignore massive amounts of contrary data and opinion.

We have already seen the barriers created between patients and their health care providers by these attitudes. How many health care providers dismiss and abuse their patients because they do not believe that these are real illnesses? And how often is this patient abuse simply provided some intellectual cover by the psychogenic advocates?

The Future of Psychogenesis for Multisystem Illnesses

I believe there is none. Psychogenesis of these illnesses is based on the shaky foundation of somatoform disorders and somatization. It is based on the nonexistent dualism between the mental/psychological/psychatric and the physical/biological/physiological. It is based on emotion-laden phrases, transparent falsehoods, logical flaws, overstated claims, and unsupported or poorly supported opinion. It is based on the failure to pose clear, testable predictions of "psychogenic theory." It is based on ignoring the existence of a genetic role in these illnesses. It is based on ignoring the long history of false psychogenic attributions of other illnesses. It is based on ignoring hundreds of studies documenting real physiological changes in multisystem illnesses. It is based on ignoring the roles of a series of short-term physiological stressors in the initiation of these illnesses. It is based on ignoring the existence of clinical studies showing that therapies producing improved biochemical function can produce measurable improvements in people suffering from these illnesses. In short, it is based on deliberate ignorance, flaws, and quicksand. Psychogenesis is like a large old building that has been set up for demolition by several dozen explosive charges designed to bring about its rapid collapse. For a split second after the charges explode, the building still appears to be there, apparently unaware that it no longer exists. I do not know how long it will take for the scientific community to realize the demise of the psychogenic view of multisystem illnesses, but it will happen.

Chapter 14

A Major New Paradigm of Human Disease?

E pluribus unum—out of many, one.

TAKE-HOME LESSONS

There are nine well-accepted paradigms of human disease. This book argues that the NO/ONOO⁻ cycle is the tenth. Based on the impact of chronic fatigue syndrome (CFS), multiple chemical sensitivity (MCS), fibromyalgia (FM), and post-traumatic stress syndrome (PTSD) on human health, as documented in Chapter 11, the NO/ONOO⁻ cycle paradigm ranks with the other three most important such paradigms in importance. It is only rivaled or eclipsed by infectious disease, ischemic cardiovascular disease, and cancer.

Whenever one proposes a new scientific paradigm, initial questions focus on how effective is it as an explanatory model and how well do the available data support it. It often shifts, then, to what other examples may fit under that paradigm. I suggest here that 14 different diseases/illnesses may be examples that fit under the NO/ONOO⁻ cycle paradigm. The criteria for possible inclusion come directly from the five principles underlying the NO/ONOO⁻ cycle, as an explanatory model. Among the 14 are several of the most important human diseases with still uncertain etiology. One needs to be skeptical about these arguments. However, the fit of a number of these 14 is surprisingly good and one can argue that each of the 14 may well fit the NO/ONOO⁻ cycle paradigm better than it fits any alternative explanation.

Explaining "Unexplained Illnesses"
© 2007 by The Haworth Press, Inc. All rights reserved.
doi:10.1300/5139_14

The NO/ONOO⁻ cycle paradigm is a major challenge to our previous understanding of medicine.

INTRODUCTION

The whole thrust of this book is that the NO/ONOO⁻ cycle mechanism is a major new paradigm of human disease that explains the properties of CFS, MCS, FM, and PTSD. If, as I have argued, this view is correct, where does this paradigm fit into the history of modern medicine? In Exhibit 14.1, I have listed the nine well-established paradigms, with the tenth listed as the NO/ONOO⁻ cycle paradigm. On occasion, in moments of perhaps misplaced confidence, I have been known to call it the tenth paradigm.

These nine or ten paradigms have been established over the past 135 years or so of medical history, and so the establishment of a new paradigm is a relatively infrequent event and a major milestone in medical science. It should be noted that some individual diseases fit under more than one paradigm. There are, for example, hormone dysfunction diseases that are a consequence of autoimmune disease or of cancer. Genetic predisposition to disease is extraordinarily common among many disease classes. The prion diseases are infectious, even though they are caused by very unusual infectious agents. If and when the nitric oxide/peroxynitrite vicious cycle paradigm is viewed as established, there may be examples that fall under this paradigm but also fall under other paradigms, as well.

EXHIBIT 14.1. Major Disease Paradigms

1. Infectious diseases
2. Genetic diseases
3. Nutritional deficiency diseases
4. Hormone dysfunction diseases
5. Allergies
6. Autoimmune diseases
7. Somatic mutation/selection (cancer)
8. Ischemic cardiovascular diseases
9. Amyloid (including prion) diseases
10. NO/ONOO⁻ cycle diseases

Dr. Claudia Miller[1] (pp. 286-290), reflecting the work of Kuhn,[2] lists four criteria for the development of a new paradigm:

1. Anomaly
2. Causality
3. Generalizability
4. Novelty

Are the observations on these four multisystem illnesses an anomaly not explained by the previously established paradigms? It can be argued that the repeated mantra that these illnesses are unexplained should be sufficient evidence that researchers in the field find that the previously established paradigms of medical science are inadequate to explain these illnesses. Certainly, attempts to determine whether CFS may be caused by a chronic infection or by an autoimmune disease have not been able to confirm any such etiology. Similarly, it is clear that MCS does not have a classic allergic etiology. So, of all groups of illnesses, one can argue that these multisystem illnesses are collectively the best candidate for a new paradigm of human disease because they are in most need of explanation. Let me remind you that, at the beginning of Chapter 1, I cited a substantial number of researchers who suggested earlier that the multiple similarities of these illnesses with each other as well as their comorbidity suggested that they probably shared a common etiologic mechanism and that we should search, therefore, for one mechanism for all four. It may be inferred from these considerations that these four multisystem illnesses, as a group, represent a substantial anomaly and that we need an etiologic mechanism for the entire group. Causality is most extensively documented by the studies of animal models implicating nitric oxide, NMDA activity, oxidative stress, and other elements of this theory as important causal elements. In Chapter 15, I will also discuss evidence from therapeutic studies in humans that provide some causal support, an area already discussed in Chapters 5 through 7. Certainly, the interpretations of the symptoms and signs of these illnesses provided in Chapter 3 and Chapters 5 to 10 provide more evidence for possible causality, as does the evidence for effectiveness of two agents lowering nitric oxide, as discussed in Chapter 6. Causality is also supported by the many initiating short-term stressors, which are known to be able to increase nitric oxide levels. Indeed, increasing nitric oxide is the only common response to this diverse group of stressors, to my knowledge. If short-term stressors do not act to initiate chronic illness via nitric oxide and its oxidant product peroxynitrite, how do they act?

The generalizability and novelty issues dominate much of this book and do not require much further discussion. Clearly, the theory is novel and it can be generalized to all four multisystem illnesses and to the Gulf War. I will also discuss other possible applications of the theory to other illnesses later in this chapter, suggesting further generalizability.

The question that will take up the majority of this chapter is whether there are other types of illnesses, in addition to the four multisystem illnesses that have dominated most of the discourse in this book, that may also fall under the fall under the tenth paradigm.

In making the claim that these four multisystem illnesses fall into a new paradigm of human disease, it is important to discuss the definition of disease and what is required to properly call a medical condition a disease.

DEFINITION OF DISEASE

In my papers on these multisystem illnesses and in the previous chapters in this book, I have tried to avoid calling them diseases but rather have called them illnesses, medical conditions, syndromes, or even disease states, but not diseases. Why is that? Clearly, one needs to ask what is a disease and how might it differ from these other terms.

Somewhat surprisingly, the definition of disease varies considerably depending on what general or medical dictionary one consults.

The medical dictionary that sits on my bookshelf[3] defines disease as: "A definite morbid process having a characteristic train of symptoms; it may affect the whole body or any of its parts, and its etiology, pathology and prognosis may be known or unknown." A second medical dictionary[4] defines disease as: "A morbid entity characterized usually by at least two of these criteria: recognized etiologic agent(s), identifiable group of signs and symptoms." These two definitions differ from each other in whether an etiologic mechanism as opposed to just a morbid process is needed to fulfill the definition. My own view is that the first of these definitions agrees more with the actual use of the term disease in medicine. Such diseases as multiple sclerosis, with its morbid process of demyelination in the brain, and Alzheimer's disease, with its morbid process involving amyloid plaque formation and neurofibrillary tangles, both lack a widely accepted overall etiology but they are both considered diseases. Still, whichever of these two definitions of disease one accepts, the case I make in this book argues that these four multisystem illnesses are diseases, albeit ones with highly variable symptoms. The morbid process and, indeed, the proposed etiology are both centered on the elements of our vicious cycle, each of which may be considered an etiologic agent.

So if we can accept as either an attractive, well-supported theory or as a working hypothesis, the view that these are diseases caused by our NO/ONOO⁻ cycle mechanism, are there other diseases that may also fit under this paradigm?

ARE THERE OTHER EXAMPLES OF NO/ONOO⁻ CYCLE DISEASES?

If there are other examples of diseases falling into our putative paradigm, how might they differ from the four multisystem illnesses? And how might we recognize possible candidates for inclusion under this paradigm? These are the two key questions that will dominate the rest of this chapter.

The answers to both of these questions will come, to a substantial extent from the five principles described for this paradigm in Chapter 1, upon which the paradigm is based:

1. Short-term stressors involved in initiating cases of multisystem illnesses act by raising levels of nitric oxide and its oxidant product peroxynitrite or possibly other cycle elements.
2. Initiation is converted into a chronic illness through the action of vicious cycle mechanisms, producing chronic elevation of nitric oxide and peroxynitrite and other cycle elements.
3. Symptoms and signs of these illnesses are generated by elevated levels of nitric oxide and/or other important consequences of the proposed mechanism, that is elevated levels of peroxynitrite or inflammatory cytokines, increased oxidative stress, superoxide, intracellular calcium levels, mitochondrial dysfunction, and NF-κB activity and elevated NMDA and vanilloid activity.
4. The basic mechanisms NO/ONOO⁻ cycle are local, and therefore there may be much difference in tissue distribution of the underlying biochemistry from one individual to another, generating, in turn, much difference in their symptoms and signs. Variation in tissue distribution may distinguish one disease from another falling under this paradigm.
5. Treatment should focus on down-regulating elements of the NO/ONOO⁻ cycle.

So we will be able to recognize possible candidates for inclusion under this putative paradigm primarily by their fit to these five principles. There may be other types of evidence that we may look for, including reported comorbidity with one or more of our multisystem illnesses.[5] But the primary type of evidence to search for in considering a particular type of illness under this putative paradigm should focus on these five principles and their consequences. In practice, the fit with these five principles will focus mainly on the search, as we have already seen in Chapters 5 through 10, for chronic illnesses with:

- short-term stressors that may be involved in initiating cases of the illness involved and have the ability to increase nitric oxide, based on known or plausible mechanisms;
- evidence for the presence in the chronic phase of the illness of elevation of several of the elements of our vicious cycle mechanism;
- evidence that the characteristic symptoms and signs of the illness may be generated by elements of the vicious cycle;
- evidence for the local nature of the mechanism, such as roles of a specific tissue in generating the pathophysiology or much variation in tissue impact from one patient to another; and
- evidence that agents predicted to down-regulate the NO/ONOO⁻ cycle biochemistry may be useful therapeutic agents.

I will discuss the issue of therapy of these candidate diseases by down-regulation of the NO/ONOO⁻ cycle here, only very briefly, because the background needed for such a discussion will be developed in Chapter 15.

How might such illness candidates differ from each other and from the four multisystem illnesses? The most obvious ways may be in terms of principle 4: They may differ from other such illnesses in terms of the tissue distribution of the underlying biochemistry. An example of this, which I will discuss briefly in the following text, is that of tinnitus, where the same basic biochemistry and physiology invoked in our vicious cycle appears to be involved, but is limited primarily to the inner ear. A second possible example that was discussed in Chapter 7 is asthma, where the biochemistry and physiology specifically impacts the bronchi of the lungs. It should be apparent to the reader that, depending on the specific tissue or tissues impacted, there could be many different types of illnesses that might fall into this putative paradigm. I would not be at all surprised if readers of this book come up with a number of possible candidates for inclusion under this paradigm that I do not discuss in this chapter, candidates characterized by possible impact in various regions of the body.

However, the variation in tissue distribution is not the only possible feature that may help distinguish one candidate medical condition from another. There may be certain candidates that are closely linked in the scientific literature to a particular stressor and may be viewed, therefore, as being distinct but may in fact be very similar to illnesses initiated by alternative stressors. I will discuss some examples of this type. Other possible candidates may be distinct because of the stage in the life cycle in which they are initiated. Still others may be distinct because of the variation of biological response to the NO/ONOO⁻ cycle, possibly because of genetic variation.

I have already suggested in earlier chapters two additional possible candidates for inclusion under this paradigm: Irritable bowel syndrome (IBS) is discussed briefly in Chapter 3, and asthma is discussed in more detail in Chapter 7. I will not consider these two any further, except to point out that they should be classified, along with other possible candidates discussed in this chapter, for *possible* inclusion under this paradigm.

There is one additional important point that needs to be considered before going on to look at possible specific candidates.

I am well aware that suggesting that there may be a dozen or more additional candidates for inclusion under this paradigm may strain credibility, in the views of many. It may be argued that it strains credibility enough to suggest a single paradigm to explain all four of these multisystem illnesses. After all, even though multiple researchers had earlier suggested two, three, or all four of these multisystem illnesses appear to share a common etiology based on their similarities with each other and their comorbidity, it still may strain credibility to suggest that there is an explanation for so many of their previously "unexplained" features sitting out there in plain sight. To suggest that a dozen or more additional illnesses, in many cases, well-accepted and well-researched diseases, may share the same etiology may be viewed as delusions of grandeur. In response to that view, I argue two things: The case for each of these should be judged on its individual merits, not on some preconceived notion. In addition, other disease paradigms have dozens of examples, with some 30 autoimmune diseases and many more types of infectious diseases and types of cancer; so why not this one?

THREE ELEMENTS OF CAUTION
AND OTHER CONSIDERATIONS

In looking for possible inclusion under this paradigm, one consideration is the role of initiating short-term stressors possibly acting via nitric oxide. This criterion may be difficult to fulfill for some illnesses. After all, there are cases of CFS, FM, and MCS where no such stressor is identifiable, and it is possible that some illnesses may present the same type of challenge in most cases rather than just in a substantial minority of cases. In some cases, the stressor involved, if any, may have occurred a long time before frank illness is apparent, making linkage difficult.

A second caution centers on evidence for vicious cycle elements in the chronic phase of illness. The various elements of our NO/ONOO⁻ cycle should be present in the chronic phase of candidate illnesses but how useful is this likely to be for determining possible inclusion under the paradigm? Most of the elements of the cycle, nitric oxide, peroxynitrite, oxidative stress, NF-κB, inflammatory cytokines, etc., are also found in a wide variety of inflammatory conditions. Given how common chronic inflammatory conditions are in medicine, it can be argued that their presence in the illness being considered for possible inclusion under this paradigm should simply be viewed as evidence that the illness is another chronic inflammatory condition, not one necessarily generated by the NO/ONOO⁻ cycle. So failure to confirm this prediction, where data are available, will lead to exclusion of a particular illness from possible inclusion under our paradigm, but confirmation may be of limited value in arguing for inclusion. That will be particularly true if there is an apparent alternative explanation for any chronic inflammation, an explanation not dependent on the NO/ONOO⁻ cycle. The reader needs to keep this particular note of skepticism in mind.

A third type of caution is that for a number of these illnesses, no fullfledged case is possible because of the limited data. In these latter cases, the argument to be made is that the explanation of the illnesses based on our on our NO/ONOO⁻ cycle appears to be the best available explanation, even if this is supported by limited data. Clearly, in these cases, the relevance of this paradigm to the specific illness should be viewed as a hypothesis that suggests a variety of future tests.

Finally, because of limitations of space available in this chapter, and my time in researching these illnesses, what I will present here is an outline of the case for possible inclusion of 12 distinct illnesses under this paradigm. It is not my goal here, to make a full-fledged case. I am not trying to convince you that I have considered all possible supportive or exclusionary data. Rather, it is my goal to state that there is a *superficial case* that can be made for each of these and that further consideration may be needed to develop a full-fledged case.

1. Tinnitus

Most cases of tinnitus are caused by dysfunction in the inner ear, causing one to "hear" sounds that do not exist—sometimes described as ringing, buzzing, roaring, or clicking in the ear. The notion here is that initiation of the NO/ONOO⁻ cycle in the cochlea of the inner ear may be the cause of most cases of tinnitus.

A similar proposal was developed by Takumida et al. in a seminal paper,[5] and as far as I can determine, their concept was developed completely independently from mine. However, Takumida et al.[5] have little to say about how a short-term nitric oxide increase may be converted into the chronic illness we know as tinnitus; so, perhaps our vicious cycle mechanism is needed to fulfill that portion of the mechanism.

In their paper, they review the evidence that five distinct short-term stressors that can initiate cases of tinnitus all have the ability to increase nitric oxide levels in the inner ear.[5] Specifically, the stressors of loud noise (acoustic overstimulation), ischemia, L-arginine injection, bacterial LPS injection, and aminoglycoside antibiotics (such as gentamycin) all can increase nitric oxide production in the inner ear and all can initiate cases of tinnitus.[5] In an animal (guinea pig) model of tinnitus, protection was produced by an inhibitor of nitric oxide synthesis, by the enzyme superoxide dismutase, and by a peroxynitrite scavenger (ebselen).[5] It follows from this that nitric oxide, superoxide, and peroxynitrite all appear to have a causal role in producing a tinnitus response in this animal model.

In the chronic phase of tinnitus, the best evidence for ongoing involvement is from studies of effective therapies, implicating particular mechanisms. In an earlier review of therapeutic approaches, Shulman[6] discussed the use of apparent protective agents including NMDA and other glutamate receptor antagonists, free radical scavengers, and other antioxidants and calcium-channel blockers. This suggests the involvement of several of our vicious cycle elements, including NMDA receptors, oxidants, and intracellular calcium. These have been confirmed by a number of more recent studies. The role of excessive NMDA activity has been confirmed by studies on the effectiveness of NMDA antagonists injected into the inner ear[7,8] and of the effectiveness of a GABA$_A$ receptor agonist,[9] which is known to lower NMDA activity. These studies also demonstrate a role for the AMPA receptors which are also stimulated by glutamate.

The effectiveness of antioxidant therapy is most convincing not for tinnitus but for the closely related Meniere's disease, where a variety of antioxidants are reported to be effective.[10,11] Studies have also implicated elevated levels of intracellular calcium in tinnitus.[12,13] It is unclear whether the studies discussed here implicating excessive superoxide and peroxynitrite in an animal model of tinnitus[5] are relevant only to the initiation phase or are also relevant to the chronic phase of the disease.

The final issue to be discussed is whether any symptoms and signs of tinnitus may be explainable through the action of elements of our vicious cycle. The cardinal symptom of tinnitus is the "hearing" of nonexistent sounds. Given the well-established role of both NMDA receptors and the AMPA/kainate glutamate receptors in the cochlear hearing mechanism in the inner ear,[14,15] this is exactly what one might expect from the role of elevated NMDA activity in our vicious cycle. Nitric oxide also has a role in the cochlea of the inner ear, but whether the nitric oxide role may help our understanding of the symptomology of tinnitus is unclear.[15]

In summary, then, the known properties of tinnitus with regard to initiation of the disease, the properties of its chronic phase, and the most characteristic symptom are all in very good agreement with the predictions of our NO/ONOO⁻ cycle mechanism. I believe that one can make a still stronger case with a more extensive consideration, and it is my intention to submit a paper with one of my former students, Sabrina Bedient, on this topic.

2. Postradiation Syndrome

Postradiation syndrome has been primarily studied among the cleanup workers and others who were exposed to substantial levels of ionizing radiation from the Chernobyl nuclear reactor accident. The symptoms of these individuals have been described in several studies and closely resemble the overlapping symptoms of multisystem illnesses described in Chapter 3. For example, Kumerova et al.[16] described the symptoms as including headache, dizziness, poor memory, prostration, lowered work ability, excessive nervousness, local pains in the bones, and disorders of the digestive system. Loganovsky[17] describes the symptoms as including persistent fatigue, odd skin sensations, bizarre feelings in bones, muscles and joints, irritability, headache, vertigo, pain in the chest area, emotional lability, lack of concentration and memory, cognitive deterioration, depression signs, and sleep disorders. Pastel[18] (p. 134) describes the symptoms as including "fatigue, sleep and mood disturbances, impaired memory and concentration and muscle and/or joint pain." The similarity of these symptoms to those of the multisytem illnesses described in Chapter 3 and elsewhere is notable.

Not surprisingly, several research groups have compared postradiation syndrome to CFS,[16-19] MCS,[19] and FM,[18] with the similarities to CFS being the most convincing.[16-19] So, we have a CFS-like chronic illness persisting a decade or more after exposure to a stressor, notably ionizing radiation. So as in the case of each of the multisystem illnesses, we have to explain both the role of the short-term stressor and the chronic nature of the subsequent illness. In addition, we need to explain the symptomatic and other (see the following text) similarities of postradiation syndrome to CFS and the other multisystem illnesses.

Ionizing Radiation Produces Activation of NF-κB
and Increases in Nitric Oxide

The first question that needs to be asked in determining whether post-radiation syndrome may fit our NO/ONOO⁻ cycle mechanism is the following: Can ionizing radiation exposure produced increases in nitric oxide? There is an extensive literature showing that ionizing radiation can activate the transcription factor NF-κB,[20-23] producing such increases even at low level radiation exposure.[22] You will recall that NF-κB can induce the inducible nitric oxide synthase (iNOS), and as expected it has been reported that ionizing radiation can produce increases in nitric oxide,[24-27] acting at least in part through iNOS induction and NF-κB.[27] So, we have still another short-term stressor that increases nitric oxide and is capable initiating chronic illness.

What About the Chronic Phase of Postradiation Syndrome?

We need to compare the predictions of our vicious cycle mechanism with the properties of the chronic phase of postradiation syndrome to determine whether they are compatible with each other. There is much less information available on the chronic phase of this illness, as compared with each of the four multisystem illnesses. However, where there is information available, it seems to be consistent with the predictions of our vicious cycle mechanism. Specifically, there is extensive evidence for oxidative stress in the chronic phase of the illness, showing that previous exposure to radiation can initiate a process leading to oxidative stress a decade or more after the radiation exposure occurred.[28-31] In addition, there are two reports of elevated levels of inflammatory cytokines during the chronic phase.[32,33] Other changes similar to those found in the multisystem illnesses have been reported including changes in immune function such as low natural killer (NK) cell function[34,35] and also chronic changes in brain physiology.[36-38]

In general, then, there is an excellent fit between the available information on postradiation syndrome and the predictions of our mechanism. Given the lack of any other attractive models of this illness, it may be inferred that the NO/ONOO⁻ cycle mechanism is the best available explanation for this previously puzzling illness.

3. Multiple Sclerosis

Multiple sclerosis (MS) is usually described as either an autoimmune disease or a disease of uncertain etiology. The pathologic hallmark of MS is the demyelination of neurons in regions of the brain and spinal cord, accompanied by inflammation and the subsequent formation of plaques, where each plaque is an area of white matter demyelination.[39-41] The autoimmune interpretation of MS has been challenged by several laboratories.[42-44] For example, Steiner and Wirguin have argued that none of the five criteria for classification as an autoimmune disease have been fulfilled in MS.[43] Barnett and Prineas[44] reported on the occurrence of lesions of recently exacerbated and deceased MS patients, which showed demyelination but no signs of autoimmune involvement. They argue that autoimmune mechanisms, where they occur in MS, may be in response to the demyelination inflammatory process rather than causing that process. The rationale for considering a possible NO/ONOO⁻ cycle mechanism for MS is dependent, then, on the apparent weakness of arguments supporting an autoimmune etiology, a weakness that is not be accepted by all experts.

As with the multisystem illnesses, cases of MS are often preceded by short-term stressors and some of the same stressors are reported to be involved in both. In MS, viral and bacterial infections may be involved in the initiation phase.[45-48] Organic solvent exposure may also be involved,[49,50] and in one review it is argued that head trauma may also be involved.[47] So, four of the initiating stressors from the multisystem illnesses that are all known to be able to increase nitric oxide may be involved in the initiation of MS. MS cases are also reported to be exacerbated by another nitric oxide-related stressor, psychological stress.[51-53] So several stressors that can act by increasing nitric oxide are implicated in initiation of cases of MS.

One of the long-known properties of MS is that it is much more common in regions of the world with little sun exposure during the winter months but is much rarer is sunnier climates.[54-56] The climatic effect occurs during roughly the first 15 years of life, and so migration to another climate after age 15 has little influence on the incidence of MS.[55,56] It has been proposed that the climatic effect is due to the action of sunlight in stimulating vitamin D synthesis in the body and that vitamin D during the first 15 years of life lowers the probability of becoming ill with MS. How might vitamin D act here? The answer is not known, but it is interesting that vitamin D is known to lower nitric oxide synthesis is some cell types.[57,58] It follows from this that some process which apparently starts the process toward the development of MS in the early years of life, years before the symptoms of MS appear, and it is possible to suggest that this early event may involve excessive nitric oxide production.

What about the chronic phase of MS? There is a substantial literature implicating most of the elements from our NO/ONOO⁻ cycle mechanism. These include nitric oxide,[59-61] peroxynitrite,[60-62] oxidative stress,[63-67] inflammatory cytokines,[68-71] NF-κB activity,[72-75] excitotoxicity including NMDA activity,[76-79] and lowered energy metabolism.[80] The permeabilization of the blood–brain barrier (BBB) in a mouse model of MS is due to elevated levels of peroxynitrite.[81] So almost all of the elements of our vicious cycle have been measured in MS and shown to be involved.

What about the cause of the most characteristic features of MS? The most characteristic feature is demyelination of the neurons of the central nervous system and such demyelination has been shown to be produced by certain reactive oxygen and nitrogen species including peroxynitrite and nitric oxide.[82-85] It follows that it is plausible that these two most central elements of the NO/ONOO⁻ cycle may produce the demyelination characteristic of MS.

In summary, the properties of MS that have been studied are in excellent agreement with the predictions of our NO/ONOO⁻ cycle. Based on this evidence, MS appears to be an example of a disease that may well fit under our paradigm.

4. Autism

Autism is characterized by early changes in development leading to lack of socialization and lack of normal verbal language skills. Both of these normally are developed by a learning process in early development and may, therefore, be explained by an early defect in learning and memory.

There are several short-term stressors that may be implicated in the autism, with each acting during the late prenatal stage or the early postnatal stage of development. These include virus infection with any of several viral agents acting both in the initiation of human cases of autism[86-93] and in animal models of autism.[93-96] Infections act to increase nitric oxide levels through the induction of iNOS, as was discussed in Chapter 5. There is a second possible type of stressor implicated in the initiation of cases of autism. The mercurial compound thimerosal, which is used as a preservative in vaccines, has been suggested to be involved in a large number of cases autism, following early vaccine injections.[97-101] Thimerosal is well documented to increase nitric oxide levels,[102-107] with those studies going back into the period where endothelial relaxing factor (EDRF) was being studied, before EDRF was identified as being nitric oxide. A third possible type of stressor, organic solvent exposure, which also can increase nitric oxide levels (Chapter 7), has also been reported to be associated with autism.[108] So we have three potential short-term stressors that may have a role in initiating cases of autism that may all act via their ability to increase nitric oxide.

What about the chronic phase of the autism? Here, the recent review by McGinnis[109] provides extensive documentation of biochemical/physiological changes in autism, as does as a review by Blaylock,[110] and I refer the reader to the references provided in those two papers. There is evidence for elevation of several of the elements in our vicious cycle mechanism in autism. These include oxidative stress monitored via a number of markers, nitric oxide, and inflammatory cyokines. While NMDA activity has not been directly implicated, there is evidence for excitoxicity including increased glutamate levels,[109,110] suggesting that NMDA activity is elevated. Finally, you may recall that mitochondrial/energy metabolism dysfunction has been shown to occur in some multisystem illnesses and is presumably caused by elevated levels of peroxynitrite, superoxide and nitric oxide (Chapter 2). Reports of mitochondrial dysfunction in autism[109] may also provide support for the involvement of our vicious cycle.

It may be argued that the characteristic features of autism may be a consequence of its initiation in early development. You will recall from Chapter 3, that learning and memory dysfunction is common in all four of the multisystem illnesses. The behavioral processes that are characteristically deficient in autism are both learned in early development and may therefore be caused by a deficiency in learning and memory that is initiated in early development. One of these is the lack of socialization in autism. It can be argued that socialization is dependent on the learning that there are other creatures out there very like ourselves, and such learning normally occurs early in development. Similarly, the development of language skills and verbal communication also normally occurs early in development. It seems reasonable, therefore, that the characteristic features of autism may be caused by the initiation of this disease early in development rather than being caused by any fundamental difference in etiology from that found in the multisystem illnesses. It should not be surprising that Miller[1] proposed that autism should be classified in the same group of illnesses as the four multisystem illnesses.

We have, then, an additional type of illness where cases appear to be initiated by a short-term stressor followed by a chronic illness and where that pattern requires a mechanistic explanation. If not via initiation of the NO/ONOO$^-$ cycle, what other explanation may apply? We have evidence for case initiation via short-term stressors raise nitric oxide levels. We have evidence for the occurrence of many of the elements of our vicious cycle in the chronic phase of the illness. And we can argue that characteristic symptoms of autism may be generated by defects in learning and memory, which may be generated in turn by elements of our vicious cycle (mainly elevated nitric oxide and NMDA activity and defects in energy metabolism, as discussed in Chapter 3). Thus, the fit with our putative paradigm is quite good.

It is my intention to write a much more detailed paper with Dr. McGinnis, making this case for publication elsewhere. In that paper, we will provide detailed documentation for the arguments outlined here and will also provide additional support of three different types:

- There are still other stressors that may act as putative initiators of autism and that may act to increase nitric oxide.
- There is at least one additional important reported sign of autism, which can be explained by the NO/ONOO⁻ cycle mechanism.
- There are several therapeutic agents reported to be useful in the treatment of autism that act to lower elements of our vicious cycle and therefore are predicted to be effective, based on the inference that autism falls under the tenth paradigm.

Autism is part of a spectrum of illnesses, called autistic spectrum disorders, with variations in symptoms and signs similar to the variation found among those suffering from the multisystem illnesses. It is plausible that this variation in symptoms in autistic spectrum disorders may be caused by variation of tissue distribution of NO/ONOO⁻ cycle biochemistry, as appears to be the case in the multisystem illnesses.

5. Overtraining Syndrome

Overtraining syndrome, sometimes referred to as underperformance syndrome, occurs not infrequently in athletes who strain their bodies with excessive exercise. The symptoms and signs of overtraining syndrome include a number of features in common with those of multisystem illnesses. These include persistent fatigue, disturbed sleep, alterations in mood state, low NK cell activity, lowered maximum oxygen utilization, and hypothalamic-pituitary-adrenal (HPA) axis dysfunction.[111-116] Prolonged rest is often seen as being an effective treatment for overtraining syndrome. The similarities between overtraining syndrome and CFS and other multisystem illnesses suggest that there may be some similarities in etiology. It has been proposed that excessive inflammatory cytokines may have a key role in overtraining syndrome,[112,117,118] but there is essentially no data to test this view.

The notion that our NO/ONOO⁻ cycle mechanism may explain the etiology of overtraining syndrome is similar to the position of Stefano et al.[119] who suggest that strenuous exercise, taken to extreme, initiates an immune and vascular proinflammatory response that they term the excessive stress response. The difference, of course, is that I would emphasize the role of the underlying inflammatory biochemistry and the NO/ONOO⁻ cycle. Interestingly, people who develop CFS are reported to often have been quite physically active,[120] suggesting a possible etiologic connection between CFS and overtraining syndrome.

There is extensive evidence showing the excessive exercise can not only produce increased oxidative stress but can also produce increases in other elements of our vicious cycle, including NF-κB activity, reactive nitrogen species including nitric oxide and inflammatory cytokine levels.[112,121-128] It seems likely, then, that oxidants produced by excessive exercise, acting through increased NF-κB activity to induce iNOS, may increase nitric oxide and other elements of our vicious cycle. There is some evidence that high-level exercise may have a role in the initiation of conventional cases of CFS as well, because CFS cases are reported to have had higher amounts of exercise before becoming ill than did controls.[129]

Unfortunately, there is essentially no biochemical data from the chronic phase of this illness, from athletes suffering from overtraining syndrome, that allows us to test the predicted presence of elements of our vicious cycle mechanism. So we have a pattern of short-term stressor followed by chronic illness in which the stressor may be able to act by increasing nitric oxide and other elements of the NO/ONOO⁻ cycle. However, the types of evidence from the chronic phase of illness, such as are described in CFS, MCS, FM, and PTSD to test for inclusion under are paradigm, are lacking for overtraining syndrome.

6. Silicone Implant Associated Syndrome

The debates on the existence and properties of silicone implant associated syndrome (SIAS) has paralleled the debate on the existence and properties of CFS, FM, and MCS, and the issues involved appear to be similar. The large study by Henneken et al.[130] provided evidence for statistically significant increases in autoimmune connective tissue diseases among those receiving silicone breast implants. However, the increase reported was small, and the statistically significant increases were see only for overall connective tissue diseases and for rheumatoid arthritis. This small increase is distinct from the much higher percentage reports from clinical observations, where these changes involve primarily changes in either symptoms often found in CFS or FM or in certain inflammatory responses. This might suggest that one should study the prevalence of multisymptom illnesses and their symptoms, among breast implant patients, rather than just the prevalence of autoimmune diseases.

That view was supported by Vasey,[131] who stated that "To clinicians who see these patients, it's clear that most of them have a fibromyalgia/chronic fatigue, peripheral neuritis, irritable bowel and bladder syndrome that has not been precisely defined." He notes a number of reports of such symptoms in symptomatic silicone breast implant patients,[131] going on to note the improvement of symptoms in some patients on removal of the implants. The study of Brown et al.[132] may be seen as important because they looked specifically at silicone implant recipients who had a rupture of their implant leading to leaked extracapsular silicone. In studying such women, they found that they had significantly higher prevalence of FM as compared to controls (odds ratio of 2.8). In a subsequent study, Brown et al.[133] (p. 293) comment that "Some studies addressing this issue of silicone breast implants and connective tissue disease specifically exclude patients with fibromyalgia from the sample or do not include the syndrome in the analysis. Case series describing fibromyalgia in patients with implants have been published, but many of these papers lack information on extracapsular silicone. . . ." There have been a number of studies specifically studying whether silicone breast implant recipients who are symptomatic, meet the criteria for either diagnosis of FM or CFS or show characteristic symptoms of these illnesses. For example, Solomon[134] described a group of symptomatic patients whose most common symptoms were chronic fatigue (77 percent) and cognitive dysfunction (65 percent), both common symptoms of multisystem illnesses. Solomon also described a number of additional symptoms, many of which may be generated by inflammation of different regions of the body. Cuellar et al.[135] reported that 54 percent of symptomatic silicone breast implant recipients met the criteria for either FM or CFS or both. Vermeulen and Scholte[136] reported that the symptoms of a group of Dutch women transplant recipients were more common in those with reported ruptured transplants including debilitating chronic fatigue, impaired memory, and multijoint pain. Most importantly, about 77 percent of these self-selected apparent transplant rupture group reported having postexertional malaise,[136] which is now considered to be the cardinal symptom of CFS. Blackburn et al.[137] reported that a majority of symptomatic patients with silicone breast implants had FM. Freundlich et al.[138] reported that 30 percent of symptomatic, referred transplant patients met the diagnostic criteria for FM, while over 70 percent reported each of three symptoms common in multisystem illnesses, fatigue, poor sleep, and arthralgia. In a small study of 11 symptomatic breast implant recipients, six met the diagnostic criteria of FM and the remaining five had symptoms of chronic fatigue syndrome.[139] In contrast to these studies, a study comparing FM prevalence in breast implant recipients versus controls found a similar incidence,[140] but that study was small, with a broad confidence interval (0.3 to 3.0).

Probably the most careful study conducted on the possible relationship between a multisystem illness and SAIS was published by Miller and Prihoda[141] on chemical sensitivity symptoms. Miller and Prihoda used a well-validated survey instrument showing a characteristic pattern of responses from MCS patients as compared with controls, with increases in symptoms on chemical exposure. In that study, both symptomatic Gulf War veterans and breast implant recipients showed very similar patterns of responses to those of MCS patients, and these were very distinct from those of controls.[141] It was shown in this study, that implant recipients reported sensitivity to a wide range of chemicals, similar to the range that MCS patients react to. From this study, it appears that symptomatic implant recipients often have MCS or an MCS-like illness.

I have no doubt that the controversy about SIAS will continue and also that further studies on the apparent connection between SIAS and CFS, FM, and MCS are needed. However, it also seems apparent that the bulk of the available evidence suggests that the more puzzling features of SIAS may be largely due to a combination of these three multisystem illnesses. Consequently, it is important to ask whether other properties of SIAS are compatible with our putative paradigm.

The usual approach that I have taken towards asking this type of question is both easier and more difficult in the case of SIAS. Clearly, I have already dealt with the question of how the symptoms of CFS, FM and MCS may be generated, so we do not need to deal with the same symptoms again when they occur in SIAS—they appear to be compatible with our paradigm. However, the division I have made between looking at the effects of short-term stressors and the properties of the chronic phase of the illness is not possible here. The stressor, exposure to the materials of a silicone implant, is a long-term one, and that makes this separation problematic. But we can still ask whether the properties of this stressor are compatible with a nitric oxide role in initiation of the illness. In addition we can ask whether the elements of our NO/ONOO⁻ cycle are found in symptomatic implant recipients. Let us take those questions one at a time.

Silicone Implant Materials, Silica and Nitric Oxide

It is possible that the initiation of SIAS may be a consequence of exposure to silica rather than silicone. As stated by Shanklin and Smalley[142] (p. 86), "Remarkably, from the earliest time, it was found necessary to add silica to silicone elastomers to obtain the material strength required for many applications. Thus from a chemical point of view, *siliconosis* is, in part *silicosis*" (italics originally present). For example, two common mixtures used for such breast implants both have about 26 percent silica.[143] There is an extensive literature showing that silica produces inflammatory responses, which include increases in nitric oxide, oxidants, NF-κB activity, iNOS induction, and inflammatory cytokine synthesis.[144-148] Consequently, there is no doubt that silica exposure can produce increases of multiple elements of our NO/ONOO⁻ cycle. There is also some evidence that silicone can produce increases in nitric oxide and oxidants,[149] but the evidence implicating silica is such responses and the apparent level of the response produced by silica makes it a much better candidate as a stressor producing a nitric oxide increase.

In the symptomatic phase of SIAS, there are three studies reporting increase inflammatory cytokine production.[137,150,151] While the other elements of the NO/ONOO⁻ cycle have apparently not been studied in symptomatic silicone transplant recipients, both increased nitric oxide and iNOS induction have been found in animal models.[149,152] So again, where we have evidence in the symptomatic phase of SIAS, it is supportive of the predictions from the tenth paradigm, but the evidence is still quite limited.

There is one other point that needs to be made here. If the primary initiator of SIAS is silica as suggested but not proven earlier in this section, the production of CFS/FM/MCS symptoms will require permeabilization of the blood-brain barrier (BBB). This is essential if silica has a central role, because many of the CFS/FM/MCS symptoms appear to be a product of dysfunction of regions of the brain and access of silica to these regions will require such permeabilization. So a weak prediction here (weak, because we have not established that silica is the most important initiating material) is that we may well see a breakdown of the BBB in symptomatic silicone transplant recipients. Clearly, if such BBB changes are found in such patients, and this has not been studied to my knowledge, such BBB changes may provide one objective criterion for diagnosis.

7. Sudeck's Atrophy

The terminology surrounding Sudeck's atrophy seems to be an exercise in confusion. It has been called reflex sympathetic dystrophy, algodystrophy, Sudeck's syndrome, and complex regional pain syndrome,[153-160] depending on the context and the symptoms that are being emphasized. It is characterized by a chronic localized illness in a limb usually, but not always, occurring after injury to that limb, producing a variety of symptoms in the limb involved including muscle and/or bone atrophy, chronic pain, muscle tremor, and/or weakness and neurological dysfunction.[153-160] The mechanism is primarily local, because the symptoms are almost always localized to a single limb that was typically damaged by a previous injury. The symptoms of Sudeck's atrophy are quite variable from one case to another, and in this sense it is similar to the multisystem illnesses.

Sudeck described this atrophy as being caused by an exaggerated inflammatory response in the limb involved, a description that is supported by more recent observations.[153,155,161] So, we have here a chronic condition that is commonly initiated by physical trauma, a stressor that can produce increased nitric oxide levels, as discussed in Chapter 8. It is also reported to be associated with and possibly initiated by both infection[162] and also organophosphorus pesticide exposure,[163] two additional stressors known to produce increases in nitric oxide. The recent study by Friedman et al.[164] described cases involving both chronic local symptoms and chronic central symptoms apparently initiated by previous organophosphorus pesticide exposure.

Other than the general observations of exaggerated inflammation, there have been few studies that may provide evidence whether elements of the NO/ONOO⁻ cycle are found in the chronic phase of Sudeck's atrophy. However, there have been several studies suggesting that excess NMDA activity may be involved and so NMDA antagonist drugs may be useful in treatment of Sudeck's atrophy.[165-168] Other pharmacological approaches to treatment that are consistent with lowering the properties of our vicious cycle mechanism, include treatment with agents that increase GABA activity (which act to lower NMDA activity)[168,169] and with antioxidant free radical scavengers.[168]

Can the symptoms be generated by elements of the NO/ONOO⁻ cycle? Clearly, pain can be as I have discussed in Chapter 3 and elsewhere. Perhaps the most characteristic symptoms involve atrophy of muscle and bone, and both of these may be explained through our vicious cycle. Muscle atrophy can be produced by excessive nitric oxide, oxidant activity, inflammatory cytokine levels, and NF-κB activity.[169,170] Bone atrophy (osteoporosis) was recently reported to be produced by chronically elevated nitric oxide levels and apparently also by excessive NMDA activity.[171]

In summary, we have in Sudeck's atrophy a condition that fits the overall pattern of short-term stressor followed by chronic illness. Clearly, the amount of data available on the mechanism of Sudeck's atrophy is distinctly limited, but where we have data, either on the initiation of cases of this illness, on the properties of the chronic phase of the illness, or on the possible mechanisms involved in symptom generation, the data fit well with predictions of the NO/ONOO⁻ cycle.

8. Postherpetic Neuralgia

Postherpetic pain also known as postherpetic neuralgia is a chronic pain response that often occurs following a herpes infection flare-up, where typically a dormant herpes virus infection becomes reactivated for a short time period. After the infection becomes dormant, again, there is often long-lasting pain subsequent to the reactivation.

Herpes viruses are known to be very active in stimulating the production of inflammatory cytokines during active infections,[172-174] so one has here the potential for a substantial nitric oxide increase in response to cytokine-mediated iNOS induction. Furthermore, because herpes viruses commonly infect neurons, the infection is located such that it may easily produce the neuropathic pain of postherpetic neuralgia.

Neuropathic pain includes the pain of secondary hyperalgesia[175-177] and involves the many components of our NO/ONOO$^-$ cycle mechanism involved in hyperalgesia including elevated nitric oxide and NMDA activity. Specifically, neuropathic pain has been shown in many studies to involve nitric oxide and peroxynitrite elevation, inflammatory cytokine elevation, NMDA activity, increased intracellular calcium levels, and vanilloid stimulation (see, for example, References 175-181). While some of these have not been explicitly studied in postherpetic pain, to my knowledge, the role of NMDA activity[182-186] and inflammatory cytokines[187-189] in generating postherpetic pain is well documented. It follows from this that two of the elements of our vicious cycle, NMDA activity and inflammatory cytokines, have roles in the generation of postherpetic pain and that others are almost certainly involved because of their known role in neuropathic pain, including nitric oxide, peroxynitrite, intracellular calcium levels, and vanilloid receptor activity.

So, we have here still another medical condition that is initiated by a short-term stressor that can increase nitric oxide, that involves in the chronic phase several of the elements of our vicious cycle, and where the NO/ONOO$^-$ cycle elements can generate the characteristic symptom of the condition, excessive pain. It follows that postherpetic pain is another good candidate for inclusion under our paradigm.

9. Chronic Whiplash-Associated Disorder

Whiplash injury to the upper spinal column is often followed by chronic excessive pain as well as other symptoms characteristic of the four multisystem illnesses. One has not only chronic pain[190,191] but also reports of memory and cognitive dysfunction,[191-193] dizziness and unsteadiness,[195] sympathetic dysfunction,[195] and anxiety and depression.[194,196] So the pattern of symptoms is quite similar to the overlapping symptoms of these multisystem illnesses described in Chapter 3. There is a report of brain injury associated with this illness,[197] again in similarity to the evidence for such injury in the multisystem illnesses from brain scan studies that were discussed in Chapter 3.

Chronic whiplash-associated disorder (CWAD) is most similar to FM, because both often appear to be initiated by physical trauma to central nervous system. Similar changes in pain processing in the spinal cord both in FM and in CWAD have been reported in a recent study,[198,199] and temporomandibular pain is often comorbid with both.[200] In similarity with FM, the NMDA antagonist ketamine has been reported to be helpful in lowering pain responses in CWAD,[201] providing evidence that excessive NMDA activity has an important role in generating the excessive pain in CWAD.

In comparison to FM or, for that matter, the other multisystem illnesses, the evidence available in CWAD is quite limited. Nevertheless, there is a superficial case to be made for its possible inclusion under our paradigm. We have a short-term stressor, physical trauma to the upper spinal column, which may generate a nitric oxide increase, as discussed in Chapter 8. Only one of the elements of our vicious cycle has been studied (NMDA activity), which appears to be elevated and to have a causal role in generating symptoms.[201] Many of the symptoms reported can each be explained, as was discussed in Chapter 3, by elements of our vicious cycle. Of course, we have the overall pattern of short-term stressor followed by chronic illness, which requires explanation.

The mechanism proposed here, is as far as I can determine, the only testable etiologic hypothesis for CWAD. All I have found in the literature as a possible alternative is some unsupported psychogenic speculation on the etiology of CWAD.

10-12. Amyotrophic Lateral Sclerosis (ALS), Parkinson's Disease, and Alzheimer's Disease

These three neurodegenerative diseases are often discussed together because of their many similarities. They are progressive, they involve extensive apoptotic neuronal cell death, and they all, as we will see, involve most of the elements of our NO/ONOO$^-$ cycle mechanism in the chronic phase. Where short-term stressors appear to have a role in the initiation of these illnesses, there are usually but not always long latency periods between exposure to the stressor and the appearance of disease symptoms. Each of them also involves certain individually characteristic features, which have significant causal roles in their overall etiology.

Both the long latency and the specific characteristic features of each of these diseases pose challenges to any advocacy of a NO/ONOO⁻ cycle etiologic mechanism. The latency can be explained through a need for a long period of apoptotic cell death after stressor exposure but before sufficient numbers of neurons have been killed and other neurological damage may have accumulated to produce the symptoms of the disease. If this is the explanation, how might the short-term stressors produce a prolonged sensitivity to apoptotic cell death? Does this involve our NO/ONOO⁻ cycle or does it involve some other mechanism? Given the difficulty in studying these latency periods, it is difficult to answer this last question, and that difficulty provides substantial weakness for any case that I can make. Still, the evidence provides some support for the role of one or more of the components of our vicious cycle during the latency period of these diseases. For example, Summers[202] (p. 673) states that "Rather it (Alzheimer's disease) is the product of free radical injury inflicted over decades after an initial insult," strongly suggesting a short-term stressor, vicious cycle type of illness pattern involving oxidative stress.

There is a second area of potential weakness for which I have at least partial answers. Each of these diseases has one or more specific characteristic features. If these diseases are to be explained as being a consequence of our NO/ONOO⁻ cycle mechanism, then each of these characteristic features must be a consequence of our vicious cycle that is *tissue specific*—that is, the feature must be a consequence of the interaction of the NO/ONOO⁻ cycle with the specific tissue elements. Examples of these specific features are the formation of amyloid plaques and hyperphosphorylated tau protein in Alzheimer's disease and the formation of Lewy bodies in Parkinson's disease. Indeed, it is possible that specific features might not only be tissue specific, but they might be tissue specific components of the NO/ONOO⁻ cycle itself. They may, in other words, contribute to the cycle, and not just be caused by the cycle. So we have another challenge in determining how these specific features may (or may not) be compatible with the NO/ONOO⁻ cycle.

I will come back to these challenges later in the sections on each of these three neurodegenerative diseases. There are a number of other observations that suggest that these three diseases share common etiologic mechanisms. For example, people in Guam and certain other tropical Pacific islands often suffer from what is known as ALS Parkinson dementia complex, a combination of all three of these diseases.[203,204] This is thought to be caused by eating cycad flour containing the neurotoxin BMAA, which, when it reacts with carbon dioxide, forms a compound that stimulates the NMDA receptors,[204,205] as well as other components of cycad flour, which also stimulate NMDA activity.[206] These observations provide support for the view that all three of these illnesses share important etiologic features, and specifically they can be initiated by excessive NMDA activity. So here is our first stressor initiating these diseases that may act through excessive nitric oxide, given the known role of NMDA receptors in increasing nitric oxide. Another observation linking two of these diseases is that sufferers with ALS often demonstrate dopamine deficiencies, a feature that is characteristic of Parkinson's disease.[207] In another linkage, the pro-oxidant APOE4 form of the APOE protein is associated with increased early incidence of all three of these illnesses.[208-210] An animal model links Alzheimer's disease and Parkinson's disease.[211]

Short-Term Stressors: In Parkinson's Disease, Alzheimer's Disease, and ALS

There are no less than nine short-term stressors that have established or suspected roles in the initiation of cases of Parkinson's disease. All nine of these are known or expected to act in ways that can increase nitric oxide levels and/or other elements of our NO/ONOO⁻ cycle. In other words, they may all plausibly act to initiate Parkinson's disease by initiating our vicious cycle mechanism. This is important because it not only increases the support for a central role of the NO/ONOO⁻ cycle in Parkinson's disease but also because it provides, for the first time, a biologically plausible mechanism for the action of all nine of these stressors in initiation of cases of this disease.

These nine stressors include organic solvent exposure[212-216] and exposure to organophosphorus and carbamate pesticides[217] and to organochlorine pesticides.[217] These are all involved in the initiation of MCS cases, as discussed in Chapter 7, and all three appear to act via distinct pathways to increase NMDA activity and presumably consequent levels of nitric oxide and peroxynitrite. The fourth class of pesticide apparently implicated in MCS, the pyrethroid pesticides, has not to my knowledge been specifically implicated in Parkinson's disease, but it should be noted that most studies of pesticides in Parkinson's disease have studied pesticides in general and have not attempted to identify specific classes of pesticides involved.[217]

Other classes of stressors include BMAA and other neurotoxins found in cycad flour, which are also consistent with an NMDA mechanism and therefore with the NO/ONOO⁻ cycle mechanism, as discussed earlier, the toxic drug MPTP,[218,219] the pesticide rotenone,[219,220] the herbicide paraquat,[217,219-221] the fungicide maneb, and certain chemically and toxicologically similar fungicides[220,221] and ionic manganese, which is implicated in cases of excessive manganese exposure in welders or from environmental sources such as well water.[222-225] So for each these six distinct types of stressors discussed in this paragraph, we need to show consistency with possible initiation of the NO/ONOO⁻ cycle in order to support our mechanism.

The toxic drug MPTP was originally implicated in the initiation of Parkinson's disease when a large number of illegal drug users came down with premature Parkinson's disease due to the presence of MPTP as an impurity in the drug they were using.[218] It has subsequently been used to induce Parkinson's-like symptoms and signs in animal models of this disease, confirming a causal role in the initiation of Parkinson's disease.[226-228] MPTP and a product derived from it inhibits what is known as complex I in the mitochondrion, leading both to decreased ATP synthesis (low energy levels) and to increased production of superoxide.[227,228] This indirectly leads to increases in nitric oxide, peroxynitrite, oxidative stress, NF-kB activity, and inflammatory cytokine activity[227-231] and thus elevates several components of the NO/ONOO⁻ cycle. The pesticide rotenone acts very much like MPTP. It also inhibits complex I activity in mitochondria and leads to consequent oxidative stress, increased nitric oxide, and lowered energy metabolism.[232,233] It is plausible, then that rotenone may act essentially like MPTP in triggering our vicious cycle. Rotenone is also used to induce Parkinson's-like symptoms and signs in animal models of the disease,[219,220,232] confirming its role as an initiator of Parkinson's disease.

The herbicide paraquat is well known to induce oxidative stress,[234,235] and it is known to stimulate NF-κB activity,[235] which will be expected to increase induction of the inducible nitric oxide synthase (iNOS), as discussed in Chapter 1. It also produces increases in peroxynitrite[229] and oxidative stress.[236] Consequently, paraquat can also act through known mechanisms to plausibly trigger the NO/ONOO⁻ cycle. The fungicide maneb is reported to act as a potent inhibitor of glutamate transport,[237] thus leading to increased activity of the NMDA receptors as well as that of other glutamate receptors. It is also reported to increase oxidative stress.[236] The role of manganese in the initiation of Parkinson's disease cases may be explained by its known role in stimulating NF-κB activity and consequent iNOS induction, nitric oxide increases, and increase inflammatory cytokine levels;[238-240] in addition, manganese is reported to increase glutamate-induced neurotoxicity.[241]

So in each of these nine stressors, known or suspected to act to initiate cases of Parkinson's disease, we have biologically plausible mechanisms through which each may trigger the NO/ONOO⁻ cycle mechanism.

This issue of *biological plausibility* is a key one in considering epidemiological evidence, such as we are considering here, whenever the role of such stressors in initiating disease is being considered based on studies of groups of people. Hennekens and Buring,[242] on p. 40 in their textbook *Epidemiology in Medicine* state "The belief in the existence of a cause and effect relationship is enhanced if there is a known or postulated biologic mechanism by which the exposure might reasonably alter risk of developing disease." It follows from this that a plausible mechanism potentially linking these nine stressors to a possible mechanism for this disease increases the strength of any epidemiological inferences that appear to link them to the disease. In other words, the fact that each of these stressors can each act to increase nitric oxide and peroxynitrite, and thus potentially initiate chronic illness through a NO/ONOO⁻ cycle mechanism, provides each of them with biological plausibility as initiators and therefore strengthens the argument for each of them in disease initiation.

This is an important general consideration and may be viewed as strengthening the case for a role of other stressors that increase nitric oxide levels in other illnesses and diseases.

Head trauma has been repeatedly reported to have an apparent role in initiating cases of Alzheimer's disease,[243-245] and head trauma is known to lead to excessive NMDA stimulation as discussed in Chapter 8, leading to increases in nitric oxide and peroxynitrite. Alzheimer's disease, like Parkinson's disease, is reported to be associated with exposure to the fungicide maneb and related dithiocarbamate fungicides.[246] So a role for both of these stressors is consistent with initiation of the NO/ONOO⁻ cycle mechanism.

For ALS, there is some evidence that organophophorus[247] and organochlorine pesticide exposures[248] have a role in initiation of disease.

The herbicide 2,4-dichlorophenoxyacetic acid (2,4-D) also appears to be implicated in initiation of some cases of ALS.[249] The herbicide 2,4-D has several known toxic mechanisms,[250] and so it is more difficult to identify any specific mode of action that may be involved in the initiation of ALS. One of these is that it acts as an uncoupler of oxidative phosphorylation in mitochondria,[250] a toxic mechanism that will act to lower ATP (energy) generation. It also acts of deplete availability of acetyl-CoA,[250] which also has important roles in energy metabolism. It is plausible, therefore that 2,4-D may lower energy metabolism; given the known effect of lowered energy metabolism in producing increased NMDA activity (discussed in Chapter 2 and Chapter 7), this may be expected to lead to increased NMDA activity and consequent increased nitric oxide and peroxynitrite. I have already discussed the role of cycad neurotoxins including BMAA in ALS. Some studies have implicated a role of physical trauma in ALS,[251] and physical trauma is another stressor that can increase nitric oxide, as discussed in Chapter 8.

Perhaps the most dramatic role for a stressor in initiation of ALS is the role of mutant forms of the copper-zinc superoxide dismutase enzyme, an enzyme that normally acts to get rid of superoxide. The mutant forms lose zinc from the enzyme much more easily than does the normal enzyme, and the mutant form plays a active role in causing this disease.[252] This is known because animals genetically engineered to produce the mutant human enzyme develop an ALS-like disease, despite the fact that they still produce normal amounts of their normal functional superoxide dismutase. This shows that it is not the lack of the normal enzyme that is involved but rather an active pathological role of the mutant enzyme. The mutant enzyme acts to generate excessive amounts of both superoxide and peroxynitrite,[252,253] and may act to initiate our NO/ONOO⁻ cycle biochemistry via these mechanisms. So, in summary, for ALS, we have five distinct types of stressors that appear to have a role in initiating the disease, and the mechanisms of all five are consistent with their acting to initiate the NO/ONOO⁻ cycle.

Chronic-Phase of Illness and Elements of the NO/ONOO⁻ Cycle

Each of the elements of our vicious cycle, with one exception, is reported to be elevated in the chronic phase of these neurodegenerative diseases.[253-275] These include oxidative stress, nitric oxide, peroxynitrite, intracellular calcium levels, NF-κB activity, inflammatory cytokine activity, superoxide levels, and excitoxicity including NMDA activity and mitochondrial dysfunction (summarized in Table 14.1). The exception is the vanilloid receptor, which has not been studied in these diseases, to my knowledge. It may

TABLE 14.1. NO/ONOO⁻ cycle elements in Alzheimer's disease, Parkinson's disease, and amyotrophic lateral sclerosis (ALS).

Vicious cycle element	References
Oxidative stress	253, 257, 258, 263, 264, 265, 268, 272, 273, 274, 275
Nitric oxide	253, 254, 255, 256, 257, 263, 264, 265, 266, 268, 270, 274, 275
Superoxide	253, 264, 265, 270, 274, 275
Peroxynitrite	253, 254, 255, 256, 264, 266, 270, 272, 275
Intracellular calcium	254, 266, 268, 271
NF-κB	258
Inflammatory cytokines	267, 269
Excitotoxicity including NMDA activity	255, 259, 260, 261, 262, 268, 270, 275
Mitochondrial dysfunction	255, 256, 259, 262, 263, 264, 266, 275

be seen from the involvement of so many cycle elements that the properties of the chronic phase of these illnesses are in excellent agreement with predictions of our vicious cycle mechanism.

The crucial sign of each of these diseases is the apoptotic cell death of neurons in the specific region of the brain impacted by them. Given the ability of peroxynitrite to induce apoptosis, as discussed in Chapter 2, such apoptotic cell death may be produced by high levels of NO/ONOO⁻ cycle activity.

Parkinson's Disease: Specific Properties

The remaining discussion of these three neurodegenerative diseases will focus on how the specific properties of the tissues involved may be expected to influence the properties and consequences of the NO/ONOO⁻ cycle in those tissues. It will consider how certain disease signs may be causally related to elements of our vicious cycle and, in one case at least, may themselves be part of that vicious cycle in the tissues involved. I will discuss one disease at a time.

Parkinson's disease is characterized by dysfunction and subsequent death of the cells producing the neurotransmitter dopamine for the brain, particularly the substantia nigra. Dopamine chemistry produces oxidative stress in these tissues and the initiation of the NO/ONOO⁻ cycle in these dopamine-producing tissues may be favored by this oxidative chemistry. Dopamine produces oxidants because it spontaneously reacts with molecular oxygen, undergoing the process of peroxidation and producing free radicals and other oxidants in the process.[253] It also is oxidized by an enzyme monoamine oxidase B, which produces the oxidant hydrogen peroxide as a product.[253] Antunes and coworkers[276] recently reviewed evidence for an additional mechanisms showing that nitric oxide can react with dopamine and its products, leading to the production of compounds that generate free radicals and other oxidants. It follows that these nitric oxide reactions may cause dopamine to lead to still more oxidative stress than is caused by its autoxidation and oxidation by monoamine oxidase. The combination dopamine reactions involving each of these three mechanisms may well exacerbate the NO/ONOO⁻ cycle in the substantia nigra and other tissues producing dopamine.

Chung et al.[277] studied the protein parkin, which has an important protective role in preventing Parkinson's disease and specifically helps prevent the formation of the intracellular structures known as Lewy bodies. They showed that parkin was modified by nitric oxide by a process known as S-nitrosylation, destroying its protective function.[277] It follows that *nitric oxide may have a key role in causing Lewy body formation* via this reaction and that Lewy body formation may therefore be a consequence of the action of the NO/ONOO⁻ cycle. This is a key observation because it provides a plausible demonstrated mechanism that may explain how Lewy bodies, characteristic features of Parkinson's disease, may be generated by nitric oxide generated by the NO/ONOO⁻ cycle.

Alzheimer's Disease: Specific Properties

Neural tissues impacted by Alzheimer's disease are characterized by two specific features: β-amyloid plaques and neurofibrillary tangles. The β-amyloid plaques have a core of aggregated protein made of β-amyloid protein. This protein is derived by protease cleavage of a larger protein called amyloid precursor protein.

It has recently been shown that the most likely protease involved in this cleavage is a protease called β-secretase or BACE1.[278] A series of recent studies have shown that oxidative stress increases both the amount of β-secretase synthesized by cells and also its activity as a protease.[279-282] It follows that oxidative stress produced as a consequence of the NO/ONOO⁻ cycle may have a key role in increasing the amount of β-amyloid protein formed and therefore the amount of β-amyloid plaques formed, thus possibly producing this characteristic feature of Alzheimer's disease.

β-Amyloid deposition, as stated earlier[283] (p. 456), "causes neuronal death via a number of possible mechanisms, including oxidative stress, excitotoxicity, energy depletion, inflammation and apoptosis." Each of these is a predicted consequence of the NO/ONOO⁻ cycle mechanism. So the question that must be asked is whether β-amyloid protein is not only a consequence of oxidative stress produced by the NO/ONOO⁻ cycle but may act, in turn, to stimulate the cycle. In other words, is β-amyloid protein an integral part of the NO/ONOO⁻ cycle in the cerebral and other tissues involved in Alzheimer's disease? β-amyloid protein has been shown to produce the following changes in neuronal cells: Increased nitric oxide, iNOS induction, increased superoxide, increased peroxynitrite, oxidative stress, excitotoxicity including increased NMDA activity, nitric oxide-mediated mitochondrial dysfunction, and increased inflammatory cytokine levels.[284-292] In other words, essentially our entire NO/ONOO⁻ cycle mechanism has been demonstrated to be induced by β-amyloid protein. So in these neuronal cells, the β-amyloid protein behaves like an important part of the cycle. It seems highly unlikely that each of these nine responses to β-amyloid protein occurs independently of each other in response to the presence of that protein. Rather, the parsimonious explanation, the explanation predicted by

Occam's razor* is that β-amyloid protein is acting simply by up-regulating the NO/ONOO- cycle, possibly by a single mechanism and that the cycle is likely to be, therefore, a central explanatory feature of Alzheimer's disease. The fact that most of the cycle elements have been found to occur in the chronic phase of this disease, and the fact that stressors initiating Alzheimer's disease may act by increasing nitric oxide (both discussed earlier), provide important further support for this inference.

The other most prominent, relatively specific correlate of Azheimer's disease is the hyperphosphorylation of a protein known as tau and the consequent formation of neurofibrillary tangles. Tau protein gets hyperphosphorylated due to the action of oxidative stress,[293-296] and of certain products of oxidative stress-related biochemistry,[295,296] nitric oxide and iNOS activity,[292] excitotoxicity including NMDA activity[297] and peroxynitrite-stimulated poly(ADP-ribose) polymerase activity.[297] So several of the elements of the NO/ONOO⁻ cycle can have causal roles in producing this response. It may produce, in turn, oxidative stress,[298] although the evidence for that is not definitive.

In summary, both of the key specific properties of Alzheimer's disease, β-amyloid protein and hyperphosphorylated tau protein, can be produced through the action of elements of the NO/ONOO⁻ cycle, providing important plausibility for a central role of the cycle in Alzheimer's disease. The β-amyloid protein appears to be an integral part of the cycle in the tissues impacted by Alzheimer's and there is some evidence that hyperphosphorylated tau protein may also be part of the cycle in these tissues. These observations may be of great importance, because they provide an attractive unifying explanatory model for the interpretation of diverse properties of Alzheimer's disease.

ALS: Specific Properties

Sanelli et al.[299] (p. 8) reported in an important study that neurofilament aggregates, an important correlate of ALS, "results in a failure of regulation of NMDA-mediated calcium influx . . . preventing . . . down-regulation of the NMDA receptor." In this way, neurofilament aggregates may produce excessive NMDA activity and may be an important part of the vicious cycle in the tissues most impacted in ALS.

---

*Occam's razor is the very old scientific principle that the simplest consistent explanation is to be preferred.

There is another observation that strongly suggests that the NO/ONOO⁻ cycle in ALS has additional elements. It has been shown that the RNA encoding the important transporter for glutamate in the brains of ALS sufferers is misspliced, leading the production of a less functional transporter.[300-302] This produces increased NMDA activity as well as activity of other glutamate receptors in ALS, thus producing still more nitric oxide and peroxynitrite. It is not clear what causes this missplicing or whether this occurs in many other neurologic diseases, but it has been reported to occur in epilepsy as well as in ALS.[302] Clearly, if this missplicing is a consequence of the NO/ONOO⁻ cycle, it follows that it is part of the vicious cycle itself in ALS.

Summary: Parkinson's, Alzheimer's, and ALS

These three neurodegenerative diseases resemble the four multisystem illnesses in two key respects: Both groups of diseases show a common pattern of initiation of cases via a short-term stressor followed by chronic illness; in addition, many of the specific stressors known or suspected to be involved in the three neurodegenerative diseases are the same as stressors implicated in the multisystem illnesses. Such stressors as organic solvent exposure, organophosphorus/carbamate, or organochlorine pesticide exposure and head trauma are implicated in both sets of diseases. These similarities suggest that they may all share a common etiology. Other stressors known or suspected to initiate these neurodegenerative diseases are also linked to nitric oxide and to other elements of our vicious cycle via well-documented mechanisms.

There are several additional key properties of these neurodegenerative diseases that are consistent with the NO/ONOO⁻ cycle mechanism. They show elevated levels of most of the elements of our vicious cycle in the chronic phase of illness. Many of these vicious cycle elements appear to have causal roles based both on animal model data and on data from therapy in humans. The apoptotic cell death found in each of them may be a consequence of elevated peroxynitrite levels. Most importantly, a series of tissue specific correlates of these illnesses are each linked to one or more elements in our vicious cycle. These include dopamine metabolism, parkin inactivation and Lewy body formation in Parkinson's disease, β-amyloid protein formation and action and tau protein hyperphosphorylation in Alzheimer's disease, neurofilament aggregates and misspliced glutamate transporter RNA in ALS. β-Amyloid protein appears to be part of the NO/ONOO⁻ cycle, and several other of these tissue-specific correlates may also be tissue-specific parts of the cycle. It is the linkage of so many of these specific correlates with elements of the NO/ONOO⁻ cycle that provides the most compelling evidence suggesting that these three neurodegenerative diseases are viable candidates for inclusion under the tenth paradigm.

THERAPEUTIC AGENTS FOR MS, PARKINSON'S, ALZHEIMER'S, AND ALS: ROLE IN DOWN-REGULATION OF THE NO/ONOO⁻ CYCLE

These four diseases, multiple sclerosis, and the three neurodegenerative diseases, Parkinson's disease, Alzheimer's disease, and ALS are all major diseases. Consequently, there have been fairly extensive studies of potential therapies and therapeutic approaches to their treatment may be analyzed to determine if they may be predicted to down-regulate the NO/ ONOO⁻ cycle. Clearly, where such down-regulation is predicted, that provides support for a possible NO/ONOO⁻ cycle etiology. While some therapies are aimed at lowering the consequences of illness, such as providing DOPA or, alternatively, dopamine agonists to treat Parkinson's disease, others, some of which are discussed in Chapter 15, may well act to lower NO/ONOO⁻ cycle mechanisms.

SUMMARIZING OTHER POSSIBLE EXAMPLES OF THE NITRIC OXIDE/PEROXYNITRITE VICIOUS CYCLE PARADIGM

I have presented 12 examples in this chapter of diseases/illnesses that may be explained by the NO/ONOO⁻ cycle paradigm, and two additional examples (irritable bowel syndrome and asthma) are presented in earlier chapters. These are each distinct from and in addition to the four multi-system illnesses that are the main focus of this book. It is interesting that, with the possible exception of MS, none of these 14 appears to be a candidate for inclusion under any of the earlier nine paradigms listed in Exhibit 14.1, but one can make at least a superficial case that each may fit under what I am calling the tenth paradigm. Even such a superficial case should make this tenth paradigm of greatly increased interest.

Of these 14 possible candidates, nine of them may be viewed as examples where a specific tissue or region of the body is impacted, possibly leading to its distinctive features (tinnitus, MS, Sudeck's atrophy, chronic whiplash injury, ALS, Parkinson's disease, Alzheimer's disease, asthma, and irritable bowel syndrome). There may be many other diseases/illnesses that may fit in this category under the tenth paradigm, but not considered in this book, given the many different tissues that may be impacted by this biochemistry. Others of the 14 differentiate themselves primarily by their being initiated by a characteristic stressor (postradiation syndrome, overtraining syndrome, and silicone implant associated syndrome). Postherpetic pain syndrome may differ from other illnesses both by having a specific stressor, herpes reactivation and specific tissue impact. One of these illnesses appears to be characterized by the state in the life cycle in which it is initiated (autism and, more generally, autistic spectrum disorders). Of these 14, it is my view that the best case for inclusion under the tenth paradigm are probably for tinnitus, MS, asthma, Alzheimer's, Parkinson's, and autism, but substantial cases may be made for several of the others. On the other hand, there are several where there is little biochemical data on the chronic phase of these illnesses but where the NO/ONOO⁻ cycle paradigm is attractive in part because of the lack of viable alternatives to explain the short-term stressor—chronic illness pattern (most notably Sudeck's atrophy, silicone implant associated syndrome, and chronic whiplash-associated syndrome).

If we can develop an approach to therapy that effectively down-regulates the proposed biochemistry and physiology of the NO/ONOO⁻ cycle and is effective in the treatment of the four multisystem illnesses, then the same therapy may be effective in treatment of these other 14 as well.

OVERALL PERSPECTIVE: THE TENTH PARADIGM

In Chapter 11, I discussed the reported prevalence of the multisystem illnesses and how their impact on human health appears to argue for the importance of the NO/ONOO⁻ cycle mechanism. If one compares this proposed paradigm with others listed in Exhibit 14.1, it may well be as important as fourth, behind only infectious disease, ischemic cardiovascular disease, and somatic mutation/selection (cancer). Such a fourth position can be supported simply based on its proposed role in explaining the etiology of the four multisystem illnesses, their prevalence, and the impact of these illnesses on human health. If even half of the 14 additional diseases/illnesses described here fall under this paradigm, the impact of this paradigm may be all the more impressive. And, as I have already stated, there may be others in addition to the 14 that should be considered for possible inclusion.

If half or more of the 14 are eventually determined to fall under this paradigm, then its role in producing an explanation for a *diversity of illnesses* will also be impressive. In terms of diversity of possible roles, the tenth paradigm may be exceeded only by infectious diseases and genetic diseases and rivaled only by autoimmune diseases.

The progression of thought in this chapter is a common one in the history of science. When one looks at areas that do not fit under established paradigms, it is the lack of fit that forces one to consider new explanatory models that may become established as new paradigms. Certainly, the previously unexplained nature of the multisystem illnesses is such that they should drive the search for such new explanatory models. Having come up with a proposed new paradigm, one often follows by asking where else that paradigm may provide enlightening explanations. That is what I tried to do in considering these fourteen diseases and illnesses.

In Chapter 3, I introduced four considerations that each favored this paradigm of human disease, and it is instructive to revisit them in the light of the proposed roles presented in this chapter.

- It is *integrative:* It integrates into a common scheme a wide variety of previously unexplained diseases/illnesses.
- It is *comprehensive:* It encompasses a wide variety of observations about these illnesses including their patterns of case initiation, both their common and unique symptoms and signs, their chronic nature, and many of the correlates of the chronic phase of these diseases.
- It is *parsimonious:* It explains by a relatively simple conceptual framework many previously unexplained observations.
- It is *fundamental:* Because it is based primarily at the biochemical level, it explains much of the complexity of these diseases through the impact of a common biochemistry on a variety of organismal functions.

Chapter 15

Therapy

TAKE-HOME LESSONS

The fifth principle of the NO/ONOO$^-$ cycle explanatory model is that diseases caused by the cycle are best treated by using agents that are expected to down-regulate NO/ONOO$^-$ cycle biochemistry. At least 30 therapeutic agents or classes of agents are available today that are expected to down-regulate cycle biochemistry. Of these 30, clinical trial studies on chronic fatigue syndrome (CFS), multiple chemical sensitivity (MCS), and/or fibromyalgia (FM) have been performed on 12, and all 12 show evidence of efficacy in treatment of these multisystem diseases or closely related illnesses. Clinical observations and/or anecdotal reports suggest that six additional agents or classes of agents are also effective in treatment. None of these reach the effectiveness of a "magic bullet," providing, in most cases, only modest improvements. Given the complexity of the NO/ONOO$^-$ cycle, this is not surprising. The question that must be raised is whether combinations of several types of these agents will be more effective than individual agents alone.

Five physicians have independently developed therapy protocols using from 14 to 18 agents or classes of agents predicted to lower the cycle biochemistry. All five report substantial improvements in their patients. The patients involved in these therapies suffer from CFS, FM, or chemical injury or unexplained chronic fatigue, and each of these types of patients show apparent substantial improvement. Two of these protocols have been tested and reported to be effective in clinical trials. It appears, therefore, that complex combinations of these agents are more effective than single agents in the treatment of these diseases.

Explaining "Unexplained Illnesses"
© 2007 by The Haworth Press, Inc. All rights reserved.
doi:10.1300/5139_15

It appears that the NO/ONOO⁻ cycle mechanism makes useful predictions on what combinations of agents are likely to be effective in the therapy of multisystem diseases.

These various trials, clinical observations, and anecdotal reports suggest that these diseases may be effectively treated by down-regulating NO/ONOO⁻ cycle biochemistry. We may be on the verge of a new era of effective therapy of this group of diseases, focusing on treatment of the underlying biochemistry rather than on symptomatic relief.

INTRODUCTION

According to our explanatory model, it is the complexity of the NO/ONOO⁻ cycle that makes treatment of these multisystem diseases so difficult. We do not have a magic bullet to treat these illnesses because of that complexity. The complexity contributes to the robustness of the etiologic mechanism, making it inherently difficult to down-regulate. In addition, although there are multiple compounds that act to scavenge peroxynitrite, the most central element in the cycle, none of them, individually or perhaps even collectively, work well enough to lower its action in vivo sufficiently to effectively prevent damage. I will suggest one possible future drug that may eventually approach magic bullet status. However, my main hope, and I think it is a promising one, is that by using a variety of agents to down-regulate the NO/ONOO⁻ cycle, we may be able to lower the cycle in multiple ways, thus producing major improvements in those suffering from these illnesses and, in some cases lowering the etiology to insignificance. This is the approach that needs to be taken to effectively treat these illnesses, in my judgement, and I am hopeful it will lead to effective treatment in many cases and possibly to a cure in some.

A number of prominent physicians have approached therapy for the multisystem diseases by treating with combinations of agents, many of which may be expected to down-regulate aspects of the NO/ONOO⁻ cycle.* These include Drs. Paul Cheney (North Carolina), Grace Ziem (Maryland), Scott Rigden (Arizona), Jacob Teitelbaum (Maryland), Sarah Myhill (United Kingdom), Gordon Baker (Washington State), David Buscher (Washington State), and Nash Petrovic (South Africa). The clinical observations of each of them suggest that combinations of agents acting to down-regulate various aspect of the cycle may be more effective than are individual agents.

---

*I am not trying to suggest that this is the reason that they have used these agents.

I will discuss a large number of individual agents before discussing what combinations may be "best guesses" for effective treatment. My own view is that we need to perform a number of clinical trials on these best guesses in order to determine their relative and absolute merits and it is tragic that foundations funding research on these illnesses have been unwilling or unable to fund such trials. Two recent reviews of "alternative" treatments for CFS[1,2] discuss quite a number of nutritional supplements that may be viewed as down-regulating the NO/ONOO⁻ cycle.

I ask the reader to keep four cautions in mind. First, I am a PhD, not an MD, and nothing in this chapter or elsewhere in this book should be viewed as medical advice. Second, this chapter is not an overall review of therapy of these illnesses, but rather is focused on agents that may act to lower aspects of the NO/OONO- cycle. Many of the therapeutic approaches taken to date have focused on symptomatic relief rather than lowering the etiology of the multisystem diseases. Third, in this chapter I will refer not only to placebo-controlled and open-lable trials but also to clinical observations and anecdotal evidence of individual sufferers. Such clinical observations and anecdotal evidence are correctly viewed as much less reliable sources of information than are data from trials, particularly placebo-controlled, double-blind trials. Because we are in need of hints from whatever source, I will discuss some clinical observations and anecdotal evidence, but I urge the reader to approach them with a high level of skepticism. The fourth caution is that, although I will discuss many different approaches to lowering the NO/ONOO⁻ cycle biochemistry, there are still others that may well be worth considering. The fact that something is not discussed here does not necessarily mean it may not be worth considering.

Most of the trials and observations suggesting effectiveness of specific agents involve CFS or FM, but with some fewer involving multiple chemical sensitivity (MCS). Therapy for post-traumatic stress disorder (PTSD) has focused on psychotherapy rather than on what I would suggest is its underlying biochemistry, so my neglect of therapy of PTSD in this chapter reflects the medical literature.

AVOIDING EXACERBATION

Physicians are urged, as part of the Hippocratic Oath, to, first, do no harm. This is also excellent advice for those who suffer from multisystem diseases, however difficult it may be to to follow this advice in practice. I have argued elsewhere that many stressors act to up-regulate the basic NO/ONOO⁻ cycle biochemistry of these diseases and act, therefore, to exacerbate not just the symptoms but also their underlying cause. There are five specific stressors that should be avoided to avoid exacerbating these diseases:

1. MCS patients should avoid, wherever possible, exposure to the chemicals that produce sensitivity responses, because such chemicals probably act to up-regulate the NO/ONOO⁻ cycle. Because such chemical exposure is produced by so many different environments, this is often very difficult to accomplish. One of many approaches is that many MCS sufferers eat mainly or only organic foods in order to avoid pesticide and other chemical exposure in their foods.

2. CFS sufferers need to avoid excessive exercise, to prevent the exacerbation through "postexertional malaise" which I have also argued upregulates the cycle biochemistry. This advice may be difficult to follow. For the most severely affected sufferers, very little such exercise may trigger postexertional malaise.

3. Many sufferers from all four of these diseases have food allergies. It is important to avoid these food allergens. I argued in Chapter 3 that this is likely to be because antibody-antigen reactions on exposure to such allergens, increase nitric oxide levels. Some physicians have put patients on a hypoallergenic diet and slowly added specific foods to determine which are well tolerated and which are not.[3] Among the allergens that many of these sufferers react to are wheat, dairy, eggs, soy, and corn (maize) products, all common dietary constituents.

4. Avoiding excitotoxins is a fourth area that may be important to "do no harm." Smith et al.[4] reported that some of their FM patients became completely asymptomatic if they avoided foods containing monosodium glutamate (MSG) and aspartame. Both of these are excitotoxins, containing glutamate;* and aspartate, respectively, and may act therefore to stimulate the NMDA receptors. Because other mixtures such as hydrolyzed vegetable protein and some things described as natural flavorings also contain substantial amounts of glutamate and aspartate, they should be avoided as well, according to Smith et al.[4] and Blaylock.[5] There have not been reports of other studies of MSG/

---

*Some have argued that, because there is limited transport of glutamate and aspartate through the blood-brain barrier, there will be little or no damage from these compounds in the brain. However, there is evidence we discussed earlier on the permeabilization of the blood-brain barrier in the multisystem diseases and even limited transport may produce excitotoxicity if the concentrations of these compounds rise precipitously.

excitoxin elimination in these diseases, to my knowledge, although the MCS patients are reported to be sensitive to MSG.[6] My feeling is that people suffering from any of these multisystem diseases should avoid these food additives whenever possible to avoid exacerbating the NO/ONOO⁻ cycle.

5. People suffering from PTSD are especially sensitive to psychological stress but others suffering from multisystem diseases may also be well advised to avoid such stress.

In general, then, all five of these factors are ones that may up-regulate the NO/ONOO⁻ cycle biochemistry and are to be avoided whenever possible, as a prelude to additional therapy.

GENERAL CONSIDERATIONS

According to our etiologic theory, therapy should be focused on the elements of the NO/ONOO⁻ cycle, on the positive feedback loops that maintain the cycle, and on important consequences of the cycle. These include excessive levels of nitric oxide, superoxide, peroxynitrite, intracellular calcium and inflammatory cytokines as well as excessive activity of the NMDA and vanilloid receptors and of NF-κB and substantial oxidative damage to mitochondrial components and to other membranes leading to selective loss of both omega-3 and omega-6 fatty acids. Each of the therapeutic approaches will be an attempt to down-regulate one or more of these aspects, so we will be returning to these different aspects repeatedly. The uncoupling of the nitric oxide synthases due to tetrahydrobiopterin depletion, as discussed in Chapter 12, may also be an important target to be minimized by therapy.

Studies of therapy of the multisystem diseases provide substantial support for the NO/ONOO⁻ cycle mechanism. Such observations are important because they strongly suggest that this etiologic theory provides useful suggestions for therapy. When I talked at the American Academy for Environmental Medicine in November 2003, there were several talks focused on therapy of MCS, CFS, and FM, using nutrients or conventional pharmaceuticals. Each of these could be interpreted in terms of down-regulating important aspects of the NO/ONOO⁻ cycle. Teitelbaum[7] talked about multiple therapeutic agents where responses are consistent with the cycle mechanism, including betaine, magnesium, α-lipoic acid, vitamin B_{12} injections, or sublingual treatment, *N*-acetyl cysteine, fish oil, vitamin C, grape seed extract, zinc, acetyl-L-carnitine, selenium, *Ginkgo biloba* extract, cat's claw, riboflavin, feverfew, and coenzyme Q10; Nicolson[8] talked about a therapy designed to reverse the mitochondrial damage in these illnesses, damage that I have argued may be caused by peroxynitrite, superoxide and nitric oxide; Gerdes[9] talked about the use of fish oil, nebulized glutathione and magnesium for treatment; Krop[10] talked about the possible use of tetracyclines, compounds that may act as both antioxidants and as antiinflammatory agents; Rea[11] talked about the use of hyperbaric oxygen therapy, a therapy that may act by improving oxidative phosphorylation despite mitochondrial deficiencies; Ionescu[12] talked about antioxidant therapy, designed to lower the oxidative damage possibly produced by peroxynitrite; LaCava[13] talked about using α-lipoic acid as a therapeutic agent for these illnesses, presumably acting as an important antioxidant; and Block[14] talked about magnesium therapy, with magnesium possibly acting to lower excessive NMDA activity. It can be seen from this that each of these eight talks on therapy using nutritional components, herbal medicines, and/or conventional pharmaceuticals can be interpreted as being consistent with the predictions of the NO/ONOO$^-$ cycle mechanism.

ANTIOXIDANT THERAPY:
A CRITIQUE OF CURRENT PRACTICES

Many of the approaches to treatment that I will discuss are centered on antioxidant therapy. However, the literature on antioxidant therapy is filled with therapy protocols that, in my judgment, are flawed. Let me give you some examples.

Many such trials have used high doses of synthetic α-tocopherol, to try to produce a favorable clinical response. Synthetic α-tocopherol is composed of eight distinct forms of vitamin E, each found in equal amounts. Only one of these eight forms is found in natural vitamin E, that being identical to natural α-tocopherol. Natural vitamin E is also composed of eight different forms found in differing amounts depending on the source, termed α-tocopherol, β-tocopherol, γ-tocopherol, and δ-tocopherol and, in addition, α-tocotrienol, β-tocotrienol, γ-tocotrienol, and δ-tocotrienol. It has been shown that high doses of either synthetic or natural α-tocopherol have the effect of lowering the levels in the body of the other tocopherols[15-18] and may also be expected lower tocotrienols, although this has not been studied. The mechanism involved is the induction of an enzyme by high levels α-tocopherol, which degrades not only other tocopherols, but also tocotrienols.[19,20] It follows that if the β, γ, or δ-tocopherols or probably any of the tocotrienols have any important functions in the body not shared by α-tocopherol, high-dose α-tocopherol supplements may make the body deficient in these functions. It has been reported that γ-tocopherol has some special antioxidant roles and that one of them is in scavenging breakdown products of peroxynitrite, especially NO_2 radical.[21-23] It follows that high-dose α-tocopherol therapy may make the body more susceptible to peroxynitrite-mediated damage, rather than less susceptible. Furthermore, it has been argued that tocotrienols are particularly important in protecting the brain from oxidative damage, being more active than tocopherols in protection from glutamate-induced neurotoxicity and possibly mitochondrial oxidative damage.[24-26]

The other issue regarding synthetic α-tocopherol is that it is possible that some of the seven unnatural forms may have some negative effect in the body. I am unaware of any literature arguing for such negative effects, but absence of evidence in not the same as evidence of absence. In any case, you may be aware of a number of clinical trials using high dose synthetic α-tocopherol, reporting no improvement in symptoms and signs with various illnesses. These have led to headlines trumpeting that vitamin E fails to improve symptoms of . . . or fails to lower the incidence of. . . . Such headlines are misleading in that they assume that all forms of vitamin E are interchangeable, differing only in their biological potency as antioxidants. My own view is that scientific studies should stop using the term vitamin E to describe such results but rather they should be described in terms of the form or forms of tocopherol and/or tocotrienol used; other combinations may produce different results. I specifically think that vitamin E used to treat these multisystem diseases should be natural vitamin E, containing γ-tocopherol to minimize peroxynitrite-mediated damage and possibly tocotrienols to minimize brain and mitochondrial damage.

There are additional potential criticisms of the antioxidant trial literature. Antioxidants such as tocopherols, vitamin C, and flavonoids all act primarily as what are known as chain breaking antioxidants, reacting with free radicals* which become nonradicals, but the antioxidants themselves are converted into free radicals. The radical produced by such reactions

---

*You may recall that free radicals all have unpaired electrons, often designated by a dot. These chain-breaking antioxidants all act to donate an electron to the free radical, but in the process the antioxidant molecule becomes a free radical itself. The consequence is that it essential that the chain breaking antioxidant be able to be converted into a nonradical by a subsequent reaction, because if it does not, it may react with molecular oxygen to generate more rather than less oxidative damage.

must itself be converted into a nonradical to stop the radical biochemistry.* Generally, this conversion involves other antioxidants, as shown in Figure 15.1. Additional antioxidants, not shown in Figure 15.1, can also be involved in conversion to nonradicals, regenerating the original antioxidant, such as dihydrolipoic acid (derived from α-lipoic) and a variety of flavonoids. This role of antioxidants in the regeneration of others means that multiple antioxidants may have synergistic effects in avoiding oxidative stress.

One of the other criticisms I have of the antioxidant trial literature is that many trials have been done with the three "antioxidant vitamins," vitamin E, vitamin C, and β-carotene (vitamin A). It makes no sense, in my judgment, to pick these three out of the much larger spectrum of antioxidants for such trials. For one thing, the reason that two of them are considered vitamins has nothing to do with their antioxidant activity. Vitamin C is a vitamin because of its role in the metabolism of the important protein collagen, not because of its antioxidant properties. β-carotene is a vitamin because it is a precursor of retinoic acid (vitamin A), not because of its antioxidant properties. β-carotene is a member of a larger group of antioxidant micronutrients, the carotenoids, several of which are more active in antioxidant properties than is β-carotene. It is true that vitamin C (ascorbate) helps regenerate vitamin E (tocopherol), as indicated in Figure 15.1, and it is definitely useful to use with forms of vitamin E because of this, but this is not a property unique to vitamin C.

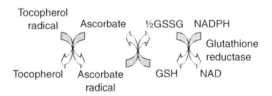

FIGURE 15.1. Regeneration of antioxidant radicals to antioxidants by reduced glutathione. Oxidized glutathione is reduced to reduced glutathione by glutathione peroxidase and NADPH. It, in turn, can regenerate ascorbate radicals to ascorbate, and ascorbate can regenerate tocopherol radicals to tocopherol. Other antioxidants, not shown here, can also be involved in these coupled, sequential antioxidant regeneration reactions, including reduced α-lipoic acid and flavonoids.

---

*Failure to convert a radical such as tocopheryl radical, derived from vitamin E or ascorbyl radical derived from vitamin C, to a nonradical can lead to a net increase in the radical biochemistry rather than a decrease. In other words, an antioxidant can have prooxidant effects, producing more oxidative damage rather than less.

There are other types of potentially synergistic interactions among antioxidants.

- Some have special properties not shared by others, such as in the ability to relatively efficiently scavenge singlet oxygen or peroxynitrite.
- Some act best in lipids such as in biological membranes but others act best in water and some can traverse both types of regions. When oxidative reactions involve both lipids and water, a common pattern, it makes sense to use more than one type of antioxidant.
- Clearly if a particular type of antioxidant is depleted in these multisystem diseases, then it makes sense to supplement with that type to restore the antioxidant pools. Many antioxidants get depleted under conditions of oxidative stress, so it makes sense to supplement (replete) them.
- Many antioxidants act to lower NF-κB activity and thus may have a role in lowering a key element in the NO/ONOO⁻ cycle.

Most of the antioxidant clinical trials have used high doses of individual antioxidants and such high doses are reported to have potential pro-oxidant effects, producing the opposite response from what is desired. Such pro-oxidant responses may be due in part to the generation of free radicals from these potential antioxidants while failing to provide adequate support for the regeneration of these free radicals back to their active antioxidant forms.

There is some empirical evidence showing the combinations of antioxidants can be effective where individual antioxidants are ineffective. Examples of this have been reported in the treatment of age-related macular degeneration, the most common form of untreatable blindness in older people. The progression of age-related macular degeneration can be effectively slowed with combinations of antioxidants,[27-32] whereas high doses of α-tocopherol alone are ineffective.[33]

So there are good arguments for constructing antioxidant clinical trials using complex mixtures of antioxidants and much of my approach here is to suggest classes of antioxidants that are good candidates for such trials, based on the known biochemistry of the elements of the NO/ONOO⁻ cycle. Logan and Wong[1] previously suggested similar complex mixtures of antioxidants for the treatment of CFS.

Antioxidants and NF-κB Activity

Many different "chain breaking" antioxidants as well as some other antioxidants have been shown to lower NF-κB activity, and this is expected to be useful in down-regulating the NO/ONOO⁻ cycle. NF-κB activity has been shown to be lowered by reduced glutathione and precursors of reduced glutathione, such as *N*-acetyl cysteine, by α-lipoic acid, by vitamin C, by α-tocopherol, by numerous phenolic antioxidants including various flavonoids, and by selenium.[34-42] Given the proposed importance of elevated NF-κB activity to the NO/ONOO⁻ cycle, these antioxidants may play a substantial role in lowering cycle activity.

Vitamin C (Ascorbate or Ascorbic Acid)

Vitamin C is an important water-soluble, chain-breaking antioxidant that is important for antioxidant therapy. My own view is that megadose vitamin C therapy may be counterproductive under certain circumstances and doses on the order of 250 mg/day may be more optimal in the treatment of these multisystem diseases. Vitamin C can act to regenerate tetrahydrobiopterin (BH4) and may act, therefore, to lower nitric oxide synthase uncoupling, another useful property. The only published clinical studies of vitamin C in these diseases were the two studies of Kodama et al.[43,44] who reported symptom improvement in CFS patients after infusion of high-dose vitamin C, and a study by Heuser and Vojdani in MCS patients,[45] showing improved immune function after vitamin C treatment.

Coenzyme Q10

Coenzyme Q10 (also known as ubiquinone or ubiquinol 10) has important functions in mitochondia and has been used as a nutritional supplement to improve mitochondrial function in a number of diseases characterized by mitochondrial dysfunction.[46-50] It is reported to have important effects both because of its role in basic mitochondrial function (in the electron transport chain) and its antioxidant activity. Several of the protective effects of coenzyme Q10 can be interpreted as being due to its scavenging of peroxynitrite breakdown products, thus leading to protection from peroxynitrite-mediated damage. For example, Lisdero et al.[51] (p. 69) state that "we have shown that increasing ubiquinol content clearly protects mitochondria from ONOO⁻ effects." In an earlier study, Schopfer et al.[52] (p. 35) showed that "Ubiquinol protected against peroxynitrite-mediated nitration of tyrosine residues in . . . mitochondrial membranes." Two sentences further down they state that "Increase in membrane-bound ubiquinol partially prevented the loss of mitochondrial respiratory function induced by peroxynitrite." The effects of coenzyme Q10 on the production and toxicity of superoxide have been mixed, with both increases and decreases being reported.[53]

An overall protective role for coenzyme Q10 has been reported in Parkinson's disease[54] and amyotrophic lateral sclerosis (ALS),[55] as well as in chemically induced neurological damage,[56] suggested that it may be protective in the related multisystem illnesses as well. Dr. David Bell[57] reports that it produces modest improvements in CFS patients, and I am aware of anecdotal reports of both modest and more substantial improvements in CFS. Lister[58] reported that coenzyme Q10 given along with Ginkgo biloba extract produced improvement in most of the FM patients studied in an open pilot study.

Coenzyme Q10 has been found to be very well tolerated in various clinical trials.[46-50,54-56,58] Because it may act to increase energy metabolism and thus down-regulate excessive NMDA activity, to scavenge peroxynitrite or its products and to have other helpful antioxidant effects, coenzyme Q10 may be expected to down-regulate the NO/ONOO⁻ cycle in three distinct ways. Coenzyme Q10 may be one of the most promising agents for treatment of multisystem illnesses, despite the fact that there have been no placebo-controlled trials studying its effects. Anecdotal reports suggest it should be taken in the morning or at mid-day, because evening doses may act to make sleeping more difficult.

Selenium

The element selenium is considered an antioxidant primarily because certain proteins that contain selenium have antioxidant functions. It has been reported that people with fibromyalgia tend to have low selenium levels[59] and Dr. Paul Cheney and Dr. Grace Ziem have found that many of their CFS and chemically sensitive patients are also low in selenium. It may be the case that multisystem illness patients in general tend to be low in selenium. Because selenoproteins have several important functions that may be deficient in such patients, it makes sense to use selenium supplements to replete their selenium pools.

Selenium only occurs in a few proteins in mammals, of which about 15 have been characterized. Four of these are selenoenzymes called glutathione peroxidases that get rid of peroxide oxidants in the cell. Others are deiodinases that are essential in making the hormone T3, the most active hormone originating in the thyroid gland. Because many people with multisystem illnesses appear to have low thyroid hormone activity, one way of improving their thyroid function may be to give them selenium supplements.

Many organic selenium compounds act as relatively strong peroxynitrite scavengers,[60] and some selenoproteins, especially a protein known as selenoprotein P,[61] act as peroxynitrite scavengers. Selenoprotein P also acts to provide selenium to many of the cells of the body[62] and is consequently an important protein in selenium nutrition. It is known that the body requires relatively high amounts of selenium in order to synthesize maximal amounts of selenoprotein P; so it follows that selenium supplements may be important in providing optimal peroxynitrite scavenging activity through the action of selenoprotein P.

Probably the best form of selenium to use as such a supplement is selenomethionine. Selenium-grown yeast, where most of the selenium is in the form of selenomethionine is also a good form for people who do not have a yeast allergy. Selenomethionine itself is a good peroxynitrite scavenger[60] as well a serving as a precursor of selenoproteins.

Selenium has also been reported to improve mood,[63] and so may be useful in lowering symptoms of depression in those suffering from these multisystem diseases.

Carotenoids As Peroxynitrite Scavengers

Carotenoids are a group of natural pigments, mostly derived from plant sources, that have unique antioxidant properties. While they act poorly as chain-breaking antioxidants, they are very active in scavenging singlet oxygen and also are quite active in scavenging peroxynitrite.[64-70] There are over 600 carotenoids that have been studied chemically, of which about a dozen are found in the human diet in sufficient quantities to be potentially physiologically important. Of these, β-carotene, lycopene (the red pigment found in tomatoes, red grapefruit, and watermelon), and lutein are the most common, making up about 60 to 70 percent of the carotenoids in the human diet. Carotenoids are yellow, orange, or red pigments that are lipid (oil or fat)-soluble, and they are absorbed most efficiently when consumed dissolved in fats. While β-carotene has been the most commonly studied, lycopene is reported to be considerably more active than β-carotene as a peroxynitrite scavenger. Lutein and its close chemical cousin zeaxanthin, may also have special roles in peroxynitrite scavenging because their chemical structure causes them to traverse biological membranes, and so they may have a special role in protecting membranes from peroxynitrite-mediated damage.

Carotenoids have been of substantial medical interest because of their properties in lowering carcinogenesis in animal models and the extensive epidemiological evidence that they may also do so in humans. However, two clinical trials using very-high-dose β-carotene supplements in smokers produced increased incidences of lung cancer rather than the expected decrease. This has led many to back away from the use of β-carotene supplements. My own view, which has been supported by subsequent studies, is that this is another example where single antioxidants when used at doses far above any likely physiological range, may produce negative effects whereas the more modest doses, particularly when used with other antioxidants, may have favorable effects.

Flavonoids

Flavonoids are a very large class of plant phenolic antioxidants, many of which may be expected to down-regulate aspects of the NO/ONOO⁻ cycle. One class of these flavonoids the anthocyanidins, has been reported to lead to improvements in FM[71] in a placebo-controlled trial and the flavonoid-containing *Ginkgo* extract was also reported to produce favorable responses when used along with coenzyme Q10 to a group of FM patients.[58] Flavonoids are also reported to produce improvements in a mouse model of CFS.[72,73] So, this may be another example where clinical trial data provide some support for the view that agents predicted to lower NO/ONOO⁻ cycle activity may be useful therapeutic agents.

Flavonoids are known to lower NF-κB activity, act as potent chain-breaking antioxidants, and have roles in regenerating other chain-breaking antioxidants after they have been converted to free radicals. Flavonoids can also act as chelators for free iron, protecting the cell from oxidative damage produced from such free iron. My own focus has been to look at flavonoids that are known to scavenge peroxynitrite and superoxide and have relatively modest pro-oxidant activities with the notion that these properties of certain flavonoids may make them good candidates as therapeutic agents in the treatment of multisystem diseases.

Most flavonoids are soluble in water, although many also have substantial solubility in lipids, as well. This allows many of them to act as antioxidants in both aqueous (water) and lipid regions of the body (the latter includes membranes). There are thousands of flavonoids and they typically fall into six classes. One of those classes is made up of the anthocyanin pigments, such as anthocyanidins and proanthocyanidins, which are colored red, purple or blue and can be detected because of their color. If plant tissue is colored purplish as in red cabbage, plums, red grapes, and many berries, for example, this is usually due to the presence of anthocyanin pigments. Many other flavonoids have a pale yellow color. There are many areas of scientific inquiry where our knowledge of flavonoids is distinctly limited. Which are best absorbed from foods? Many of the flavonoids are conjugated to sugars, but many of these may be modified in bacteria in the gastrointestinal (GI) tract, but how extensive such modifications may be and what their physiological consequences may be is still largely unexplored. How different flavonoids concentrate into different tissues in the body is largely unknown.

There is a large literature showing that a variety of flavonoids act as peroxynitrite scavengers and as superoxide scavengers, and some of them, at least, also act as nitric oxide scavengers. Two studies reviewed the activity of fairly diverse flavonoids as peroxynitrite scavengers,[60,74] and a large number of studies have focused on specific plant extracts or specific flavonoid chemicals. A green tea flavonoid,[75] citrus flavonoid,[76] and one[77] or several components of dark-colored grapes, and grape seed extract[78] are reported to act as peroxynitrite scavengers. *Ginkgo biloba* extract flavonoids are reported to scavenge peroxynitrite,[79] have long been known to be strong superoxide scavengers,[80] and are reported to also scavenge nitric oxide.[81]

Green tea flavonoids have not only been shown to scavenge peroxynitrite,[75] but also superoxide[83-85] and nitric oxide.[85] Soy and olive extracts have been shown to scavenge superoxide,[86,87] as have hawthorn extracts.[88] Anthocyanin pigments from blueberry and purple/black rice are potent superoxide scavengers.[89]

There are still other activities reported for flanonoids that may be predicted to influence the NO/ONOO⁻ cycle activity. A number of flavonoids have been reported to inhibit xanthine oxidase activity.[90] The xanthine oxidase inhibition will not only lower the generation of superoxide by one such mechanism (predicted to be favorable) but also may lower the generation of uric acid from purines (predicted to be unfavorable). The flavonoid silymarin from milk thistle extract not only scavenges peroxynitrite but also is reported to increase the synthesis of the enzyme superoxide dismutase,[60] both being potentially favorable effects.

Given the many different flavonoids with potentially NO/ONOO⁻ cycle down-regulation activity, it is difficult to determine what combination of these may be most effective in the treatment of multisystem diseases. My own feeling is that combinations of flavonoids with both relatively high scavenging activity in vitro and a long history of safety, relatively low cost, ability to produce improvements in central nervous system diseases, and efficacy in humans and animal models for the treatment other diseases are to be preferred as potential agents to treat multisystem diseases.

One of the properties of flavonoids is that they are typically absorbed rapidly in foods but are also excreted rapidly by the kidneys. Because of this, they typically reach peak blood levels about two hours after consumption and, by four hours, have dropped to less than half of peak levels. Consequently, it may be desirable to consume flavonoids several times per day.

Reductive Stress—A Fascinating Puzzle

Those of you who are interested in looking at difficult puzzles may find this particularly interesting. Two Hungarians, Ghyczy and Boros (G & B), wrote a fascinating paper on what they call reductive stress—stress to cells caused by excessive amounts of the reductant NADH relative to its oxidized form NAD.[92] NADH is a reduced compound that introduces what are called reducing equivalents into the electron transport chain of the mitochondrion. It is needed for oxidative energy metabolism, generating energy in the form of ATP. While this is important in order to use oxygen to generate energy, an excessively high ratio of NADH/NAD causes problems that G & B have called reductive stress.[92] Reductive stress in not the opposite of oxidative stress; rather, it tends to cause oxidative stress.[92] Reductive stress occurs in diabetics or in alcoholics because of the generation of excessive reducing equivalents and therefore excessive NADH from excessive glucose sugar or excessive alcohol.[92] It can also be caused by oxygen deprivation of tissues, where there is insufficient oxygen to oxidize the NADH effectively. What G & B show in their review is that a group of chemically similar compounds, having methyl groups attached to positively charged nitrogens or sulfurs, helps by a still partially undefined mechanism to allay reductive stress. These methylated compounds include such compounds as choline and phosphatidyl choline, betaine, carnitine, and S-adenosyl methionine.[92] This pattern of activity suggests that these compounds act because of their chemistry to allay reductive stress because they all have chemical similarities, whereas the normal biochemistry of carnitine is distinct from the others. This raises an important question of how can these methylated compounds relieve reductive stress through their chemistry?

You may be wondering how reductive stress may be related to the multisystem illnesses? You may recall from Chapter 2 that peroxynitrite and to a lesser extent nitric oxide can act to lower the activity of the electron transport chain in the mitochondrion, and this will be expected, in turn, to produce reductive stress by lowering the ability of mitochondria to oxidize NADH. Is there evidence that reductive stress occurs in the multisystem illnesses? There is no direct evidence to my knowledge, but there is some indirect evidence.

Felipo and coworkers, scientists in Valencia Spain, have published a series of papers showing that a group of methylated compounds similar those discussed by G & B protected mammalian tissues from much of the toxicity caused by excessive NMDA activity.[93-97] Among the compounds studied by the Spanish group was D-carnitine, a biochemically inactive version of L-carnitine. The fact that D-carnitine was active in such protection provides convincing evidence that these compounds are acting because of their chemistry, not their biochemistry, because D-carnitine is biochemically inactive and even antagonizes the normal biochemistry of L-carnitine. Because excessive NMDA activity appears to be involved in the multisystem illnesses and because such excessive NMDA activity is a key element of the NO/ONOO⁻ cycle, I would expect reductive stress to occur in the multisystem diseases. These results suggest that any of these methylated compounds may be useful agents in the treatment of multisystem diseases.

Ghyczy and Boros and an additional collaborator published a paper in the prestigious *FASEB Journal,* reporting that mitochondria under reductive stress produced something that reacts with such methylated compounds to produce methane gas.[98] They argue that these methylated compounds are all chemically similar, containing electrophilic methyl groups, and that these methyl groups are reacting with some toxic compound generated by reductive stress, relieving much of the toxicity of reductive stress while producing methane gas as a product. We do not know yet what toxic compound in the mitochondria these methylated compounds may be reacting with.

Is there evidence that methylated electrophilic compounds are useful therapeutic agents in the treatment of multisystem illnesses? There is evidence in the case of FM and CFS that *S*-adenosyl methionine (sometimes abbreviated SAMe or SAM) is useful,[99] with five out of seven studies of *S*-adenosyl methionine treatment of FM patients reporting improved symptoms including lessened pain. I am aware of several anecdotal reports of improvement in CFS patients in response to *S*-adenosyl methionine, some of whom report it seems to be most effective taken in the morning. L-Carnitine[101] and the related compound acetyl-L-carnitine are reported to be useful in clinical studies.[102] The carnitine/acetyl carnitine are likely to involve an another mechanism in addition to relieving reductive stress and will be considered in the section of this chapter immediately following.

My best candidate among these electrophilic methylated compounds to be used as an agent to relieve reductive stress is the compound betaine,* also known as trimethylglycine. The reason that it is my best candidate, despite the fact that there is no clinical data on efficacy, is that it is cheap, it is found in high concentrations in common foods[100] such as marine shellfish, spinach, and beets (the name betaine comes from the scientific name for beet, *Beta vulgaris*). It is synthesized in the human body from choline and it can be used to generate *S*-adenosyl methionine in the body, but is much

---

*Betaine is pronounced *bay*-tah-een or *bee*-tah-een, but is often mispronounced *bee*-tayn.

more stable than and cheaper than *S*-adenosyl methionine. Betaine is often sold as trimethylglycine (TMG) and is also sold as betaine hydrochloride (or betaine HCl). This latter form, betaine hydrochloride, is sold to provide stomach acid for improved stomach function for people who are deficient in the production of stomach acid. It is not recommended to people with multisystem diseases unless those people are also deficient in stomach acid.

Carnitine and Acetyl-Carnitine

Clinical trial data show that carnitine and acetyl-carnitine may be useful in the treatment of multisystem diseases[101,102] as well as other clinical studies showing positive responses in other diseases. Aberrations of carnitine metabolism have been reported in CFS.[103,104] It is known that L-carnitine (the biologically active form of carnitine) has a special role in lowering what is known as the mitochondrial phase transition, with the phase transition leading, in turn, to apoptotic cell death. Thus, L-carnitine has a special protective role in mitochondria. Acetyl-L-carnitine, which is more active than L-carnitine[105] possibly for reasons that will be discussed shortly, has been shown to have both antioxidant effects in the mitochondrion and to have several other favorable effects.[105] The well-documented function of L-carnitine in the cell is to transport fatty acids from fats into the mitochondrion for subsequent oxidation, allowing the mitochodria to produce energy in the form of ATP from the oxidation of the fatty acids. It is difficult to see how this well-documented role could lead to lowered oxidative stress, improved general mitochondrial function and lowered mitochondrial membrane phase transition. It seems unlikely that the reductive stress puzzle, discussed earlier, is the main explanation either. So, how can we explain these favorable effects of L-carnitine or acetyl-L-carnitine supplementation?

The explanation may be due, in part, to a second potential consequence of transporting fatty acids into the mitochondrion. It is known that the inner mitochondrial membrane has a special lipid compound making up much of its structure called cardiolipin. The fatty acids making up much of the structure of cardiolipin are over 90 percent polyunsaturated omega-6 fatty acids.[106-108] This has two important consequences. First, it makes the cardiolipin unusually sensitive of oxidation (a process known as lipid peroxidation), thus destroying the structure of the cardiolipin and the integrity of the inner membrane. If the integrity of the inner membrane is destroyed, the ability of the mitochondrion to generate energy in the form of ATP is also destroyed. Because this oxidative sequence is presumably initiated by superoxide and because increased superoxide production by the mitochondrion is part of the NO/ONOO⁻ cycle mechanism, we can predict that increased cardiolipin oxidation will be found in multisystem diseases. The second important consequence of this biochemistry is that because all of these polyunsaturated fatty acids in humans must come from our foods because we are unable to synthesize them, they must be transported into the mitochondrion by L-carnitine in order to be used to regenerate the cardiolipin in the inner membrane. So, I would argue that the most likely interpretation of the favorable effects of L-carnitine here is to allow the transport of these fatty acids into the mitochondrion. This in turn, will allow increased cardiolipin levels and the restoration of the mitochondrial inner membrane integrity. That restoration may also be expected to lower superoxide production in the mitochondrion and thus have antioxidant effects.

There is one last puzzle to consider: Why is acetyl-L-carnitine more effective as a nutritional supplement than is L-carnitine?[109] The answer seems to be that most of the L-carnitine taken orally ends up in the urine, being excreted by the kidney before it can be transported into cells and specifically before it is transported through the blood-brain barrier. It is reported that acetyl-L-carnitine is transported more efficiently than is L-carnitine, allowing it to be used more efficiently.[109,110]

Other Approaches to Regenerating the Mitochondrial Inner Membrane

Nicolson and coworkers have published a number of clinical studies reporting that a proprietary mixture designed to allow regeneration of the mitochondrial inner membrane produces favorable clinical responses in a group of chronically fatigued patients[8,111,112] with substantially lessened fatigue, suggesting that this approach may be useful for CFS and other multisystem disease patients. The proprietary mixture contains phospholipids, glycolipids, and antioxidants. The phospholipids presumably act as precursors for the cardiolipin of the mitochondrial inner membrane, but it is not clear to me how the glycolipids may act. The phospholipids known to act as precursors of cardiolipin are found in lecithin, so that lecithin supplements* may be useful here.

Hydroxocobalamin (Vitamin B₁₂) and Other Approaches to Lowering Nitric Oxide

The use of hydroxocobalamin, a known nitric oxide scavenger, in lowering nitric oxide levels in multisystem diseases and the favorable responses

---

*Many multisystem disease patients are allergic to soy or egg products, so these should probably not use soy or egg lecithin supplements.

to such treatment was discussed in Chapter 6. I think this is one of the most promising approaches to treatment, although it again falls short of the magic bullet. The question is what approach should be used to raise hydroxocobalamin levels. The usual approach is to use intramuscular (IM) injections. However, hydroxocobalamin nasal spray is reported to give substantial therapeutic responses as well as substantial B_{12} blood levels,[113] presumably because the nasal mucosa are leaky, allowing efficient absorption of the hydroxocobalamin through that route. Alternatively, Dr. Grace Ziem with her chemically sensitive patients finds that inhaled, nebulized hydroxocobalamin is clinically effective in unpublished studies, again apparently because of the leakiness of the lung epithelia. The studies of using sublingual B_{12} have been mixed, with one suggesting somewhat improved uptake[114] but another showing no increase in sublingual B_{12} absorption compared with oral B_{12}.[115] So, the leakiness of the epithelia under the tongue may be insufficient to allow efficient B_{12} absorption via that route.

The absorption of B_{12} orally is limited by two factors. Intrinsic factor, the glycoprotein, which normally serves to increase B_{12} absorption in the GI tract, has limited capacity and thus is unable to allow efficient B_{12} absorption of high-dose supplements because its capacity is saturated at much lower levels. In addition, the GI tract epithelia are relatively tight, not allowing the efficient absorption of B_{12} over and above that absorbed through the action of intrinsic factor. It is estimated in the scientific literature that absorption independent of intrinsic factor is 1 percent or less of the total B_{12} ingested.

Folate (Folic Acid)

The B vitamin folate was suggested for CFS therapy by Werbach,[2] noting that high-dose folate was reported to be effective in the treatment of a group of patients with easy fatigability and minor neurological symptoms.[116] In contrast to this, a low-dose, short-term folate supplement study of CFS patients showed no significant improvement.[117] I am aware of a number of anecdotal reports where CFS patients stated that they experienced improved symptoms with folate supplements.

How might folate supplements be expected to produce improvements in multisystem disease patients? Folate is known to decrease the uncoupling of nitric oxide synthase (NOS) activity,[118-121] thus lowering the production of NOS-dependent superoxide that was discussed in Chapter 12. This decreases the production of peroxynitrite derived from NOS activity. Part of this activity of folate is through the action of 5-methyltetrahydrofolate, which acts, in turn, to regenerate tetrahydrobiopterin (BH4)[122-124] that has been oxidized by peroxynitrite (you may recall that the uncoupling of NOS activity is largely caused by BH4 depletion). An alternative mechanism has been supported by the work of Hyndman et al.[125] who reported that 5-methyltetrahydrofolate binds to the eNOS form of nitric oxide synthase in place of BH4, decreasing the enzyme uncoupling.

Are there any other ways to restore BH4 levels? BH4 (tetrahydrobiopterin) supplements have been used in a number of animal studies and in at least one human experimental study.[126] Another approach may be to use hydrogen peroxide, which is reported to induce increased BH4 synthesis but does not cause its degradation.[127] I have been skeptical about the use of hydrogen peroxide therapy for multisystem disease patients because of the damaging oxidative activity of hydrogen peroxide, but there may well be a positive response to hydrogen peroxide that may be worth considering.

Folate may have a special role in the treatment of patients who are unavoidably exposed to formaldehyde because its reduced form, tetrahydrofolate, can act to scavenge formaldehyde.

Before leaving the discussion of folate and multisystem diseases, I want to call your attention to an interesting pattern. I have suggested the use of three agents that are known to lower homocysteine levels, betaine, vitamin B_{12}, and folate, and suggest a the use of a fourth such agent, vitamin B_6 (see the following text), for possible treatment of these multisystem diseases. However, the main rationale for their use in treatment of these diseases has nothing to do with homocysteine levels. Each of them is suggested here because of distinct biochemistry unrelated to their effect on homocysteine. Still, they may be expected to have favorable effects on ischemic heart disease and other diseases by lowering homocysteine, and homocysteine was recently reported to produce partial NOS uncoupling.

Vitamin B_6 : Pyridoxine and Pyridoxal Phosphate

The role of excessive glutamate stimulation and specifically, that of excessive NMDA activity in multisystem diseases opens up additional types of potential therapies. You may recall that glutamate is the most important stimulatory neurotransmitter in the brain and its effects are partially counteracted by GABA (γ-amino butyric acid), the most important inhibitory neurotransmitter in the brain. It is important, for proper brain function and to avoid excitotoxicity, to have a balance between glutamate and GABA. GABA acts to lower glutamatergic activity and specifically lowers NMDA receptor activity.

The importance of this balance is emphasized by the fact that GABA is directly produced from glutamate through the action of the enzyme glutamate decarboxylase. It follows that insufficient glutamate decarboxylase activity leads to excitotoxicity. The enzyme glutamate decarboxylase requires the presence of a cofactor, pyridoxal phosphate, which is derived from the several forms of vitamin B_6, collectively called pyridoxine. It follows that vitamin B_6 helps protect the nervous system from some of the effects of excessive glutamate by converting some of that glutamate to GABA.

The protective role of vitamin B_6 in minimizing excitotoxicity has long been known. For example it has long been known that vitamin B_6 lowers Chinese restaurant syndrome[128]—the effect of monosodium glutamate sometimes used in Chinese restaurant foods. Similarly, it protects neurons in cell culture from the effects of glutamate.[129]

I would like to tell you about a personal experience that I had that may convey some of the potential importance of anecdotal reports. I have been in occasional e-mail contact with Diane Dawber, who wrote a book about multisystem diseases.[130] She has suffered from FM and MCS and has worked diligently to find answers that work for her in terms of therapy. Some time ago, she contacted me and told me that she and two other women who formed a small *ad hoc* therapy group in Toronto, had found that oral pyridoxal phosphate seemed to be helping the three of them with their illnesses, whereas the usual forms of vitamin B_6 had little effect. Pyridoxal phosphate differs from one of the forms of B_6 by having a phosphate group on it (that is by being phosphorylated). I emailed her saying that I was skeptical about their observations, stating that oral pyridoxal phosphate should not be more effective than regular B_6 because of several reasons: One is that the GI tract has substantial amounts of enzymes known as phosphatases, which remove phosphate groups, and this should convert pyridoxal phosphate into the pyridoxal form of B_6. Furthermore, I stated that most phosphorylated compounds are not transported across the outer membranes of cells and that this should prevent pyridoxal phosphate from being taken up into the blood from the GI tract, and if it were taken up, should prevent it from being taken up into cells where it could effect their biochemistry. In response to this, Diane Dawber challenged me, saying that pyridoxal phosphate was working for the three of them and I should figure out how it was working.

When I looked into the scientific literature, I found that, although the generalizations I outlined to her are often correct, pyridoxal phosphate *is an exception to all of them* and that there is at least one other partial exception. Pyridoxal phosphate can get through the GI tract intact, it can be taken up into the blood, and it can subsequently be taken up into cells (and presumably be transported as well through the blood brain barrier). So, I was completely wrong about that. There are examples where oral pyridoxal phosphate is more effective than other forms of B_6.[131,132] It is quite possible, therefore, that pyridoxal phosphate nutritional supplements may be more effective in the treatment of multisystem diseases than are other forms of B_6.

It should be noted that pyridoxal phosphate has many roles in amino acid biochemistry, and so lowering effects of excessive glutamate may not be the only useful role here. However, the role in allowing glutamate decarboxylase to perform its function is predicted to be the most direct effect on the NO/ONOO⁻ cycle.

Riboflavin and FMN

The B vitamin riboflavin resembles vitamin B_6 in having several important functions, having a certain key role in energy metabolism in addition to other functions. I will focus on the function of riboflavin in the regeneration of the central antioxidant reduced glutathione. Reduced glutathione is oxidized when it is used as an antioxidant in the body, being converted to oxidized glutathione. In order for it to function further, the oxidized glutathione must be reduced back to reduced glutathione by the enzyme glutathione reductase. The enzyme glutathione reductase contains an essential cofactor containing riboflavin known as FAD. It is well known that glutathione reductase levels are decreased in mammals that are even marginally deprived of riboflavin;[133-135] so marginal riboflavin deficiencies can lead to lessened availability of the important antioxidant reduced glutathione. There are some clinical observations that multisystem disease patients are more commonly deficient in riboflavin than are controls, suggesting that riboflavin supplements may be useful.

Some people have advocated the use of riboflavin 5'-phosphate (often known as FMN, the direct precursor of FAD) as a supplement rather than just riboflavin itself. Riboflavin 5'-phosphate is transported into the blood from the GI tract (like pyridoxal phosphate), does circulate in the blood, and is taken up into cells. However, I am unaware of any clinical studies showing that riboflavin 5'-phosphate supplements are more effective than riboflavin itself, and so it is not clear to me whether this is necessary for optimal repletion of the active forms of riboflavin.

Migraine headaches are often comorbid with multisystem diseases, and there is a substantial literature showing that riboflavin is useful in the treatment of migraine headache sufferers.

Other B Vitamins

Supplements of other B vitamins, including niacin and thiamine, may also be of some value based on their roles in energy metabolism, given the defects in energy metabolism that have been shown to occur in CFS and FM. The B vitamin biotin is known to be depleted when α-lipoic acid is used as a supplement; so supplements of biotin are probably useful for patients treated with α-lipoic acid.

Reduced Glutathione and Glutathione Precursors

Reduced glutathione has often been described as the most important antioxidant produced in the body. It is made up of three amino acids, cysteine, glutamate and glycine, and it is generally thought that under most conditions, the amino acid cysteine is the one most likely to be rate limiting in its synthesis. When it is used as an antioxidant in vivo, it is oxidized from reduced glutathione, often designated GSH, to oxidized glutathione, often designated GSSG. The GSSG can be reduced back to two molecules of GSH, as was discussed under the riboflavin section above, through the action of the enzyme glutathione reductase.

Tissues under oxidative stress become severely depleted of GSH for two reasons. The first is that there is often insufficient glutathione reductase activity to efficiently reduce the GSSG back to GSH, either because of insufficient enzyme or insufficient reductant (NADPH) or both. Second, when a cell accumulates large amounts of GSSG, it transports much of the GSSG out of the cell, where it gets degraded. Clearly transport and degradation of GSSG prevents its being reduced back to GSH. Consequently, oxidative stress can lead not only to a loss of GSH but also of total glutathione (GSH + GSSG), thus preventing short-term restoration of the GSH. In this way, short-term oxidative stress can be converted into long-term oxidative stress. Recovery of the tissue may require not only restoration of GSH pools in the cells of the tissue but also improved reduction of GSSG to GSH. Both of these may be essential to recovery of tissues suffering the consequences of elevated levels of free radicals and/or other oxidants such as peroxynitrite. Physicians treating patients with multisystem diseases, such as those discussed in the introduction to this chapter, have often focussed on the first of these but have often not treated to improve the second.

The reports of oxidative stress in all four of the multisystem diseases suggest that sufferers may have glutathione depletion. Droge and Holm[136] inferred that CFS patients may be deprived of reduced glutathione based on depletion of its cysteine precursor, and Bounous and Molson[137] inferred glutathione depletion in CFS based on other considerations; these inferences were confirmed by the study of Manuel y Keenoy et al.[176]

Oral reduced glutathione is apparently broken down in the GI tract and is not, therefore, absorbed intact.[138] However, there are transport mechanisms by which reduced glutathione can be taken up into cells[139,140] and also transported across the blood-brain barrier[141,142] so that, if reduced glutathione can be gotten into the blood, it should be transported into cells of the brain and elsewhere, where it may lower oxidative stress. Several physicians in the Puget Sound region of Washington State and also Dr. Grace Ziem in Maryland and some others[9] have used either reduced-glutathione nasal spray or nebulized, inhaled reduced-glutathione solution to treat patients with multisystem diseases. They report that such patients often experience rapid improvement of symptoms, suggesting that the reduced glutathione traverses the leaky epithelia in the nose or lungs, and gets taken up into cells where it can improve their biochemistry. So there are unpublished clinical observations suggesting that these may be useful ways of approaching reduced glutathione therapy.

What about the use of possible precursors of glutathione synthesis to increase the synthesis of reduced glutathione in patient tissues? The obvious precursor to use is l-cysteine, the common rate-limiting precursor in the synthesis of reduced glutathione. However, cysteine in known to produce excitotoxicity by acting mainly through excessive NMDA stimulation.[143,144] Furthermore, when cysteine gets oxidized to cystine, cystine can also produce excitotoxicity. Cystine is well known to be a substrate for a glutamate/cystine exchanger so that excessive cystine in the brain will exchange with intracellular glutamate, thus leading to increased extracellular glutamate and consequent excitotoxicity.[145,146] The basic strategy for restoring glutathione levels is to provide something that produces a modest but prolonged increase in cysteine/cystine by serving as a precursor for cysteine or cystine, thus preventing a high concentration of cysteine or cystine and thus minimizing any excitotoxicity.

There have been several physicians who have used whey protein preparations to possibly accomplish this goal.[147-150] Whey protein is a cysteine-rich protein, which can be broken down over time in the GI tract, and thus supply cysteine, which can be used to synthesize more reduced glutathione.

Another approach that has been used with other types of diseases is to use the compound N-acetyl cysteine (NAC) as a precursor of cysteine, which can, in turn, allow increased glutathione synthesis. NAC has been a well-tolerated supplement used to increase glutathione synthesis for over 50 years.[153] However, some people with multisystem diseases may not tolerate NAC well, possibly because of a combination of sensitivity to excitotoxins due to excessive NMDA activity and perhaps rapid hydrolysis of NAC to release cysteine. So, NAC should probably be used with care here and then perhaps only at low doses.

What about the use of agents to improve the reduction of GSSG back to GSH (reduced glutathione)? I have already discussed the use of riboflavin to try to increase such glutathione reduction. A second agent, α-lipoic acid is discussed in the following section, acts to increase GSSG reduction, and has other favorable effects as well.

α-*Lipoic Acid*

α-Lipoic acid is a wide-ranging antioxidant,[151-157] acting in part through its reduced form dihydrolipoic acid and its derivatives α-lipoamide and dihydrolipoamide. It acts directly or indirectly to scavenge free radicals and other reactive oxidants, including peroxynitrite, singlet oxygen, superoxide, peroxyl radicals, and the breakdown products of peroxynitrite.[151-158] Dihydrolipoic acid can regenerate other antioxidants by reducing oxidized and free radical forms of such antioxidants as glutathione, tocopherols, vitamin C, and flavonoids.[152-157] For example dihydrolipoic acid can reduce oxidized glutathione to reduced glutathione.[158,159] It is this last mechanism, regenerating reduced glutathione from oxidized glutathione, that maintains the glutathione pools, an important function as discussed in the preceding section of this chapter. α-Lipoic acid is known to be able to cross the blood–brain barrier and it is useful, therefore, in the treatment of some neurodegenerative diseases.[156] α-Lipoic acid is reported to be an effective therapeutic agent in the treatment of diabetes and its complications, diseases characterized by mitochondrial dysfunction, immunological dysfunction, excessive exercise, cardiovascular disease and neurodegenerative diseases.[151-157] All of these features suggest that it may be useful in the lowering of the NO/ONOO⁻ cycle and the treatment of multisystem diseases, as previously suggested by Logan and Wong[1] and by Werbach.[2]

Magnesium

The most obvious link between magnesium and the NO/ONOO⁻ cycle is the role of magnesium ions in lowering NMDA activity. As discussed in Chapter 2, magnesium deficiency causes the NMDA receptors to by hypersensitive to stimulation. There is a second possible link: magnesium has a universal role in bioenergetics because the energy currency of the cell, ATP, is bound to and functions with magnesium bound to it. Marginal magnesium deficiencies are known to be widespread in the United States and many other parts of the world, suggesting that severity of multisystem illnesses and probably increased prevalence may be controlled, in part, by magnesium.

Magnesium consumption in the United States and other Western country diets has declined substantially over the past century, and so a large number of people are currently marginally magnesium deficient.[160-172] The marginal magnesium deficiencies have been shown to have roles in cardiovascular diseases, insulin resistance and type 2 diabetes, hypertension, kidney dysfunction, and asthma.[162-169] Deficiencies also have roles in a number of neurological diseases and conditions, such as in stress responses, tension headache and migraine, latent tetany, and anxiety,[170-172] and influence EEG patterns.[173,174] These neurological changes in response to marginal magnesium deficiency may be the ones most relevant to the multisystem diseases.

The possible role of magnesium in multisystem diseases has focussed on two questions: Are patients with these illnesses more likely to be magnesium deficient than are controls? What effects do magnesium supplements, either oral or injected, have on the symptoms of these multisystem diseases? These have often been viewed as linked questions, because researchers have often assumed that, if the patients are not more magnesium deficient than controls, they should not respond to magnesium supplements. However, given how common marginal magnesium deficiencies are in the general population, there is no necessary linkage between responsiveness and lowered magnesium status compared with controls. The evidence on magnesium deficiency, compared with controls, is mixed, with some studies reporting such deficiency but others not, and so I will focus, instead, on the trial data.

A placebo-controlled study was performed by Cox and coworkers on a group of CFS patients, showing a statistically significant improvement of magnesium supplemented patients versus controls.[175] Subsequently, a number of other studies have been reported on magnesium therapy in CFS. Manuel y Keenoy et al.[176] reported that two measures of oxidative stress in CFS-like patients, the rate of production of fluorescent lipid peroxidation products and vitamin E levels both improved significantly with magnesium therapy. Clague et al. reported[177] significant improvement of fatigue in CFS patients with magnesium treatment. Seelig, in her review on magnesium and CFS,[178] suggested that magnesium may act to lower NMDA activity, in line with the suggested mechanism at the beginning of this section. Kurup and Kurup[179] found low levels of magnesium in CFS patients as well as elevated NMDA activity, again supporting a possible linkage between the two.

In an FM study, Russell et al.[180] showed a statistically significant improvement in all three primary outcome measures of pain and tenderness during a six-month-long open-label portion of their trial. An earlier study by Abraham and Flechas of FM patients reported lessened pain after treatment with magnesium malate.[181]

Magnesium supplements have been widely used in the treatment of these multisystem diseases. I believe that all eight of the physicians discussed in the second paragraph of the introduction, use magnesium supplements as part of their therapy. At the 2003 AAEM meeting focused on these diseases, of the eight talks on nutritional and/or pharmaceutical agents that might be useful in therapy, four[7-9,14] discussed using magnesium supplements. One of these[14] titled her talk "First Do No Harm, Next Try Magnesium." I think that magnesium is one of the most promising agents for treatment of multisystem diseases, but like other such agents, it produces modest responses and may be best used in a complex, combination therapy.

Zinc, Manganese, and Copper: Components of Superoxide Dismutases

Superoxide dismutases (SODs) are key enzymes that convert superoxide into hydrogen peroxide and molecular oxygen. SODs allow organisms to live in oxygen-containing environments owing to the toxicity of superoxide produced from molecular oxygen. SODs in mammals come in three distinct forms: mitochondrial manganese SOD, cytoplasmic copper–zinc SOD, and also an extracellular copper–zinc SOD. Because each of these contains one or more metal ions, the availability of these ions may have a role in determining the ability of the body to synthesize these important enzymes. There is evidence that zinc,[182,183] copper,[184,185] and manganese deficiencies can produce oxidative stress and that part of this stress may be produced by the lowered ability to synthesize the SODs.[186-188] Consequently, it is possible that supplementing with these three metals may help lower the levels of superoxide, an important element of the NO/ONOO$^-$ cycle.

However, doses of such supplementation may be a bit tricky. Excessive levels of both copper and manganese, because of the transition metal chemistry of these free ions, can produce oxidative stress. Even excessive zinc can have negative effects, one of which is that it acts to lower copper levels. So, in general, I would suggest using only modest doses of zinc, copper, or manganese supplements, to prevent any toxic effects of excessive levels.

NMDA Antagonists

There are a large number of drugs and potential future drugs that act as NMDA antagonists that may be current or future therapeutic agents for the treatment of multisystem illnesses. These may act, along with magnesium supplements to lower excessive NMDA and vitamin B$_6$ activity in multisystem diseases. Among the NMDA antagonists that should be currently considered, in my view, are the the over-the-counter drug dextromethorphan, the drug memantine, which is now approved for chronic use in the treatment of Alzheimer's patients, and the drugs ketamine and flupirtine, which have been studied in FM.

There have been a large number of studies reporting that NMDA antagonists are effective in lowering pain in FM,[189-199] with most of these using the drug ketamine but with a study reporting effectiveness with the drug flupirtine[195] and another with dextromethorphan.[199] This large total number of studies collectively involving three different NMDA antagonists provides convincing evidence for a role of excessive NMDA activity in FM. Clinical observations suggest that such NMDA antagonists are helpful in the treatment of CFS as well.[179,200]

NMDA receptors were first implicated in MCS by Dr. Donald Dudley.[201] Dudley observed that, when MCS patients were reacting to a chemical exposure, if they take some dextromethorphan in an hour or so, it often reverses the sensitivity symptoms. This approach has been followed by a number of physicians in the Puget Sound region of Washington State, observing similar clinical responses to those reported by Dudley. I have talked with six MCS patients who have tried this approach, and five of them have confirmed these observations. One, a young woman who developed MCS after pesticide and organic solvent exposure, reported some remarkable responses. After she was apparently chemically exposed, she reported severe headache, like someone "was beating on my head with a baseball bat." After taking dextromethorphan, an hour later she was fine.

Some MCS patients, I estimate about 10 percent from physician's clinical observations, cannot tolerate the normal dosage of dextromethorphan, but some of these can both tolerate and get clinical relief from doses of half to a quarter of the normal adult dose. Drug sensitivities are common in people with MCS, possibly from combinations of blood-brain barrier breakdown and nitric oxide-mediated inhibition of cytochrome P450 drug metabolism, providing a possible explanation for this sensitivity to dextromethorphan. Many of the MCS patients take their dextromethorphan in the over-the-counter cough suppressant liquid drug Delsym, although others have taken a liquid cough suppressant designed for children. Most cough suppressants containing dextromethorphan contain other active ingredients, but in the United States there are several brands sold over the counter that contain no other active ingredients.

One last clinical observation may be relevant to the role of NMDA receptor hyperactivity in multisystem diseases. Dr. Jonathan Wright reports (personal communication) that low-dose lithium appears to be helpful to his multisystem disease patients, and lithium is reported to lower NMDA activity.[202,203]

Riluzole

Riluzole is a drug that acts as a sodium-channel blocker and indirectly lowers glutamate release, thus lowering both NMDA activity and also other glutamate-dependent (non-NMDA) activity. It has a role, therefore, in lowering excitoxicity. Riluzole is the only drug approved for the treatment of ALS, producing a significant, but modest, lengthening of survival.[204,205] It is also effective in the treatment of a mouse ALS model.[206] It shows promise for the possible treatment of Huntington's disease,[207,208] Parkinson's disease,[209] and spinal cord trauma.[210] Given that excessive excitotoxicity and NMDA activity are elements in the NO/ONOO⁻ cycle and that excessive NMDA activity has been reported in all four of the multisystem diseases, riluzole may be a promising drug for the treatment of those diseases as well.

Taurine

Taurine is an unusual amino acid that has antioxidant properties and also acts as neurotransmitter. Taurine levels are reported to be low in CFS,[211] MCS,[212] and FM.[213]

Taurine scavenges the oxidant hypochlorous acid,[214] and the product of this reaction, taurine chloramine, lowers NF-κB activity and iNOS induction,[215,216] each an important element of the NO/ONOO⁻ cycle.

Taurine's various activities as a neurotransmitter are also expected to down-regulate the cycle. You may recall that glutamate is the most active excitatory neurotransmitter in the brain, stimulating NMDA and also non-NMDA receptors but that GABA is the most important inhibitory neurotransmitter in the brain, acting to lower the NMDA receptor sensitivity to stimulation. Taurine has certain properties similar to those of GABA. Taurine acts to stimulate the synthesis of GABA[217] but is transported readily across the blood-brain barrier, allowing taurine supplements to act effectively in the brain.[218] Taurine stimulates several inhibitory receptors including GABA(A) and glycine receptors,[219-224] leading to lowered NMDA activity.[224] It also acts to lower intracellular calcium levels,[225] and thus lowers nitric oxide synthesis. All of these are expected to produce lowered NO/ONOO⁻ cycle activity, and given the lowered levels of taurine reported in CFS, MCS, and FM,[211-213] it makes sense to replete the pools of taurine.

Before leaving this topic, it should be pointed out that the drug gabapentin acts via a different target mechanism to produce lowered excitatory activity and lower NMDA activity.[226,227]

Uric Acid (Urate) and Inosine

Uric acid (urate) is an antioxidant compound that is found in human blood at relatively high concentrations.[230] It has been shown to be an important peroxynitrite scavenger[231-235] and prevents peroxynitrite-mediated breakdown of the blood-brain barrier.[236] It also lowers the uncoupling of nitric oxide synthases that is produced by peroxynitrite-mediated oxidation of tetrahydrobiopterin.[232] Consequently, uric acid may be a useful compound in the prevention of peroxynitrite-mediated damage, and these are all expected to be important effects in protecting the body by down-regulating the NO/ONOO⁻ cycle in these multisystem diseases. Uric acid levels are often low in a number of inflammatory diseases. Conversely, high uric acid levels may be protective. An apparent example of this is where the disease gout, which is characterized by elevated uric acid levels, and multiple sclerosis (MS) appear to exclude each other—people with gout essentially never come down with MS,[237,238] suggesting that the elevated levels of uric acid in gout protect people from succumbing to MS. I have been unable to find any data on whether gout tends to protect people from multisystem diseases.

Uric acid itself cannot be taken orally in order to raise systemic uric acid levels because the uric acid is metabolized to other compounds by the bacteria in the GI tract. However, the purine-containing compound inosine can be taken to raise systemic uric acid levels, because it is absorbed intact into the body and then metabolized to produce uric acid.[239] Consequently, inosine can be used to raise uric acid levels, but also to possibly provide partial protection from MS,[240] traumatic spinal cord injury,[241] nerve damage in diabetes,[242] graft rejection,[243] and ischemic brain injury.[244]

While the use of inosine to raise uric acid levels will probably be helpful, based on the clinical observations just mentioned, it may also, however, have some negative effects. Inosine and other purines are converted to uric acid via the action of the enzyme xanthine dehydrogenase/xanthine oxidase. When xanthine oxidase activity is involved, superoxide is generated as a product, as discussed in Chapter 1. So, it is not completely clear whether the net effect of using inosine supplements will be favorable or not.

Inosine, acting as a precursor of uric acid, *may* be a promising agent for the treatment of multisystem diseases, and it is unfortunate, in my view, that there have been no trials specifically testing its efficacy.

It should be noted that the breakdown of ribonucleic acid (RNA) will also generate uric acid, and so RNA supplements may be useful to raise uric acid levels.

Long-Chain Omega-3 Fatty Acids

Polyunsaturated fatty acids are much more susceptible to lipid peroxidation than are other fatty acids, and consequently they tend to be depleted whenever organisms suffer from chronic oxidative stress. The long-chain omega-3 fatty acids, sometimes referred to as DHA and EPA, are the most susceptible to such oxidation because they have the greatest number of unsaturated bonds. Therefore, DHA and EPA are the most susceptible to being depleted during oxidative stress. There have been three studies reporting deficiencies in these long-chain omega-3 fatty acids in CFS,[245-247] and in my first paper on CFS, I suggested that this was probably caused by elevated peroxynitrite levels and consequent oxidative stress.[248] DHA and EPA have special roles in brain membranes and in brain function, and so it may be important to replete them in order to restore brain function.

Three CFS studies, using supplements containing such long-chain omega-3 fatty acids (commonly found in fish oils), have reported that such supplementation produces lessened symptoms in CFS,[247,249,250] and a fourth study reported improvement in FM.[251] One study failed to see any improvement in CFS,[252] but this study used the often-questioned Oxford criteria for CFS and may be flawed for that reason.

In addition to possible improved brain function, repleting long-chain omega-3 fatty acids may be helpful for another reason. Supplements containing these fatty acids have been shown to lower iNOS induction[253-256] by lowering NF-κB activity.[257] iNOS induction and NF-κB activity are both important elements of the NO/ONOO⁻ cycle and lowering them should act, therefore, to down-regulate cycle activity.

Long-chain omega-3 fatty acids found in fish oils may be still another useful nutritional supplement that lower NO/ONOO⁻ cycle activity and have been reported in four studies to produce improvements in multisystem disease sufferers.

Agents That Lower NF-κB Activity

NF-κB activity, is down-regulated by a large number of antioxidants, so it is not clear to me that we need to have additional agents that lower such activity as part of a treatment protocol that includes these antioxidants. However, I am aware of several anecdotal reports of improvement in response to treatment with cat's claw, an herbal that lowers NF-κB activity. Furthermore, Teitelbaum[7] includes both cat's claw and also feverfew, another such herbal in his treatment protocol for CFS and FM. There is a lot of research being done on potential pharmaceuticals that lower NF-κB activity, so it is likely that, in the future, additional agents will become available that produce this response.

Azelastine is a drug currently used to treat asthma and allergies. It is known to lower NF-κB activity[258,259] and may be an attractive candidate for the treatment of multisystem diseases. Another such drug is the compound parthenolide,[260-263] the main active component in feverfew and certain other herbals that lower NF-κB activity. Cat's claw, an herbal derived from a Peruvian Amazon basin plant is also active in lowering NF-κB activity.[264,265] It should be noted, however, that Foster and Tyler[266] report that cat's claw comes in two types, only one of which will contain substantial amounts of the component lowering NF-κB activity.

Each of these may have possible roles in the treatment of these multisystem diseases.

Curcumin

Curcumin is the main pigment providing the yellow color in tumeric, the yellow component of curry powders. Curcumin is chemically similar to the flavonoids, being a polyphenolic antioxidant. It acts as a chain-breaking antioxidant and lowers NF-κB activity and stimulates the synthesis of reduced glutathione.[267] Curcumin is reported to be quite active as a peroxynitrite scavenger,[268,269] and it also complexes with copper or manganese ions to form a superoxide dismutase (SOD) mimic[270-272]—that is, it forms a complex that metabolizes superoxide in the same way as do the enzymes known as superoxide dismutases. This combination of activities may make curcumin or the spice tumeric, an attractive candidate as a possible therapeutic agent for the treatment of multisystem diseases.

Algal Supplements and Antioxidant Therapy

It has been reported that supplements of the alga *Chlorella* produced clinical improvement in a study of FM patients.[273,274] I am also aware of anecdotal reports of improvement by both CFS and MCS sufferers taking blue-green algal supplements. While the efficacy of neither of these algal supplements has been definitively shown, it may still be worth asking how they may act, if they are effective. Both *Chlorella*[275-279] and blue-green algae[279-281] are very rich in antioxidants, including carotenoids and vitamin

C, and in the case of blue-greens, the antioxidants known as phycocyanins. In contrast, the content of other components that may be helpful seem to be too low to explain any efficacy, because relatively small amounts of these algae have been given as a nutritional supplement. The blue-green algal phycocyanins are reported to be potent peroxynitrite scavengers.[282,283]

The antioxidants present in these algae might conceivably be used as a base for adding other nutritional supplements in compounding a formula that might be expected to down-regulate the NO/ONOO⁻ cycle.

Hyperbaric Oxygen Therapy

Hyperbaric oxygen therapy, typically placing patients in pressure chambers at a modest increase in atmospheric pressure using 100 percent oxygen, has been reported to produce improvements in patients with FM[284] and with CFS.[285] Several physicians have clinical observations suggesting that this is helpful for MCS patients as well, including Rea,[10] Ziem, and Heuser.

I have been concerned with the possible exacerbation of oxidative stress by hyperbaric oxygen, because it is well known that both hypoxia (too little oxygen) and hyperoxia (too much) can produce oxidative stress. Consequently, it is my opinion, that any hyperbaric oxygen therapy should only be performed in patients who are also treated with a variety of antioxidants. Still, the observations of improvement with this therapy are intriguing, leading one to ask how might it act?

There are two *distinct types* of mechanisms by which hyperbaric oxygen therapy might be expected to lower NO/ONOO⁻ cycle biochemistry. The most obvious of these is to increase delivery of oxygen to the tissues and therefore to increase mitochondrial energy metabolism. Nitric oxide is well known to inhibit the enzyme cytochrome oxidase, the enzyme that uses molecular oxygen for energy metabolism in the mitochondrion. Oxygen will compete with nitric oxide, and therefore increased oxygen will have the effect of lowering the inhibition produced by nitric oxide. There is a second possible, albeit related expected, reason why increased oxygen delivery to the tissues may be expected to stimulate mitochondrial energy metabolism in these multisystem diseases. The release of oxygen from hemoglobin in the blood is highly regulated, with oxygen being selectively released in the tissues in most need*—these are the same tissues that are metabolizing most rapidly and therefore producing the most carbon dioxide. However,

---

*The mechanisms here are described in most biochemistry and medical biochemistry textbooks—they involve the increased release of oxygen from hemoglobin produced by carbon dioxide and by the lowered pH produced by carbon dioxide.

both peroxynitrite and nitric oxide lower the ability of the electron transport chain of the mitochondria to consume oxygen and therefore produce carbon dioxide. So, one can see here a bit of a vicious cycle—lowered metabolism due to peroxynitrite and nitric oxide leads to lessened oxygen release from hemoglobin, which leads to still lower metabolism. Hyperbaric oxygen will be expected to provide increased oxygen to the tissues and therefore allow the tissues to produce both energy and carbon dioxide at a higher rate, thus stimulating oxygen release from hemoglobin.

There is an additional possible mechanism by which hyperbaric oxygen may also be useful. Hyperbaric oxygen is known to lead to increased tissue production of hydrogen peroxide.[286-288] Hydrogen peroxide, as was discussed earlier in the chapter, will induce increased tetrahydrobiopterin synthesis[127] and therefore may decrease uncoupling of the nitric oxide synthases.

Minocycline

A number of tetracycline antibiotics, including minocycline, are reported to have both antioxidant and anti-inflammatory properties, including the scavenging of peroxynitrite or its breakdown products.[289-292] However, minocycline appears to be the most promising of these for the treatment of multisystem diseases because it is a more active antioxidant than some other tetracyclines[292] and because it readily traverses the blood–brain barrier,[293,294] thus having increased access to the brain. Minocycline is reported to lower iNOS induction[295] and to protect neurons from excessive NMDA activity.[292,296] It is also reported to protect neurons from excessive nitric oxide.[295] Minocycline has been shown to lead to prolonged survival of animal models of amyotrophic lateral sclerosis[297,298] and Huntington's disease.[299] These observations suggest that minocycline may be among the more promising conventional pharmaceuticals for the treatment of multisystem illnesses not only because of its antioxidant activity but also because of its ability to lower elements of the NO/ONOO⁻ cycle.

Food As Therapy

We have been taught to look at foods as sources of carbohydrates, fats, and proteins and also of a few minerals, vitamins, and fiber. These are the only things that we get nutritional information about on food containers, suggesting that these are the only things that are important. However, there is a growing scientific literature on the importance of other components of foods that may be relevant to recovering from not only multisystem dis-cases but from other diseases as well. I have talked about some of these earlier in this chapter but want to reconsider them and others in a dietary context. Antioxidants, minerals such as zinc, manganese, copper, and selenium can all be obtained from nutritional supplements, but supplements should be used to support an already basically healthful diet, not to substitute for one. Other components such as phospholipids are needed to help restore brain and mitochondrial function, and both omega-3 and omega-6 fatty acids are also involved in these as well. There are components of foods that we can make in our bodies, but not in adequate amounts, such as choline/phosphatidyl choline; these are consequently needed in our foods, as well. Each of these—minerals, antioxidants, and phospholipids and also many vitamins and much fiber— are removed in our highly processed foods, and while a few may be added during "enrichment," this does not compensate for the many that are still largely deficient. So, one approach that has often been repeated is to stick to whole foods wherever possible, hence not missing the many components of life.

In the second section of this chapter, I suggested that sufferers from these diseases avoid foods that they have become allergic to in order to avoid exacerbating their illnesses. MCS sufferers may be well advised to eat mainly organic foods to avoid exposure to pesticides. Organic foods may also be desirable because they are reported to have increased levels of several important minerals and also some other nutrients.

In addition to the three principles discussed—eat whole foods, avoid food allergens and consider organic foods—three other principles need to be emphasized:

1. There are certain foods that stand out as highly nutritious, not just for specific nutrients, but almost across the board. These are foods that contain plant or animal tissues that are rapidly growing or with high energy metabolism or that are key storage tissues where the organism stores important nutrients. Some of them, like plant seeds, are all three. There are certain groups of organisms such as the leguminous plants that are particularly nutritious—beans, lentils, peas, and their close relatives often stand out as having nutritious seeds. Rapidly growing plant tissues such as leafy greens, asparagus, broccoli, and green onions all have more nutrients than do related, but more slowly growing, tissues. Animal tissues that are energetic or rapidly growing tend to be more nutritious, such as heart tissue and shellfish. Liver is a key storage organ, but unfortunately, liver also accumulates many toxins and so may be undesirable for that reason. Yeasts including nutritional yeasts are among the most nutritious of all foods, not surpris-

ingly because they grow so rapidly. *Chlorella* and other microalgae are also very nutritious for the same reason as yeast and add high-level antioxidants into the mix. Rapidly growing tissues and cells tend to be rich in nucleic acids, RNA and DNA, which have purines in their structure. When purines are consumed and degraded, they produce uric acid, a key antioxidant and peroxynitrite scavenger, providing still another reason to favor these as foods. Pennington[300] provides a partial list of foods rich in purines, including many seafoods and organ meats, asparagus, spinach, whole grain foods, and wheat germ, legumes, and mushrooms.

2. We need a balance between omega-3 and omega-6 fatty acids and most, but not all, of our diets are imbalanced with excessive levels of omega-6s and too few long-chain omega-3s. Omega-6 fatty acids tend to be proinflammatory because of their role as precursors of inflammatory regulatory molecules known as eicosanoids and may have important roles in exacerbating the inflammatory biochemistry in multisystem diseases. Omega-3 fatty acids tend to be anti-inflammatory. Both of these are essential; so neither are inherently good or bad but a substantial imbalance in the diet can have major consequences. The long-chain omega-3s are most important and are obtained in the diet mostly from seafood, particularly cold-water-grown seafood. We do consume shorter-chain omega-3s in foods such as canola oil, walnuts, and flaxseed with smaller amounts in soy oil, but our ability to convert these to the longer-chain omega-3s (DHA and EPA) is *distinctly limited.* These long-chain omega-3s have special roles in brain function, as well as being precursors for anti-inflammatory eicosanoids. However, the omega-6s are also essential, and the most common omega-6 fatty acid, linoleic acid, has a special role in the regeneration of cardiolipin in mitochondria. All these omega-3 and omega-6 fatty acids are susceptible to lipid peroxidation, becoming rancid and therefore toxic. They should be stored away from light in as cool a place as possible. I store my canola oil in the refrigerator and buy walnuts shortly after harvest and store them in the freezer so as to minimize such oxidation.

3. Antioxidant levels in some plant foods may be 100 times or more higher than in other plant foods, and such excellent sources of antioxidants should be kept in mind. This variation is particularly extreme in the case of carotenoids, which are found in very high levels in such foods as deep green vegetables, and ripe, deeply colored foods such as tomatoes, red peppers, winter squash, and sweet potatoes. The anthocyanin pigment flavonoids can also be seen from their intense

purplish color in ripe fruits such as blueberries and other deeply colored berries, colored plums, red cabbages, and onions. Many of the flavonoids are particularly concentrated in and near the peels of fruit, as can be seen from the color of the peels and nearby tissues. Other more lightly colored flavonoids are found in high amounts of tea, onions, apples, and soy products. The spice tumeric has high amounts of the antioxidant curcumin and paprika is very rich in carotenoids, whereas a number of herbs are rich in flavonoids.

If you are a sufferer of one of more of these multisystem diseases, you need to think of foods as important therapeutic agents. While I do not want to add to your burdens in surviving from day to day, orienting your diet to give your body what it needs may be essential to any recovery.

Creatine

The compound creatine has been widely used as a nutritional supplement by certain groups of athletes. It has an important role of storing energy in brain and muscle tissues, in the form of creatine phosphate. Creatine has been shown to prolong survival of ALS animal models.[298] It appears to stimulate the transport of glutamate into glial cells, thus lowering the excitotoxicity produced by glutamate.[301] Creatine has been shown to lower NMDA-mediated excitotoxicity.[302,303]

Creatine is a well-tolerated nutritional supplement that may have some promise as an agent in lowering NO/ONOO⁻ cycle biochemistry in the treatment of multisystem diseases.

Ebselen

Ebselen is a synthetic organic selenium compound currently under testing as a potential drug, which has also been studied intensively under laboratory conditions. Ebselen is a potent peroxynitrite scavenger.[60,74,75,304] It acts as a glutathione peroxidase mimic, substituting for the enzyme glutathione peroxidase in getting rid of organic peroxides.[60,304] Ebselen acts as a free radical scavenger.[304,305] It lowers excessive pain under some circumstances, including pain caused by excessive vanilloid activity.[306] It protects organisms and cells from excessive NMDA activity.[307] Ebselen is a neuroprotective agent in spinal cord injury.[308] It acts to regenerate chain-breaking antioxidants after they have acted as antioxidants.[309,310] These diverse properties of ebselen suggest that, if it is approved for human use, it may well approach magic bullet status in the therapy of multisystem diseases. In my judgement, it is the most attractive possible therapeutic agent to lower

NO/ONOO⁻ cycle activities among the possible conventional pharmaceuticals currently being evaluated for possible human use.

SOD Mimics

The enzyme superoxide dismutase converts two molecules of the free radical superoxide into one molecule of molecular oxygen, the form of oxygen found in the atmosphere and also one molecule of hydrogen peroxide (H_2O_2). In this way, it gets rid of superoxide radicals. There are a number of relatively low molecular weight compounds that act as SOD mimics, performing the same reaction as SOD. These may be able to lower the toxicity of superoxide in the body if they themselves are sufficiently nontoxic to be used in this way. Many of these SOD mimics are porphyrin compounds,[311] somewhat similar in structure to the heme in hemoglobin, usually with manganese at their center, although some do have iron instead of manganese.[312] These SOD mimics have been shown to improve the survival of cells deficient in SOD such as SOD-deficient neurons[313] or SOD-deficient bacteria.[314] The most impressive feat to date is that one SOD-mimic, when given to ALS transgenic mice, increased survival about threefold when given at the onset of symptoms.[315] While these are interesting molecules and are very useful in studying mechanisms in cell culture or in experimental animals, I suspect we are a long way from establishing them as useful drugs for human use.

Agents That Lower Vanilloid Activity

Of the elements of the NO/ONOO⁻ cycle, the vanilloid receptor is the least studied in the general scientific literature. However, there is evidence for excessive vanilloid activity in both FM[316-318] and in MCS.[319] The compound capsazepine has long been known to act as a relatively specific vanilloid antagonist, but it has not been developed as a drug for human use. Nor have other specific vanilloid antagonists been approved for human use.

Prolonged or repeated exposure to low levels of many but not all vanilloid agonists lead to lowered vanilloid activity. Such treatment can be used, therefore, to test for vanilloid roles in biological responses. This was done in an FM study where a skin cream containing capsaicin, the classic vanilloid agonist, was shown to lower pain sensitivity.[320] This sort of approach is not a practical one to try to systemically lower vanilloid activity. Perhaps the only current practical way to systemically lower such activity is to use *Panax ginseng* extracts because ginsenosides found in this herbal preparation have been reported to lower vanilloid activity.[321,322] It should be noted, however, that materials are often sold as *Panax ginseng* extracts that are not what they claim to be,[266] and so one would need to have a reliable source before considering such treatment.

There is one other area of study that may or may not be relevant to attempts to lower vanilloid activity. The over-the-counter drug guaifenesin has been touted by Dr. Paul St. Amand as being effective in the treatment of FM, and others have argued that it may also be effective in CFS. However, I believe that the interpretation of the proposed action of guaifenesin that St. Amand has argued to his patients and has been posted on several Web sites is inconsistent with established biochemical principles. Furthermore, a placebo-controlled trial by Bennett et al.[323] on guaifenesin effects in FM patients showed no significant improvement over placebo. Despite both of these, I have heard enough anecdotal reports of efficacy that I am not yet ready to completely discard the notion that guaifenesin may be a useful therapeutic agent for these multisystem disease.

Guaifenesin is sold as a cough suppressant (antitussive agent), and it is well known that stimulating the vanilloid receptor in the upper respiratory tract with capsaicin produces cough responses. Furthermore, a recent study[324] reported that guaifenesin greatly lowered coughing in response to capsaicin treatment. This study suggests but does not prove that guaifenesin may be a vanilloid antagonist blocking the responses of the vanilloid receptor.

Carnosine

Carnosine (not to be confused with carnitine) is an unusual antioxidant[325,326] that acts as an antiglycation agent—it reverses some of the damage produced by excessive sugar to proteins. Carnosine concentrates in the brain and in certain muscle, particularly heart muscle, and may therefore be particularly useful in protecting those tissues. It is reported to act as a peroxynitrite scavenger,[327,328] and may therefore be useful in the treatment of multisystem illnesses. Carnosine has been used in a clinical study of autism[329] with significant favorable results.

TRH

TRH, thyrotropin-releasing hormone, has been reported by Dr. Gordon Baker in clinical observations, to lower symptoms of MCS when used as a nasal spray. Dr. Baker asked me about this, wondering whether the responses he was seeing to TRH were consistent with the NO/ONOO$^-$ cycle. The TRH mechanism here may be due to the known effect of TRH in lowering NMDA activity[330-332] and consequently lowering glutamate-stimulated nitric oxide synthesis.[333]

SUMMARY: INDIVIDUAL AGENTS
AND CLASSES OF AGENTS

The evidence suggesting efficacy of the various agents and classes of agents, in multisystem diseases, is summarized in Exhibit 15.1. There are

EXHIBIT 15.1. Summary of Individual Agents

Agent or class of agents	Clinical trial data or clinical observation/ anecdotal reports
Tocopherols/Tocotrienols	Anecdotal reports
Vitamin C (ascorbic acid)	Clinical trial data
Selenium	None
Carotenoids	None
Flavonoids	Clinical trial data
Reductive stress relieving agents	Clinical trial data
L-Carnitine/Acetyl-L-carnitine	Clinical trial data
Mitochondrial regeneration agents	Clinical trial data
Hydroxocobalamin/B_{12}	Clinical trial data
Folic acid	Clinical trial data
Vitamin B_6/pyridoxal phosphate	Anecdotal report
Riboflavin	None
Other B vitamins	None
Glutathione/glutathione precursors	Clinical observations
α-Lipoic acid	None
Magnesium	Clinical trial data
SOD minerals/zinc,manganese, copper	None
NMDA antagonists	Clinical trial data
Riluzole	None

Taurine	None
Inosine/uric acid	None
Long chain omega-3 fatty acids	Clinical trial data
Agents that lower NF-κB activity	Anecdotal reports
Curcumin	None
Algal supplements	Clinical trial data
Hyperbaric oxygen	Clinical trial data
Minocycline and other tetracyclines	Clinical observations
Creatine	None
Ebselen	None
Lowered vanilloid activity	None
Carnosine	None
TRH	Clinical observation

32 such agents or classes, of which two, ebselen and SOD mimics, are still in the stages of possibly being approved for use as pharmaceuticals, and so not surprisingly, we have no data on efficacy of these two in multisystem diseases. Of the other 30, the efficacy of 12 is supported by clinical trial data and six additional are supported by clinical observations and/or anecdotal reports. Although these multisystem diseases have suffered from having little clinical trial study, there is still a substantial amount of evidence suggesting that a dozen of these agents have measurable efficacy in the treatment of these diseases. Consequently, even though the conventional medical view is that there is no effective treatment for these diseases based on nutritional or pharmaceutical therapy, that conventional wisdom is challenged by a number of clinical studies reporting favorable responses that are consistent with a NO/ONOO⁻ cycle mechanism. Six additional agents have been used by multiple physicians as part of their complex treatment protocols for multisystem disease but have no literature of efficacy as individual agents. These six are selenium, riboflavin, other B vitamins, α-lipoic acid, SOD minerals, and taurine.

You may have noted that there have been a number of studies, mentioned earlier, where agents down-regulating the NO/ONOO⁻ cycle have shown efficacy in the treatment of ALS, Parkinson's, Alzheimer's, and MS. These diseases were all suggested to be possible NO/ONOO⁻ cycle diseases in Chapter 14, and these observations are consistent with that suggestion.

There is no question that, based on the standards of much better studied and better funded diseases, the data available on treatment of these multisystem diseases are sparse and certainly less convincing than one would like. Nevertheless, the data that is available challenges the view that these diseases are not treatable other through the treatment of symptoms. The pattern of evidence is consistent with the NO/ONOO⁻ cycle mechanism, the only proposed mechanism for the etiology of this group of diseases. I will pursue these issues further in considering complex treatment protocols developed by specific physicians.

CFS TREATMENT PROTOCOLS OF FOUR PHYSICIANS

In the treatment of CFS, there are a certain number of physicians who have used all of their knowledge of biological mechanism together with their own clinical observations to try to come up with treatment protocols that help their patients.* Each of the four discussed in the following text have focused on treatment protocols that use 14 or more agents that can be viewed as down-regulating the NO/ONOO⁻ cycle. I am not suggesting that they have all come to this because of the NO/ONOO⁻ cycle, although I know that two of the four that I will discuss here have been influenced to some extent by this mechanism. Rather, I am suggesting that it is probably not a coincidence that each of these protocols has focused on many agents that are expected to down-regulate the cycle. In this discussion, I will only discuss those agents, in their treatment protocols, that can be viewed as down-regulating the cycle rather than discussing the minority of agents that do not have obvious connections with elements of the cycle.

Dr. Paul Cheney

Dr. Cheney starts his protocol[149,334] by trying to avoid things that exacerbate the NO/ONOO⁻ cycle mechanism, some of the same things that I discussed in the second section (avoid exacerbation) of this chapter. Specifically he suggests attenuating GI tract problems by such strategies as going on a low food allergen diet, minimizing environmental chemical exposure and also inflammatory diseases, such as around the teeth. He uses many

---

*Much of the material in the rest of the chapter is derived from the author's Web site.

agents that lower NO/ONOO⁻ cycle biochemistry. The agents that I list are followed, in some cases, by comments on how they may act—those comments are mine, not Cheney's.

- High dose hydroxocobalamin (B_{12}) injections—nitric oxide scavenger.
- Whey protein—glutathione precursor.
- Guaifenesin—vanilloid antagonist?
- NMDA blockers.
- Magnesium—lowers NMDA activity.
- Taurine—antioxidant and acts to lower excitotoxicity including NMDA activity.
- GABA agonists—GABA acts as an inhibitory neurotransmitter to lower NMDA activity—these include the drug neurotin (gabapentin).
- Histamine blockers—mast cells which release histamine are activated by both nitric oxide and vanilloid stimulation (Chapter 7) and may therefore be part of the cycle mechanism.
- Betaine hydrochloride (HCl)—Betaine lowers reductive stress; the hydrochloride form should only be used in those with low stomach acid. Betaine (trimethylglycine) is also listed separately in the protocol description.

Antioxidants and anti-inflammatories listed as follows:

- Flavonoids, including "bioflavonoids," olive leaf extract, organic botanicals, and hawthorn extract.
- Vitamin E (forms not listed).
- Coenzyme Q10—acts both as antioxidant and to stimulate mitochondrial function.
- α-lipoic acid.
- Selenium.
- Omega-3 and Omega-6 fatty acids.
- Melatonin—as an antioxidant.
- Pyridoxal phosphate—improves glutamate/GABA ratio.
- Folic acid—lowers uncoupling of nitric oxide synthases.

You can see that Cheney prescribes for his patients a total of 18 distinct agents or classes of agents, each of which can be viewed as down-regulating aspects of the NO/ONOO⁻ cycle. I would argue that this in not just coincidental and that it argues in support of the NO/ONOO⁻ cycle mechanism.

Dr. Jacob Teitelbaum

Teitelbaum has published placebo-controlled trial data supporting the efficacy of one version of his protocol,[7,335] something none of these other physicians has done. I am going to describe a recent version of his complex protocol, focusing on what may be considered the central parts of the protocol, the parts described as "nutritional treatments" and "mitochondrial energy treatments."

- Daily energy B-complex—B vitamins including high dose B_6, riboflavin, thiamine, niacin and also folic acid. These fall into four categories that I have listed earlier in the chapter.
- Betaine hydrochloride (HCl)—lowers reductive stress; hydrochloride form should only be taken by those deficient in stomach acid.
- Magnesium as magnesium glycinate and magnesium malate—lowers NMDA activity—often uses magnesium injections.
- α-Lipoic acid—important antioxidant helps regenerate reduced glutathione.
- Vitamin B_{12} IM injections, 3 mg injections (does not state whether this is hydroxocobalamin)—may act as potent nitric oxide scavenger.
- Eskimo fish oil—excellent source of long-chain omega-3 fatty acids. Lowers iNOS induction, is anti-inflammatory.
- Vitamin C.
- Grape seed extract (flavonoid).
- Vitamin E, natural—does not state whether this includes γ-tocopherol or tocotrienols.
- Physician's protein formula, used as glutathione precursor.
- Zinc—antioxidant properties and copper/zinc superoxide dysmutase precursor.
- Acetyl-L-carnitine—important for restoring mitochondrial function.
- Coenzyme Q10—both important antioxidant properties and stimulates mitochondrial function.

If you consider that the oral B vitamins fall into four categories listed earlier in the chapter, Teitelbaum uses a total of 17 agents or classes of agents that are predicted to down-regulate the NO/ONOO⁻ cycle, in the core part of his treatment protocol.

Dr. Garth Nicolson

Dr. Nicolson is an interesting scientist who started his scientific career developing the famous Singer/Nicolson fluid mosaic model of biological membranes, a model that is described in essentially all of the standard biochemistry textbooks. He and his colleagues have published on open-label trials of a complex mixture known as NT factor, a proprietary mixture that is designed to improve mitochondrial and thus energy metabolism function. The trials have been on a group of older patients with unexplained chronic fatigue, and so there is some question whether these patients have CFS. Nevertheless, Nicolson and coworkers[8,336,337] report statistically significant improvements not only in fatigue but in several other changes often found in multisystem disease patients, affective/meaning, sensory, and cognitive/mood. The NT factor components were presumably designed to improve mitochondrial function, but as we shall see shortly, may be equally effective in lowering much of the NO/ONOO⁻ cycle biochemistry. Unfortunately, there is no detailed description of the concentrations of the components of the NT factor proprietary mixture. The mixture contains the following components that are predicted to lower NO/ONOO⁻ cycle biochemistry:

- Polyunsaturated phosphatidyl choline—predicted to lower reductive stress.
- Other phosphatidyl polyunsaturated lipids—this and the phosphatidyl choline are predicted to help restore the oxidatively damaged mitochondrial inner membrane.
- Magnesium—lowers NMDA activity, may aid in energy metabolism.
- Taurine—antioxidant activity and lowers excitoxicity including NMDA activity.
- Artichoke extract—as flavonoid source?
- Spirulina—blue-green alga is a concentrated antioxidant source.
- Natural vitamin E—does not tell us whether this includes γ-tocopherol or tocotrienols.
- Calcium ascorbate—vitamin C.
- α-Lipoic acid—important antioxidant, key role in regeneration of reduced glutathione, but also has role in energy metabolism.
- Vitamin B_6—balance glutamate and GABA levels, lowers excitotoxicity.
- Niacin—role in energy metabolism.

- Riboflavin—important in reduction of oxidized glutathione back to reduced glutathione; also has important role in mitochondrial function.
- Thiamin—role in energy metabolism.
- Vitamin B_{12}—as nitric oxide scavenger?
- Folic acid—lowers nitric oxide synthase uncoupling.

The way I have categorized these earlier in the chapter, these agents fall into 15 distinct categories of agents expected to lower NO/ONOO⁻ cycle biochemistry.

Dr. Neboysa (Nash) Petrovic

Dr. Petrovic is a physician in South Africa who has developed his own protocol for CFS treatment that also involves numerous agents predicted to down-regulated NO/ONOO⁻ cycle biochemistry. Dr. Petrovic does not detail his treatment protocol on his own Web site.[339] The protocol description I am using here is from an earlier version of a Web site set up by Lorrie Rivers,[340] a former patient of Dr. Petrovic. According to that earlier information, Petrovic's protocol includes the following:

- Valine and isoleucine—branched-chain amino acids known to be involved in energy metabolism in mitochondria, and may be expected, therefore, to stimulate energy metabolism; modest levels may also lower excitotoxicity.
- Pyridoxine (B_6)—improves balance between glutamate and GABA, and lowers excitotoxicity.
- Vitamin B_{12} in the form of cyanocobalamin—cyanocobalamin is converted to hydroxocobalamin in the human body but the latter form will be more active as a nitric oxide scavenger since it does not require such conversion.
- Riboflavin—helps reduce oxidized glutathione back to reduced glutathione.
- Carotenoids (α-carotene, bixin, zeaxanthin and lutein)—lipid (fat)-soluble peroxynitrite scavengers.
- Flavonoids (flavones, rutin, hesperetin, and others).
- Ascorbic acid (vitamin C).
- Tocotrienols—forms of vitamin E reported to have special roles in lowering effects of excitotoxicity.
- Thiamine (aneurin)—B vitamin involved in energy metabolism.
- Magnesium.

- Zinc.
- Betaine hydrochloride (HCl)—lowers reductive stress; hydrochloride form should only be used by those deficient in stomach acid.
- Essential fatty acids including long chain omega-3 fatty acids.
- Phosphatidyl serine—reported to lower iNOS induction.[341,342]

So, according to this information, the Petrovic protocol includes 14 different agents or classes of agents predicted to lower NO/ONOO⁻ cycle biochemistry. These include two types that I have not considered previously in this chapter, the branched-chain amino acids valine and isoleucine, which are known to stimulate energy metabolism in mitochondria, and also phosphatidyl serine, which is reported to lower iNOS induction and thus lower nitric oxide levels.

AN ATTEMPT TO ASSEMBLE A "BEST GUESS" TREATMENT FOR MULTISYSTEM DISEASES

My own attempt to assemble a best guess treatment dates from a meeting that I attended about two and a half years ago, at this writing, a meeting that was also attended by Dr. Grace Ziem of Maryland. After we had both talked, Dr. Ziem asked me to propose a treatment protocol based on the NO/ONOO⁻ cycle mechanism. I went home and worked on such a protocol for several weeks and sent it to Dr. Ziem.

Ziem had already been using certain approaches outlined earlier in the chapter to treat her chemically injured patients. She was using nebulized, inhaled reduced-glutathione and also treated some patients with hyperbaric oxygen therapy (up to 1.5 atm), and she advocated environmental controls to minimize chemical exposure for all chemically injured patients. Many of her patients had low levels on laboratory testing of such important nutrients as vitamin B_{12}, coenzyme Q10, α-lipoic acid, riboflavin, B_6, magnesium, folate, selenium, copper, manganese, and zinc, and she recommended nutritional supplements to replete those who tested low in these nutrients. She was finding that this therapy was providing observable improvement in her patients, but this improvement was, as described in a personal communication, "modest and not rapid." She ascribed most of the improvement to the environmental controls minimizing chemical exposure and to the nebulized glutathione.

Dr. Ziem's patients are chemically injured, many with known initiating exposures. Some are apparently chemically injured where chemical initiation is not documented but is inferred from tests, symptoms and physical examination. Many of these patients have heightened sensory response, such as to light, sound, or touch. She feels that most of her chemically injured patients meet the diagnosis for toxic encephalopathy, arguing that this is both a more complete and more accurate diagnosis than is MCS.* Dr. Ziem makes clear on her Web site[343] that she feels the likely etiology of her patients who often suffer from reactive airways disease involves the NO/ONOO⁻ cycle and specifically the part of the cycle centered on neural sensitization.

The initial therapy that I proposed was entirely based on oral nutritional supplements, in part because Dr. Ziem wanted the therapy to avoid conventional synthetic pharmaceuticals. She states that "Drugs don't cure chemical injury." After discussion with a number of other scientists, she added nebulized, inhaled reduced-glutathione and hydroxocobalamin, and we have made certain changes to the oral supplements as well. The current protocol (and we view this as a work in progress) is as follows:

1. Nebulized, inhaled reduced glutathione
2. Nebulized, inhaled hydroxocobalamin (some use sublingual)
3. Mixed, natural tocopherols including γ-tocopherol
4. Buffered vitamin C
5. Magnesium as malate
6. Four different flavonoid sources: *Ginkgo biloba* extract, cranberry extract, silymarin, and bilberry extract
7. Selenium as selenium-grown yeast
8. Coenzyme Q10
9. Folic acid
10. Carotenoids including lycopene, lutein, and β-carotene
11. α-Lipoic acid
12. Zinc (modest dose), manganese (low dose) and copper (low dose)
13. Vitamin B$_6$ in the form of pyridoxal phosphate
14. Riboflavin 5'-phosphate (FMN)
15. Betaine (trimethylglycine)

Patients are advised to use environmental controls to reduce exposure to volatile organic solvents, pesticides and other irritant chemicals wherever possible. The therapeutic agents are not a substitute for avoidance of irritant chemicals, but rather are only effective in these chemically injured patients

---

*Dr. Ziem critiques the use of the term MCS, arguing that it was initially proposed without testing patients for a possible diagnosis of toxic encephalopathy. She expresses other concerns about the MCS diagnosis on her Web site.[343]

when used along with environmental controls. There are a number of observations that Ziem has made to optimize the protocol for specific patients, which are discussed on her Web site.[343] For example, she finds that her most severely chemically injured patients need to be started on much lower doses of the glutathione and α-lipoic acid, increasing exposure as they see initial improvement. The therapeutic agents were compounded by Key Pharmacy in Kent, Washington, which has been calling it their "neural sensitization protocol." Key Pharmacy has a Web site that lists its e-mail address and phone number, and consequently further information can be easily obtained.

Dr. Ziem reports four distinct observations about her patients:

1. The majority of her patients suffering from reactive airways were placed on this protocol during the first half of 2004, and almost all of them were on it or most of it by spring 2005. Patients coming back to see her report consistent improvement of their symptoms, including respiratory symptoms, fatigue, cognitive function, and usually migraine. Improvements were well above those seen with her previous treatment approach.
2. Historically, Dr. Ziem has gotten many emergency calls each summer from patients who have become very ill from nearby pesticide spraying. In the summer of 2004, she did not receive any such calls from her patients on the protocol. In the summer of 2005, she received only one such call from a patient on the protocol who was directly exposed to pesticide spray.
3. Two of her patients reported being completely asymptomatic, something she had not seen before. These were, however, still controlling their environment to minimize exposure and still on the protocol.
4. Patients seem to be improving at such a rapid rate that many are no longer coming in regularly to see her. She is now able to take new patients at 10 to 15 times the previous rate. In order to assess the progress of the patients who are no longer coming in, Mr. Jim Seymour has contacted 30 such patients, and all 30 report substantial improvement in their symptoms. However, the majority of them are not on the complete protocol, reporting that they are unable to be on all of it for financial reasons. Seymour's subjective assessment is that those on the complete protocol have seen much greater improvement than have those on only part.

As of the beginning of 2006, two additional agents are being added to the oral part of the protocol, acetyl-L-carnitine and taurine. We are considering adding one or two flavonoid-containing extracts that scavenge superoxide.

Dr. Ziem states, in a personal communication, that "I consider the protocol to be the most significant medical advance ever for chemical injury, but it is not a substitute for environmental controls. It does gradually allow patients to be in social environments with fewer symptoms and less severe exacerbation."

There are three factors that should be considered about Ziem's observations:

1. The previous physicians reported improvements in CFS patients or those suffering from CFS-like illness and, in the case of Teitelbaum, in CFS and FM. Ziem finds that a similar protocol works well with chemically injured patients, as well. Such chemical injury patients are often thought to be more difficult to treat than are CFS or FM patients. There is a literature reporting some complete recovery in some CFS and FM patients, but there is no similar literature regarding chemically injured patients.

2. The Pall/Ziem (PZ) protocol is entirely based on agents chosen for their ability down-regulate NO/ONOO$^-$ cycle biochemistry. The protocol of Teitelbaum and to some extent that of Cheney contain several agents that are not obviously linked to NO/ONOO$^-$ biochemistry. The PZ protocol provides the clearest evidence that a set of agents chosen for their ability to lower this biochemistry can be effective in the treatment of this class of diseases.

3. Ziem's observations suggest that comorbid diseases such as airways disease (asthma) and migraine also respond to this protocol. This suggests these diseases may respond to it in other sufferers, as well.

THERE ARE OTHERS

Other physicians have used multiple agents predicted to down-regulate NO/ONOO$^-$ cycle biochemistry to treat these diseases, including Scott Rigden (Arizona), Sarah Myhill (United Kingdom), and Gordon Baker (Washington State). Rigden's protocol was published[3] and can, therefore, be compared by the reader with the five described here. Each of these use fewer such agents but may still have substantial effectiveness. I have been working with Dr. Stephen Levine, president and founder of Allergy Research Group on an over-the-counter version of these protocols, designed to down-regulate the NO/ONOO$^-$ cycle. The protocol is called the multisystem formula and contains 19 classes of agents listed in Exhibit 15.1. We expect it to be both relatively effective, convenient, and inexpensive and information on it can be accessed at: www.allergyresearchgroup.com

TREATMENT NOW?

Biologically plausible mechanisms, as discussed in Chapter 4, are viewed as key features in support of epidemiological evidence. We have seen earlier in this chapter, that individual agents and groups of agents predicted to down-regulate NO/ONOO⁻ cycle biochemistry have been repeatedly reported in both clinical trials and in clinical observations to produce distinct and wide ranging improvements in people sufferering from multisystem diseases. The interconnection between mechanism and observation here is clearly important for two reasons.

1. The biological plausibility of the mechanisms of action of these agents provides increased plausibility to the trial data and the clinical observations supporting their efficacy.
2. Conversely, the clinical trial data, clinical observations, and anecdotal evidence provide substantial support for the NO/ONOO⁻ cycle mechanism. In other words, the mechanism is validated, to a substantial extent by the apparent efficacy of the therapies.

How, then, should we view this area based on the perspective of evidence-based medicine. In one of the most highly cited papers published on evidence-based medicine,[344] David Sackett makes the following points:

- Evidence-based medicine is not restricted to randomized trials and meta-analysis. It involves tracking down the best external evidence with which to answer our clinical questions.
- And if no randomized trial has been carried out for our patients predicament, we follow the trail to the next best external evidence and work from there.
   The practice of evidence-based medicine means:
   1. Integrating individual clinical expertise with the best available clinical evidence from systematic research.
   2. The more thoughtful identification and compassionate use of individual patients' predicaments, rights and preferences in making clinical decisions about their care.
- Evidence-based medicine is not "cookbook" medicine. It requires a bottom-up approach that integrates the best external evidence with clinical expertise and patient-choice.

There is no question that we need much more clinical trial data to compare and define the efficacy of combinations of agents designed to down-regulate NO/ONOO⁻ cycle biochemistry. But the question that faces both physicians and sufferers today is: Do we treat now based on the current evidence for effectiveness of the similar protocols of these five physicians and based on evidence of the efficacy of many of these individual agents? We have, after all, tens of millions of people around the world with multisystem diseases whose suffering may be alleviated by these treatment protocols. The individual agents and, in the hands of these physicians at least, the groups of agents, are reported to be very well tolerated by most these patients and we have, no effective alternative therapies to alleviate their abundant suffering.

So, my answer to that question is yes. Indeed it is my hope that changing the perception of medical professionals on the treatability of these diseases will lead to much more rapid diagnosis and treatment and consequent improve prognosis. Clinical observations have consistently suggested that substantial improvements are much more likely in newly occurring cases than in those who have been ill for many years previously. It is possible, therefore, that early diagnosis and treatment will not only prevent unnecessary suffering but also improve long-term prognosis.

I have no doubt that others will contest the view that we should move now to treatment with multiple agents down-regulating NO/ONOO⁻ cycle biochemistry. Reasonable people may differ on this. What I think is clear is that not asking the question is indefensible.

Chapter 16

Overview

My motives in publishing are the following: I wish to spread among men all that makes intellectual relationships and freedom of thought possible, so that it may be passed from mouth to mouth; the rest, with discernment and common sense will be accomplished by hand. Verily, I am setting in motion something with which others shall experiment.

Sir Francis Bacon

It is possible to know when you are right, way ahead of checking all the consequences. You can recognize truth by its beauty and simplicity.

Richard Feynman

In Chapter 1, I promised you a theory of these multisystem illnesses. I stated that it is the pattern of evidence that may (or may not) lead you to find that the NO/ONOO⁻ cycle mechanism has merit. My goal here is not to reiterate the pattern of evidence but to focus on whether this vision gives important insights into these illnesses—important, long-sought explanations. But before doing that, I wish to provide a useful perspective by discussing the role of theory* in biology and in science in general.

Most philosophers of science have an idealized view of science, a view that does not correspond very well to the way science is actually done in the life sciences. It has been stated that in science one proposes theories, suggests tests of those theories, and, if one performs those tests and they come

---

*The theory I am referring to here includes all types of explanatory models and is distinct from experiment or observation that may be used to test such theories.

Explaining "Unexplained Illnesses"
© 2007 by The Haworth Press, Inc. All rights reserved.
doi:10.1300/5139_16

out differently than predicted, one rejects the theory. That is the conventional view, one that was developed largely in the context of physics, where very precise predictions can often be made and tested. In the life sciences, and this is rarely recognized, this view does *not* correspond to the way science actually functions in analyzing the broadest theoretical constructs. Let me give you an example.

In Mendelian genetics taught in every basic biology and genetics text, there are two laws of inheritance proposed by Gregor Mendel in the 1860s. Those two laws* are presented as the basis of the theory of genetics. And yet, those laws rarely work well and there have been many thousands of tests of those laws that should have led to our rejecting them. These laws are inconsistent with such phenomena as linkage on chromosomes, or of multigenic inheritance where large numbers of genes are responsible for a particular trait. Mendels's laws demand complete stability of genes—that is, they are inconsistent with mutation or genetic transposition (jumping genes). They are inconsistent with genes that strongly influence survival and therefore produce very different ratios of progeny from those predicted. They do not work in bacteria and, in fact, in many other organisms. They do not work with sex-linked traits or with unstable trinucleotide repeats, which are found in many of the most studied human genetic traits. So Mendel's laws should have been rejected many thousands of times based on the conventional view of science, and yet they are taught in every textbook of basic genetics.

Why is this? There are several reasons. First of all, behind Mendel's laws are some other concepts—that genes determining biological inheritance are separate and distinct from the properties that they influence-that genotype is distinct from phenotype. Genes do segregate and recombine with each other in certain ways, but those ways vary considerably in different situations. Furthermore, the expression of those genes is often more complex than the simple dominance-recessiveness relationship described by Mendel. In other words, biology is inherently very complex but the basic insights of Mendel hold up well even when his laws do not. Those basic *insights* have revolutionized our explanations of the living world even though the quantitative tests of his *laws* should have led to our rejecting them over a century ago.

This essential conflict between the simple views of the philosophers of science and the inherent complexities of the living world has led to the love/hate relationship between life scientists and theory. On the one hand,

---

*Mendel's laws are known as the law of segregation and law of independent assortment.

the staggering diversity of observations in the life sciences demands theories to help us make sense out of this almost incomprehensible complexity. On the other hand, theories are much more difficult to test because of this complexity. When does an experiment give results that should lead to our rejecting the theory and when does it simply provide evidence that the theory is not sufficiently complex to reflect the inherent complexities of life? Still, we have no choice in the matter. Without theory, there is no science and the main role of observation and experiment is to allow us to formulate and test theory, however difficult the interpretation of such tests may be. To a greater extent than most of us realize, the tests of a theory in the life sciences often come not just from specific experimental tests but, as is true with Mendelian inheritance, with the explanations and insights they provide into the complexities of biology. The challenge to a scientist or thoughtful lay person trying to look at these insights is how to objectively assess their importance without "falling in love" with the theory and thus destroying one's objectivity. That is a major challenge and in the face of this challenge—I would simply say that you do the best you can.

COMPARISON WITH ANOTHER PARADIGM

The last great theoretical synthesis in medical science was the serial somatic mutation/selection model of cancer, which was developed about a quarter century ago. I would like to compare the NO/ONOO⁻ cycle explanatory model now with the cancer model, as it existed circa 1980. This cancer model was based, to a great extent, on several types of observations. It was based on some observations arguing that most carcinogens are mutagens; however, this was a difficult argument to make because of the many distinct types of genetic end points that were involved in carcinogenesis, because of the variable metabolism of potential carcinogens in different tissues leading to active or inactive compounds, and because some compounds that act in the overall process of carcinogenesis act to stimulate cell growth or by stimulating epigenetic mechanisms as opposed to genetic mechanisms. Nevertheless, the focus on specific mutant genes having a positive role in carcinogenesis (oncogenes) and others having a negative role in carcinogenesis (tumor suppressor genes) allowed scientists to produce convincing evidence for genetic mechanisms in specific types of cancer. And these studies, in turn, allowed scientists to integrate other mechanisms, such as chromosomal rearrangement mechanisms, gene amplification mechanisms, viral carcinogenesis mechanisms, mechanisms that selectively stimulate the growth of precancer cells, and epigenetic mechanisms into the overall explanatory model. The solidity of the data implicating certain genes in certain specific types of cancer allowed one to use their role as the base for a conceptual framework that could be used to integrate these other factors. That conceptual framework, in turn, could be used to make sense of the staggering diversity one sees in different types of cancer.

So how does the NO/ONOO⁻ cycle compare with the serial somatic mutation/selection model of cancer? I am not saying that the roles of nitric oxide, peroxynitrite, and NMDA receptors are as well documented in these multisystem diseases as were the roles of specific genes in cancer. Certainly, the roles of such oncogenes such as ras or myc or the that of the tumor suppressor gene *p53* in certain forms of cancer was more convincingly established 25 years ago than is the causal role of nitric oxide, peroxynitrite, or NMDA receptors in multisystem diseases now. Yes, we do have evidence from animal models and from humans, but the studies specifically aimed at testing NO/ONOO⁻ cycle roles in these diseases are just starting. Yes, we do have evidence that several short-term stressors may act to increase nitric oxide synthase activity, but again, such studies on the mechanisms of action of short-term stressors are only beginning to be focused on the issue of their possible role in initiating the NO/ONOO⁻ cycle.

Nevertheless, as an explanatory model, the NO/ONOO⁻ cycle has at least as much power as did the serial somatic mutation/selection model of cancer. It takes a series of individually well-documented biochemical and physiological mechanisms and develops a mechanism that provides detailed explanations for each of the following:

1. It provides explanations for the etiology of not just one but all four of these multisystem diseases.
2. It explains their chronic nature.
3. It explains how cases of each can be initiated by 12 diverse and distinct stressors.
4. It explains the diverse biochemical and physiological properties of the chronic phase of these diseases.
5. It explains how 18 different agents or groups of agents may produce reported improvements and how the treatment protocols of five different physicians may lead to major improvements in sufferers.
6. It explains 16 of the shared symptoms and signs of these diseases, symptoms and signs that have repeatedly been described as being previously unexplained.
7. It explains the symptoms that are specific for each type of disease, symptoms that can be explained by the influence of the NO/ONOO⁻ cycle on specific tissues.

8. It explains their high comorbidity with each other.
9. It explains their high comorbidity with such well-accepted diseases as tinnitus, asthma, migraine, lupus, and rheumatoid arthritis.
10. It explains 11 distinct puzzling features of multiple chemical sensitivity (MCS), only one of which was adequately explained previously.
11. It explains the properties of animal models of chronic fatigue syndrome (CFS), MCS, and post-traumatic stress disorder (PTSD), each of which provides evidence, in turn, supporting a NO/ONOO⁻ cycle etiology.
12. It explains the stunning qualitative and quantitative variation in symptoms from one patient to another.

We had no previous etiologic theory that explained any one of these, let alone all 12. I fully acknowledge that I am not an objective observer here. But I do not see how anyone can see the extraordinary fit between observation and explanation and the equally extraordinary previous lack of adequate explanation without coming to the conclusion that the NO/ONOO⁻ cycle theory is at least the etiologic theory of preference for these four diseases. It has no rivals. When one adds that it explains 14 additional diseases/illnesses including eight common and well-accepted diseases, many of them almost effortlessly, it is difficult to ignore its power as an explanatory model.

The fit between this explanatory model and so many distinct but related previously puzzling areas of medicine is the most persuasive evidence for its validity. The NO/ONOO⁻ cycle mechanism has great explanatory power and that explanatory power argues, in the absence of any empirical evidence to the contrary, that it has great merit.

THREE SETS OF PRINCIPLES

In the writing of this book, I have listed three sets of principles that have allowed us to focus on the major issues of the NO/ONOO⁻ cycle. It is worthwhile revisiting these in this overview chapter of the book.

The first of these, presented in Chapter 1, contains the five principles upon which the NO/ONOO⁻ cycle is based:

1. Short-term stressors that initiate cases of multisystem illnesses act by raising nitric oxide synthesis and consequent levels of nitric oxide and its oxidant product peroxynitrite.

2. Initiation is converted into a chronic illness through the action of vicious cycle mechanisms, through which chronic elevation of nitric oxide and peroxynitrite and other cycle elements is produced and maintained.
3. Symptoms and signs of these illnesses are generated by elevated levels of nitric xide and/or other important consequences of the proposed mechanism, i.e., elevated levels of peroxynitrite or inflammatory cytokines, oxidative stress, and elevated NMDA and vanilloid receptor activity.
4. Because the compounds involved, nitric oxide, superoxide, and peroxynitrite, have quite limited diffusion distances in biological tissues and because the mechanisms involved in the cycle act at the level of individual cells, the fundamental mechanisms are local.
5. Therapy should focus on down-regulating NO/ONOO⁻ cycle biochemistry.

The second is the set of four principles listed early in Chapter 14 were from Dr. Claudia Miller's paraphrasing of Kuhn's principles for consideration of a theory as a new paradigm:

1. *Anomaly:* Clearly the fact that these four multisystem diseases are repeatedly described as unexplained shows that they fail to fit the currently accepted disease paradigms, and therefore are anomalous.
2. *Causality:* Causality is less firmly established. The main evidence for causality is from animal model studies, from the fit with the symptoms and signs of these illnesses, from the link to short-term stressors that can increase nitric oxide or other cycle elements (i.e., superoxide), from the roles of certain specific genes in determining susceptibility, and from therapy via agents that also are predicted to lower the elements of the cycle.
3. *Generalizability:* The NO/ONOO⁻ cycle can be generalized not only to these four multisystem diseases but quite possibly to 14 additional diseases/illnesses. It may be among the most generalizable disease paradigms among the 10 discussed in Chapter 14.
4. *Novelty:* Clearly, this is a novel mechanism for human disease, although it shares, with a few other examples, the role of a vicious cycle.

The third set of four principles was discussed in Chapters 3 and 14, which may be the most important in assessing overall merit:

1. It is *integrative:* It integrates into a common scheme a wide variety of previously unexplained diseases/illnesses.
2. It is *comprehensive:* It encompasses a wide variety of observations about these diseases including their patterns of case initiation, their chronic nature, many of their shared and unique symptoms and signs of the chronic phase of these diseases. It also explains the reported efficacy of over a dozen distinct agents. Each of these four aspects has previously challenged explanation and the combination of all four has been a much larger challenge.
3. It is *parsimonious:* It explains by a relatively simple conceptual framework many previously unexplained observations.
4. It is *fundamental:* Because it is based primarily at the biochemical level, it explains much of the complexity of these diseases through the impact of a common biochemistry on a variety of organismal functions.

CAN YOU HELP?

For those of you who think the NO/ONOO⁻ cycle theory has merit, I need your help. The process of science requires that theories receive critical scrutiny in order to test their merit, but this theory has not received sufficient interest or scrutiny to date. I have received invitations to give major addresses to international scientific meetings, but this is just the beginning of the needed process. There are many barriers to this process. The NO/ONOO⁻ cycle is sufficiently complex that simple laziness may be expected to constrain attention and scrutiny. There are many others.

One of the little secrets of science is that if the process of science is successful, we scientists are continually in the process of making ourselves obsolete. If we have established something, it is time to move on. Many of us have become comfortable with this challenge but many have not, placing a barrier to progress—it is easier to continue to do what we have been doing by ignoring insights that suggest we need to progressively change our approach. In the health sciences, there seems to be a special barrier because of a high-level role of "authority" in making what are presumably scientific decisions—it often seems that one individual or group is continually waiting for a group in authority to tell them it is alright to consider or establish a new viewpoint. This is unlike other areas of science, where most scientists take pride in thinking for themselves. So, for example, the new paradigm for gastric ulcers as an infectious disease took about 10 years to be accepted after the evidence supporting it was very strong, despite the fact that it pro-

vided a simple and effective treatment for this disease. How much more difficult will this be for this putative paradigm, given the complexities of
multisystem diseases? How long will it take before claims that these illnesses are unexplained will be commonly challenged? How long will it take
before the predictions of the NO/ONOO⁻ cycle will lead further therapeutic trials that may, in turn, establish effective treatment of the millions
suffering from these diseases? And how many millions will needlessly
suffer because of the inertia of "the system"?

There are other barriers. This putative paradigm was developed with no
support from the NIH or and CDC, despite their role as leaders in medical
science support. Indeed, the lack of support from the NIH for research on
MCS is a disgrace, given the high prevalence of this illness in the population,
and can only be rationalized based on the view that it is not a real illness.
The support for CFS or fibromyalgia (FM) research has been marginal at
best. One should not ignore the roles of major economic interests that have
a vested interest in maintaining the view that these are not real illnesses, let
alone real diseases. These economic interests can have major roles in influencing the science and science funding. Neglect from the NIH, CDC, and
certain foundations with claimed interest in CFS or FM breeds further neglect, given that the alternative may be to admit that they have been less
than diligent in their duties to support and, in the case of foundations, to
publicize important developments. Such neglect from the NIH is not unusual. For example, when the Nobel Prize was given to Stanley Prusiner for
his work on the prion theory of disease, it was commented that this work
was mostly supported by foundations and was long neglected by the NIH.
And some foundations have been reticent to follow in the wake of the
March of Dimes, which, having helped to prevent polio, was in the difficult
situation of either having to go out of business or finding another disease to
support-they ended up supporting research on birth defects, an area of
research that is sufficiently diverse that they will never have to worry about
preventing or curing all of them.

I do *not* ask for and indeed do *not* want uncritical acceptance. Rather,
what is needed is appropriate attention and scrutiny, as well as appropriate
challenge to previously repeated dogma. To the extent that you can encourage the process of science, I need your help.

Kuhn, in his famous book, *The Structure of Scientific Revolutions,* observed that new scientific paradigms have most often been developed by
people who are new to a field, providing novel insights not shared by more
established authorities. Such insights by outsiders are often initially rejected, in part because they come from outsiders. I am a person new to this
field, having only turned my attention to it in early 1998 and published my

first paper in this area in January of 2000. Kuhn observed that[1] (p. 64) "Novelty emerges only with difficulty, against a background provided by expectation." I would hope that knee-jerk rejection, which has initially greeted other new insights, not be the predominant initial response to this one. However, most proposed new paradigms turn out to be wrong, and so skepticism is much needed. It is my hope that this will be healthy skepticism, which is fundamental to all good science.

The need for good science here is far from academic. There are tens of millions of people whose lives are severely impacted by these diseases and they are depending on us, whether they know it or not, to do the right thing.

References

Chapter 1

1. Miller CS. Are we on the threshold of a new theory of disease? Toxicant-induced loss of tolerance and its relationship in addiction and abdiction. *Toxicol Ind Health* 1999;15:284-294.

2. Buchwald D, Garrity D. Comparison of patients with chronic fatigue syndrome, fibromyalgia, and multiple chemical sensitivities. *Arch Int Med* 1994;154: 2049-2053.

3. Ziem G, Donnay A. Chronic fatigue, fibromyalgia, and chemical sensitivity: overlapping disorders. *Arch Intern Med* 1995;155:1913.

4. Donnay A, Ziem G. Prevalence and overlap of chronic fatigue syndrome and fibromyalgia syndrome among 100 new patients. *J Chronic Fatigue Syndr* 1999; 5(3/4):71-80.

5. Clauw DJ, Crousos GP. Chronic pain and fatigue syndromes: overlapping clinical and neuroendocrine features. *Neuroimmunomodulation* 1997;4:134-153.

6. Yunus MB. Central sensitivity syndromes: a unified concept for fibromyalgia and other similar maladies. *J Indian Rheumatism Assoc* 2001;8(1):27-33.

7. White KP, Speechley M, Harth M, Ostbye T. Co-existence of chronic fatigue syndrome with fibromyalgia in the general population - A controlled study. *Scand J Rheum* 2000;29:44-51.

8. Rowat SC. Integrated defense system overlaps as a disease model: with examples for multiple chemical sensitivity. *Env Health Perspect* 1998;106(Suppl 1): 85-109.

9. Clauw D. Fibromyalgia associated syndromes. *J Musculoskeletal Pain* 2002; 10(1/2):201-214.

10. Wessely S, Nimnuan C, Sharpe M. Functional somatic syndromes: one or many? *Lancet* 1999;354:936-939.

11. Aaron LA, Buchwald D. A review of the evidence for overlap among unexplained clinical conditions. *Ann Intern Med* 2001;134:868-881.

12. Lipschitz EL. Chronic fatigue syndrome and posttraumatic stress disorder. *JAMA* 2001;286:916-917.

13. Cohen H, Neumann L, Haiman Y, Matar MA, Press J, Buskila D. Prevalence of post-traumatic stress disorder in fibromyalgia patients: overlapping syndromes of post-traumatic fibromyalgia syndrome? *Semin Arthritis Rheum* 2002;32: 38-50.

Explaining "Unexplained Illnesses"
© 2007 by The Haworth Press, Inc. All rights reserved.
doi:10.1300/5139_17

14. Friedman MJ. Neurobiological sensitization models of post-traumatic stress disorder: their possible relevance to multiple chemical sensitivity syndrome. *Toxicol Ind Health* 1994;10:449-462.

15. Pall ML. Common etiology of posttraumatic stress disorder, fibromyalgia, chronic fatigue syndrome and multiple chemical sensitivity via elevated nitric oxide/peroxynitrite. *Med Hypoth* 2001;57:139-145.

16. The Iowa Persian Gulf Study Group. Self-reported illness and health status among Gulf War veterans–a population-based study. *JAMA* 1997;227:238-245.

17. Kipen MH, Hallman W, Kang'H, Fiedler N, Natelson BH. Prevalence of chronic fatigue and chemical sensitivities in Gulf War Registry Veterans. *Arch Environ Health* 1999;54:313-318.

18. Nicolson GL, Nicolson NL. Gulf War illnesses: complex medical, scientific paradox. *Med Confl Surviv* 1998;14:156-165.

19. Hodgson MJ, Kipen HM. Gulf War illnesses: causation and treatment. *J Occup Environ Med* 1999;41:443-452.

20. Baker DG, Mendenhall CL, Simbartl LA, Magan LK, Steinberg JL. Relationship between posttraumatic stress disorder and self-reported symptoms of Persian Gulf War veterans. *Arch Intern Med* 1997;157:2076-2078.

21. Pall ML. Elevated, sustained peroxynitrite levels as the cause of chronic fatigue syndrome. *Med Hypoth* 2000;54:115-125.

22. Behan PO, Goldberg DP, Mowbray JF, eds. Postviral Fatigue Syndrome, *Br Med J*, vol 47. Edinburgh: Churchill Livingstone;1991.

23. Bell, DS. *The Doctor's Guide to Chronic Fatigue Syndrome*. Reading, MA: Addison-Wesley;1995.

24. Komaroff AL. Clinical presentation of chronic fatigue syndrome. *Ciba Foundation Symp* 1993;173:43-54.

25. Mowbray JF, Yousef GE. Immunology of postviral fatigue syndrome. *Br Med Bull* 1991;47:886-894.

26. Behan PO, Bakheit AMO. Clinical spectrum of postviral fatigue syndrome. *Br Med Bull* 1991;47:793-808.

27. Natelson BH, Lange G. A status report on chronic fatigue syndrome. *Environ Health Perspect* 2002;110(suppl 4):673-677.

28. Englebienne P, DeMeirleir K, eds. *Chronic Fatigue Syndrome: A Biological Approach*. Boca Raton: CRC Press;2002.

29. Rea T, Russo J, Katon W, Ashley RL, Buchwald D. A prospective study of tender points and fibromyalgia during and after an acute viral infection. *Arch Intern Med* 1999;159:865-870.

30. Massarotti EM. Lyme arthritis. *Med Clin North Am* 2002;86:297-309.

31. Daoud KF, Barkhuizen A. Rheumatic mimics and selected triggers of fibromyalgia. *Curr Pain Headache Rep* 2002;6:284-288.

32. Vassilopoulos D, Calabrese LH. Rheumatic manifestations of hepatitis C infection. *Curr Rheumatol Rep* 2003;5:200-204.

33. Buskila D, Gladman DD, Langevitz P, Urowitz S, Smythe HA. Fibromyalgia in human immunodeficiency virus infection. *J Rheumatol* 1990;17:1202-1206.

34. Wolfe F. Fibromyalgia. *Rheum Dis Clin North Am* 1990;16:681-698.

35. Waylonis GW, Perkins RH. Post-traumatic fibromyalgia. A long term follow-up. *Am J Phys Med Rehabil* 1994;73:403-412.

36. Greenfield S, Fitzcharled MA, Esdaille JM. Reactive fibromyalgia syndrome. *Arthritis Rheum* 1992;35:678-681.

37. Aaron LA, Bradley LA, Alacon GS, et al. Perceived physical and emotional trauma as precipitating events in fibromyalgia. Associations with health care seeking and disability status but not pain severity. *Arthritis Rheum* 1997;40:453-460.

38. Al-Allaf AW, Dunbar KL, Hallum NS, Nosratzadeh B, Templeton KD, Pullar T. A case-control study examining the role of physical trauma in the onset of fibromyalgia syndrome. *Rheumatology* 2002;41:450-453.

39. Buskila D, Neumann L, Vaisberg G, Alakalay D, Wolfe F. Increased rates of fibromyalgia following cervical spine injury. A controlled study of 161 cases of traumatic injury. *Arthritis Rheum* 1997;40:446-452.

40. Neumann L, Zeldets V, Bolotin A, Buskila D. Outcome of posttraumatic fibromyalgia: a 3-year followup of 78 cases of cervical spine injuries. *Semin Arthritis Rheum* 2003;32:320-325.

41. Ashford NA, Miller C. *Chemical Exposures: Low Levels and High Stakes.* New York: John Wiley and Sons, Inc;1998.

42. Sorg BA. Multiple chemical senstivity: Potential role for neural sensitization. *Crit Rev Neurobiol* 1999;13:283-316.

43. Johnson A, ed. Casualties of Progress. MCS Information Exchange, Brunswick, ME; 2000.

44. Miller CS, Mitzel HC. Chemical sensitivity attributed to pesticide exposure versus remodeling. *Arch Environ Health* 1995;50:119-129.

45. Rea WJ. *Chemical Sensitivity.* Vol. 1, Boca Raton: Lewis Publishers;1992.

46. American Psychiatric Association. *Diagnostic and Statistical Manual of Mental Disorders* 4th ed. DSM-IV. Washington, DC: American Psychiatric Press; 1994.

47. Pall ML. Elevated peroxynitrite as the cause of chronic fatigue syndrome: Other inducers and mechanisms of symptom generation. *J Chronic Fatigue Syndr* 2000;7(4):45-58.

48. Pall ML. Common etiology of posttraumatic stress disorder, fibromyalgia, chronic fatigue syndrome and multiple chemical sensitivity. *Medical Hypoth* 2001; 57:139-145.

49. Pall ML, Satterlee JD. Elevated nitric oxide/peroxynitrite mechanism for the common etiology of multiple chemical sensitivity, chronic fatigue syndrome and posttraumatic stress disorder. *Ann NY Acad Sci* 2001;933:323-329.

50. Pall ML. NMDA sensitization and stimulation by peroxynitrite, nitric oxide and organic *FASEB J* 2002;16:1407-1417.

51. Pall ML. Elevated nitric oxide/peroxynitrite theory of multiple chemical sensitivity: central role of N-methyl-D-aspartate receptors in the sensitivity mechanism. *Environ Health Perspect* 2003;111:1461-1464.

52. Pall ML, Anderson JH. The vanilloid receptor as a putative target of diverse chemicals in multiple chemical sensitivity. *Arch Environ Health* 2004;59: 363-375.

53. Wallis RA, Panizzon KL, Girard JM. Traumatic neuroprotection with inhibitors of nitric oxide and ADP-ribosylation. *Brain Res* 1996;710:169-177.

54. Stoll G, Jander S, Schroeter M. Detrimental and beneficial effects of injury-induced inflammation and cytokine expression in the nervous system. *Adv Exp Med Biol* 2002;513:87-113.

55. Wada K, Chatzipanteli K, Busto R, Dietrich WD. Role of nitric oxide in traumatic brain injury in the rat. *J Neurosurg* 1998;89:807-818.

56. Lewen A, Matz P, Chan PH. Free radical pathways in CNS injury. *J Neurotrauma* 2000;17:871-890.

57. Khaldi A, Chiueh CC, Bullock MR, Woodward JJ. The signficance of nitric oxide production in the brain after injury. *Ann NY Acad Sci* 2002;962:53-59.

58. Obrenovitch TP, Urenjak J. Is extracellular glutamate the key to excitotoxicity after brain injury? *J Neurotrauma* 1997;14:677-698.

59. Khaldi A, Chiueh CC, Bullock MR, Woodward JJ. The significance of nitric oxide production in the brain after injury. *Ann NY Acad Sci* 2002;962:53-59.

60. Lynch DR, Dawson TM. Secondary mechanisms in neuronal trauma. *Curr Opin Neurol* 7:1994;510-516.

61. Palmer GC. Neuroprotection by NMDA receptor antagonists in a variety of neuropathologies. *Curr Drug Targets* 2001;2:241-271.

62. Gebhardt F, Nussler AK, Rosch M, Pfetsch H, Kinzl L, Bruckner UB. Early posttraumatic increase in production of nitric oxide in humans. *Shock* 1998;10:237-242.

63. Wotta DR, El-Fakahany E. Muscarinic receptor-mediated activation of nitric oxide synthase. *Drug Dev Res* 1997;40:205-214.

64. McKinney M. Muscarinic receptor subtype-specific coupling to second messengers in neuronal systems. *Prog Brain Res* 1993;98:333-340.

65. van Zwieten PA, Doods HN. Muscarinic receptors and drugs in cardiovascular medicine. *Cardiovasc Drugs Ther* 1995;9:159-167.

66. Okere CO, Kaba H, Higuchi T. Importance of endogenous nitric oxide synthase in the rat hypothalamus and amygdala in mediating the response to capsaicin. *J Comp Neurol* 2000;423: 670-686.

67. Wu J, Lin Q, McAdoo DJ, Willis WD. Nitric oxide contributes to central sensitization following intradermal injection of capsaicin. *Neuroreport* 1998;9:589-92.

68. Rinder J. Sensory neuropeptides and nitric oxide in nasal vascular regulation. *Acta Physiol Scand* 1996;(Suppl 632):1-45.

69. Akiba Y, Guth PH, Engel E, Nastaskin I, Kaunitz JD. Acid-sensing pathways of rat duodenum. *Am J Physiol* 1999;277:G268-74.

70. Suzuki T, Wada S, Tomizawa N, et al. A possible role of nitric oxide formation in the vasodilation of rabbit ear artery induced by topically applied capsaicin analogue. *J Vet Med Sci.* 1998;60:691-697.

71. Hou M, Uddman R, Tajti J, Kanje M, Edvinsson L. Capsaicin receptor immunoreactivity in the human trigeminal ganglion. *Neurosci Lett.* 2002;330:223-226.

72. Kamei J, Tanihara H, Igarashi H, Kasuya Y. The effects of N-methyl-D-aspartate antagonists on the cough reflex. *Eur J Pharmacol* 1989;168:153-158.

73. Coderre TJ, Melzack R. Central neural mediators of secondary hyperalgesia following heat injury in rats: neuropeptides and excitatory amino acids. *Neurosci Lett* 1991;131:71-74.

74. Dougherty PM, Willis WD. Enhanced responses of spinothalamic tract neurons to excitatory amino acids accompany capsaicin-induced sensitization in monkey. *J Neurosci* 1992;12:883-894.

75. Dray A. Neurophacological mechanisms of capsaicin and related substances. *Biochem Pharmacol* 1992;44:611-615.

76. Andersen OK, Felsby S, Nicolaisen L, Bjerring P, Jensen TS, Arendt-Nielsen L. The effect of Ketamine on stimulation of primary and secondary hyperalgesia area induced by capsaicin—a double blind, placebo-controlled, human experimental study. *Pain* 1996;66:51-62.

77. Sethna NF, Liu M, Gracely R, Bennett GJ, Max MB. Analgesic and cognitive effects of intravenous ketamine-alfentanil combinations versus either drug alone after intradermal capsaicin in normal subjects. *Anesth Analg* 1998;86:1250-1256.

78. Mitsikostas DD, Sanchez del Rio M, Waeber C, Moskowitz MA, Cutrer FM. The NMDA receptor antagonist MK-801 reduces capsaicin-induced c-fos expression within rat trigeminal nucleus caudalis. *Pain* 1998;76:239-248.

79. Kawamata T, Omote K, Toriyabe M, Kawamata M, Namiki A. Involvement of capsaicin-sensitive fibers in spinal NMDA-induced glutamate release. *Neuroreport* 2001;12:3447-3450.

80. Palazzo E, de Novellis V, Marabese I, et al. Interaction between vanilloid and glutamate receptors in the central modulation of nociception. *Eur J Pharmacol* 2002;439:69-75.

81. Heresco-Levy U, Javitt DC. The role of N-methyl-D-asparate (NMDA) receptor-mediated neurotransmission in the pathophysiology and therapeutics of psychiatric syndromes. *Neuropharmacol* 1998;8:141-152.

82. McEwen BS. Possible mechanisms for atrophy of the human hippocampus. *Mol Psychiatry* 1997;2:255-262.

83. Chambers RA, Bremner JD, Moghaddam B, Southwick SM, Charney DS, Krystal JH. Glutamate and post-traumatic stress disorder: toward a psychobiology of dissociation. *Semin Clin Neuropsychiatry* 1999;4:274-281.

84. Miserendino MJ, Sananes CB, Melia KR, Davis M. Blocking of acquisition but not expression of conditioned fear-potentiated startle by NMDA antagonists in the amygdala. *Nature* 1990;345:716-718.

85. Goldstein LE, Rasmussen AM, Bunney BS, Roth RH. Role of the amygdala in the coordination of behavioral, neuroendocrine and prefrontal cortical monoamine responses to psychological stress in the rat. *J Neurosci* 1996;16:4787-4798.

86. Goldstein LE, Rasmussen AM, Bunney BS, Roth RH. The NMDA glycine site antagonist (+)-HA-966 selectively regulates conditioned stress-induced metabolic activation of the mesofrontal cortical dopamine but not serotonin systems: a behavioral, neuroendocrine and neurochemical study. *J Neurosci* 1994;14:4937-4950.

87. Adamec RE, Burton P, Shallow T, Budgell J. NMDA receptors mediate lasting increases in anxiety-like behavior produced by the stress of predator exposure—

implications for anxiety associated with posttraumatic stress disorder. *Physiol Behav* 1999;65:723-737.

88. Gould E, Cameron HA. Early NMDA blockade impairs defensive behavior and increases cell proliferation in the dentate gyrus of developing rats. *Behav Neurosci* 1997;111:49-56.

89. Shors TJ, Elkabes S, Selcher JC, Black IB. Stress persistently increases NMDA receptor-mediated binding of [3H]PDBu (a marker for protein kinase C) in the amygdala and re-exposure to the stressful context reactivates the increase. *Brain Res* 1997;750:293-300.

90. Laudanno OM, Cesolari JA, San Miguel P, Bedini OA. A role of inducible nitric oxide synthase in acute gastric mucosal damage in stress in rats. *Acta Gastroenterol Latinoam* 1996;26:221-224.

91. Behan PO. Chronic fatigue syndrome as a delayed reaction to chronic low-dose organophosphate exposure. *J Nutr Environ Med* 1996;6:341.

92. Kennedy G, Abbot NC, Spence V, Underwood C, Belch JJ. The specificity of the CDC-1994 criteria for chronic fatigue syndrome: comparison of health status in three groups of patients who fulfill the criteria. *Ann Epidemiol* 2004;14:95-100.

93. Wood GC, Bentall RP, Gopfert M, Edwards RH. A comparative psychiatric assessment of patients with chronic fatigue syndrome and muscle diseases. *Psychol Med* 1991;21:619-628.

94. Dobbins JG, Natelson BH, Brassloff I, Drastal S, Sisto S-A. Physical, behavioral, and psychological risk factors for chronic fatigue syndrome: a central role for stress? *J Chronic Fatigue Syndr* 1995;1:43-58.

95. Taylor RR, Jason LA. Chronic fatigue, abuse-related traumatization, and psychiatric disorders in a community-based sample. *Social Sci Med* 2002;55: 247-256.

96. Klimas NG, Morgan R, Salvato F, et al. Chronic fatigue syndrome and psychoneuroimmunology. In: Schneiderman N, McCabe P, Baum A, eds. *Stress and Disease Progression: Perspectives in Behavioral Medicine.* Hillsdale, NJ: Lawrence Erlbaum, Assoc.;1992:121-137.

97. Sorg BA, Prasad BM. Potential role of stress and sensitization in the development and expression of multiple chemical sensitivity. *Environ Health Perspect* 1997;105(Suppl)2:467-471.

98. Bell IR, Baldwin CM, Russek LGS, Schwartz GER, Hardin EE. Early life stress, negative paternal relationships, and chemical intolerance in middle-age women: support for a neural sensitization model. *J Women's Health* 1998;7: 1135-1147.

99. Harvey AG, Brewin CR, Jones C, Kopelman MD. Coexistence of posttraumatic stress disorder and traumatic brain injury: Towards a resolution of the paradox. *J Int Neuropsychological Soc* 2003;9:663-676.

100. Shalev AY. Acute stress reactions in adults. *Biol Psychiatry* 2002;51: 532-543.

101. Boisset-Pioro MH, Esdaile JM, Fitzcharles MA. Sexual and physical abuse in women with fibromyalgia syndrome. *Arthritis Rheum* 1995;38:235-241.

102. Racciatti D, Vecchiet J, Ceccomancini A, Ricci F, Pizzigallo E. Chronic fatigue syndrome following a toxic exposure. *Sci Total Environ* 2001;270:27-31.

103. Chester AC, Levine PH. Concurrent sick building syndrome and chronic fatigue syndrome. *Clin Infect Dis* 1994;18(suppl 1):S43-S48.

104. Abdel-Rahman A, Shetty AK, Abou-Donia MB. Disruption of the blood-brain barrier and neuronal death in cingulated cortex, dentate gyrus, thalamus and hypothalamus in a rat model of Gulf-War syndrome. *Neurobiol Dis* 2002;10:306-326.

105. Abdel-Rahman A, Abou-Donia SM, El-Masry EM, et al. Stresss and combined exposure to low doses of pyridostigmine bromide, DEET and permethrin produce neurochemical and neuropathological alterations in cerebral cortex, hippocampus and cerebellum. *J Toxicol Env Health* 2004;676:163-192.

106. Piette J, Piret B, Bonizzi G, et al. Multiple redox regulation in NF-κB transcription factor activation. *Biol Chem* 1997;378:1237-1245.

107. Baeuerle PA, Henkel T. Function and activation of NF-κB in the immune system. *Ann Rev Immunol* 1994;12:141-179.

108. Janssen-Heininger YM, Poynter ME, Baeuerle PA. Recent advances towards understanding redox mechanisms in the activation of nuclear factor kappa B. *Free Radic Biol Med* 2000;28:1317-1327.

109. Cooke CL, Davidge ST. Peroxynitrite increases iNOS through NF-κB and decreases prostacyclin synthase in endothelial cells. *Am J Physiol Cell Physiol* 2002;282:C395-C402.

110. Rieber P, Baeuerle PA. Reactive oxygen intermediates as apparently widely used messengers in the activation of the NF-kappa B transcription factor and HIV-1. *EMBO J* 1991;10:2247-2258.

111. Akira S, Kishimoto T. NF-IL6 and NF-κB in cytokine gene regulation. *Adv Immunol* 1997;65:1-46.

112. Baeuerle PA, Baichal VR. NF-κB as a frequent target for immunosuppressive and anti-inflammatory molecules. *Adv Immunol* 1997;65:111-137.

113. Roebuck KA. Regulation of interleukin-8 gene expression. *J Interferon Cytokine Res* 1999;19:429-438.

114. Palanki MS. Inhibitors of AP-1 and NF-κB mediated transcriptional activation: therapeutic potential in autoimmune diseases and structural diversity. *Curr Med Chem* 2002;9:219-227.

115. Xie QW, Kashiwabara Y, Nathan C. Role of transcription factor NF-kappa B B/Rel in induction of nitric oxide synthase. *J Biol Chem* 1994;269:4705-4708.

116. Asehoune K, Strassheim D, Mitra S, Kim JY, Abraham E. Involvement of reactive oxygen species in Toll-like receptor 4-dependent activation of NF-κB. *J Immunol* 2004;172:2522-2529.

117. Bai Y, Onuma H, Bai X, et al. Persistent nuclear factor-kappa B activation in Ucp2$^{-/-}$ mice leads to enhanced nitric oxide and inflammatory cytokine production. *J Biol Chem* 2005;280:19062-19069.

118. Snyder AR, Morgan WF. Differential induction and activation of NF-kappa B transcription complexes in radiation-induced chromosomally unstable cell lines. *Environ Mol Mutagen* 2005;45:177-187.

119. Zheng X, Zhang Y, Chen YQ, et al. Inhibition of NF-κB stabilizes gadd45-alpha mRNA. *Biochem Biophys Res Commun* 2005;329:95-99.

120. Goldhaber JI, Qayum MS. Oxygen free radicals and excitation-contraction coupling. *Antioxid Redox Signal* 2000;2:55-64.

121. Chakraborti T, Das S, Mondal M, Roychoudhury S, Chakraborti S. Oxidant, mitochondria and calcium: an overview. *Cell Signal* 1999;11:77-85.

122. Lounsbury KM, Hu Q, Ziegelstein RC. Calcium signaling and oxidant stress in the vasculature. *Free Rad Biol Med* 2000;28:1362-1369.

123. Zaidi A, Michaelis ML. Effects of reactive oxygen species on brain synaptic plasma membrane Ca(2+)-ATPase. *Free Radic Biol Med* 1999;27:810-821.

124. Schoneich C, Viner RI, Ferrington DA, Bigelow DJ. Age-related chemical modification of the skeletal muscle sarcoplasmic reticulum Ca-ATPase of the rat. *Mech Ageing Dev* 1999;107:221-231.

125. Muriel P, Sandoval G. Hepatic basolateral plasma high-affinity Ca^{2+}-ATPase is inhibited by nitric oxide and peroxynitrite anion. *J Appl Toxicol* 2000; 20:435-439.

126. Gutierrez-Martin Y, Martin-Romero FJ, Henao F, Gutierrez-Merino C. Synaptosomal plasma membrane Ca(2+) pump activity inhibition by repetitive micromolar $ONOO^-$ pulses. *Free Radic Biol Med* 2002;32:46-55.

127. Choudhary G, Dudley SC Jr. Heart failure, oxidative stress, and ion channel modulation. *Congest Heart Fail* 2002;8(3):148-155.

128. Grover AK, Kwan CY, Samson SE. Effects of peroxynitrite on sarco/endoplasmic reticulum Ca^{2+} pump isoforms SERCA2b and SERCA3A. *Am J Physiol Cell Physiol* 2003;285:C1537-C1543.

129. Mattson MP. Free radicals, calcium, and the synaptic plasticity-cell death continuum: emerging roles of the transcription factor NF kappa B. *Int Rev Neurobiol* 1998;42:103-168.

130. Lewis RS. Calcium oscillations in T-cells: mechanisms and consequences for gene expression. *Biochem Soc Trans* 2003;31:925-929.

131. MacMillan-Crow LA, Crow JP, Kerby JP, Beckman J, Thompson JA. Nitration and inactivation of manganese superoxide dismutase in chronic rejection of human renal allografts. *Proc Natl Acad Sci USA* 1996;93:11853-11858.

132. MacMillan-Crow LA, Crow JP, Thompson JA. Peroxynitrite-mediated inactivation of manganese superoxide dismutase involves nitration and oxidation of critical tyrosine residues. *Biochemistry* 1998;37:1613-1622.

133. McCord JM, Roy RS. The pathophysiology of superoxide: roles of inflammation and ischemia. *Can J Physiol Pharmacol* 1982;60:1346-1352.

134. McCord JM. Oxygen-derived free radicals in postischemic tissue injury. *N Engl J Med* 1985;312:159-163.

135. Atlante A, Gagliardi S, Minervini GM, et al. Glutamate neurotoxicity in rat cerebellar granule cells: a major role for xanthine oxidase in oxygen radical formation. *J Neurochem* 1997;68:2038-2045.

136. Berry CE, Hare JM. Xanthine oxidoreductase and cardiovascular disease: molecular mechanisms and pathophysiological implications. *J Physiol* 2003;555: 589-606.

137. Meneshian A, Bulkley GB. The physiology of endothelial xanthine oxidase: from urate metabolism to reperfusion injury in inflammatory signal transduction. *Microcirculation* 2002;9:161-175.

138. Kosenko E, Venediktova N, Kaminsky Y, Montoliu C, Felipo V. Sources of oxygen radicals in brain in acute ammonia intoxication in vivo. *Brain Res* 2003; 981:193-200.

139. Amaya F, Oh-hashi K, Naruse Y, et al. Local inflammation increases vanilloid receptor 1 expression within distinct subgroups of DRG neurons. *Brain Res* 2003;963:190-196.

140. Ganju P, O'Bryan JP, Der C, Winter J, James IF. Differential regulation of SHC proteins by nerve growth factor in sensory neuronse and PC12 cells. *Eur J Neurosci* 1998;10:1995-2008.

141. Dai Y, Iwata K, Fukuoka T, et al. Phosphorylation of extracellular signal-regulated kinase in primary afferent neurons by noxious stimuli and its involvement in peripheral sensitization. *J Neurosci* 2002;22:7737-7745.

142. Zhou Y, Li GD, Zhao ZQ. State-dependent phosphorylation of epsilon-isozyme of protein kinase C in adult rat dorsal root ganglia after inflammation and nerve injury. *J Neurochem* 2003;85:571-580.

143. Distler C, Rathee PK, Lips KS, Obreja O, Neuhuber W, Kress M. Fast Ca^{2+}-induced potentiation of heat-activated ionic currents requires camp/PKA signaling and functional AKAP anchoring. *J Neurophys* 2003;89:2499-2505.

144. Vellani V, Mapplebeck S, Moriondo A, Davis JB, McNaughton PA. Protein kinase C activation potentiates gating of the vanilloid receptor VR1 by capsaicin, protons, heat and anadamide. *J Physiol* 2001;534:813-825.

145. Ustinova EE, Schultz HD. Activation of cardiac vagal afferents by oxygen-derived free radicals in rats. *Circ Res* 1994;74:895-903.

146. Schultz HD, Ustinova EE. Capsaicin receptors mediate free radical-induced activation of cardiac afferent endings. *Cardiovascular Res* 1998;38:348-355.

147. Chen J, Daggett H, De Waard M, Heinemann SH, Hoshi T. Nitric oxide augments voltage-gated P/Q-type Ca(2+) channels constituting a putative positive feedback loop. *Free Radic Biol Med* 2002;32:638-649.

148. Canossa M, Giordano E, Capello S, Guanieri C, Ferri S. Nitric oxide down-regulates brain-derived neurotrophii factor secretion in cultured hippocampal cells. *Proc Natl Acad Sci USA* 2002;99:3282-3287.

149. Banan A, Fields JZ, Zhang Y, Keshavarzian A. iNOS upregulation mediates oxidant-induced disruption of F-actin and barrier intestinal monolayers. *Am J Physiol Gastrointest Liver Physiol* 2001;280:G1234-G1246.

150. Hallen K, Olgart C, Gustafsson LE, Wiklund NP. Modulation of neuronal nitric oxide release by soluble guanylate cyclase in guinea pig colon. *Biochem Biophys Res Commun* 2001;280:1130-1134.

151. Chen JX, Berry LC, Tanner M, et al. Nitric oxide donors regulate nitric oxide synthase in bovine pulmonary artery endothelium. *J Cell Physiol* 2001;186:116-123.

152. Yuhanna IS, MacRitchie AN, Lantin-Hermoso RL, Wells LB, Shaul PW. Nitric oxide (NO) upregulates NO synthase expression in fetal intrapulmonary artery endothelial cells. *Am J Respir Cell Mol Biol* 1999;21:629-636.

153. McVeigh GE, Hamilton P, Wilson M, et al. Platelet nitric oxide and superoxide release during development of nitrate tolerance: effect of supplemental ascorbate. *Circulation* 2002;106:208-213.

154. Reuter U, Chiarugi A, Bolay H, Moskowitz MA. Nuclear factor-kappa B as a molecular target for migraine therapy. *Ann Neurol* 2002;51:507-516.

155. Reuter U, Bolay H, Jansen-Olesen I, et al. Delayed inflammation in rat meninges: implications for migraine pathophysiology. *Brain* 2001;124:2490-2502.

156. Kaesemeyer WH, Ogonowski AA, Jin L, Caldwell RB, Caldwell RW. Endothelial nitric oxide synthase is a site of superoxide synthesis in endothelial cells treated with glyceryl nitrate. *Br J Pharmacol* 2000;131:1019-1023.

157. Pardutz A, Krizbai I, Multon S, Vecsie L, Scoenen J. Systemic nitroglycerine increases nNOS levels in rat trigeminal nucleus caudalis. *Neuroreport* 2000; 28:3071-3075.

158. Abou-Mohamed G, Kaesemeyer WH, Caldwell RB, Caldwell RW. Role of L-arginine in the vascular actions and development of tolerance to nitroglycerin. *Br J Pharmacol* 2000;130:211-218.

159. Rachmilewitz D, Stamler JS, Karmeli F, et al. Peroxynitrite-induced rat colitis—a new model of colonic inflammation. *Gastroenterol* 1993;105:1681-1688.

160. Rachmilewitz D, Karmeli F, Okon E, et al. Experimental colitis is ameliorated by inhibition of nitric oxide synthase activity. *Gut* 1995;37:247-255.

161. Chao CC, De La Hunt M, Hu S, Close K, Peterson PK. Immunologically mediated fatigue: a murine model. *Clin Immunol Immunopathol* 1992;64:161-165.

162. Sheng WS, Hu S, Lamkin A, Peterson PK, Chao CC. Susceptibility to immunologically mediated fatigue in C57BL/6 versus Balb/C mice. *Clin Immunol Immunopathol* 1996;81:161-167.

163. Sheng WS, Lin JC, Apple F, Hu S, Peterson PK, Chao CC. Brain energy stores in C57BL/6 mice after C. parvum injection. *Neuroreport* 1999;10:177-81.

164. Sheng WS, Hu S, Ding JM, Chao CC, Peterson PK. Cytokine expression in the mouse brain in response to immune activation by Corynebacterium parvum. *Clin Diagn Lab Immunol* 2001;8:446-448.

165. Ambs S, Ogunfusika MO, Merriam WG, Bennett WP, Billiar TR, Harris CC. Up-regulation of inducible nitric oxide synthase expression in cancer-prone p53 knockout mice. *Proc Natl Acad Sci USA* 1998;95:8823-8828.

166. Urban MO, Gebhart GF. Supraspinal contributions to hyperalgesia. *Proc Natl Acad Sci USA* 1999;96:7687-7692.

167. Willis WD. Role of neurotransmitters and sensitization of pain responses. *Ann N Y Acad Sci* 2001;933:142-156.

168. Ferreira SH. The role of interleukins and nitric oxide in the mediation of inflammatory pain and its control by peripheral analgesics. *Drugs* 1993;46(suppl 1):1-9.

169. Liu L, Simon SA. Modulation of IA currents by capsaicin in rat trigeminal ganglion neurons. *J Neurophysiol* 2003;89:1387-1401.

170. Sung CS, Wen ZH, Chang WK, et al. Intrathecal interleukin-1β administration induces thermal hyperalgesia by activating inducible nitric oxide synthase expression in the rat spinal cord. *Brain Res* 2004;1015:145-153.

171. Tegeder I, Niederberger E, Schmidt R, et al. Specific inhibition of I-kappa B kinase reduces hyperalgesia and neuropathic pain models in rats. *J Neurosci* 2004; 24:1637-1645.

172. Sakaue G, Shimaoka M, Fukuoka T, et al. NF-kappa B decoy suppresses cytokine expression and thermal hyperalgesia in a rat neuropathic pain model. *Neuroreport* 2001;12:2079-2084.

173. Chan CF, Sun WZ, Lin JK, Lin-Shiau SY. Activation of transcription factors nuclear factor kappa B, activator protein-1 and octamer factors in hyperalgesia. *Eur J Pharmacol* 2000;402:61-68.

174. Nicholson B. Gabapentic use in neuropathic pain. *Acta Neurol Scand* 2000; 101:359-371.

175. Saegusa H, Kurihara T, Zong S, et al. Suppression of inflammatory and neuropathic pain symptoms in mice lacking N-type Ca^{2+} channel. *EMBO J* 2001; 20:2349-2356.

176. Distler C, Rathee PK, Lips KS, et al. Fast Ca^{2+}-induced potentiation of heat-activated ionic currents requires camp/PKA signaling and functional AKAP anchoring. *J Neurophysiol* 2003;89:2499-2505.

177. Isaev D, Gerber G, Park SK, Chung JM, Randik M. Facilitation of NMDA-induced currents and Ca^{2+} transients in the rat substantia gelatinosa neurons after ligation of L5-L6 spinal nerves. *Neuroreport* 2000;11:4055-4061.

178. McRoberts JA, Coutinho SV, Marvizon JC, et al. Role of peripheral N-methyl-D-aspartate (NMDA) receptors in visceral nociception in rats. *Gastroenterology* 2001;120:1737-1748.

179. Caterina MJ, Leffler A, Malmberg AB, et al. Impaired nociception and pain sensation in mice lacking the capsaicin receptor. *Science* 2000;288:306-313.

180. Di Marzo V, Blumberg PM, Szallasi A. Endovanilloid signaling in pain. *Curr Opin Neurobiol* 2002;12:372-379.

181. Sachs D, Cunha FQ, Poole S, Ferreira SH. Tumor necrosis factor-α, interleukin-1β, and interleukin-8 induce persistent mechanical nociceptor hypersensitivity. *Pain* 2002;96:89-97.

182. Schafers M, Sorkin LS, Sommer C. Intramuscular injection of tumor necrosis factor-α induces muscle hyperalgesia in rats. *Pain* 2003;104:579-588.

183. Obreja O, Rathee PK, Lips KS, Distler C, Kress M. IL-1β potentiates head activated currents in rat sensory neurons: involvement of IL-1R1, tyrosine kinase and protein kinase C. *FASEB J* 2002;16:1497-1503.

184. Wang ZQ, Porreca F, Cuzzocrea S, et al. A newly identified role for superoxide in inflammatory pain. *J Pharmacol Exp Ther* 2004;309:869-878.

185. Tal M. A novel antioxidant alleviates heat hyperalgesia in rats with experimental painful peripheral neuropathy. *Neuroreport* 1996;7:1382-1384.

186. Liu T, Knight KR, Tracey DJ. Hyperalgesia due to nerve injury-role of peroxynitrite. *Neuroscience* 2000;97:125-131.

187. Ridger VC, Greenacre SA, Handy RL, et al. Effect of peroxynitrite on plasma extravasation, microvascular blood flow and nociception in the rat. *Br J Pharmacol* 1997;122:1083-1088.

188. Donnay A. On the recognition of multiple chemical sensitivity in medical literature and government policy. *Int J Toxicol* 1999;18:383-392.

189. Donnay A. Carbon monoxide as an unrecognized cause of neurasthenia: a history. In Penney D, ed. *Carbon Monoxide Toxicity.* Boca Raton, Florida: CRC; 2000:231-260.

190. Keller RH, Lane JL, Klimas N, et al. Association between HLA class II antigens and the chronic fatigue immune dysfunction syndrome. *Clin Infect Dis* 1994; 18(Suppl 1):S154-S156.

191. Rowe PC, Barron DF, Calkins H, Maumenee IH, Tong PY, Geraghty MT. Orthostatic intolerance and chronic fatigue associated with Ehlers-Danlos syndrome. *J Pediatr* 1999;135:494-499.

192. Buchwald D, Herrell R, Ashton S, et al. A twin study of chronic fatigue. *Psychosom Med* 2001;63:936-943.

193. Torpy DJ, Bachmann AW, Grice JE, et al. Familial corticosteroid-binding globulin deficiency due to a novel null mutation: association with fatigue and relative hypotension. *J Clin Endocrinol Metab* 2001;86:3692-3700.

194. Aaron LA, Herrell R, Ashton S, et al. Comorbid clinical conditions in chronic fatigue: a co-twin study. *J Gen Intern Med* 2001;16:24-31.

195. Pellegrino MJ, Waylonis GW, Sommer A. Familial occurrence of primary fibromyalgia. *Arch Phys Med Rehabil* 1989;70:61-63.

196. Buskila D, Neumann L, Hazanof I, Carmi R. Familial aggregation in the fibromyalgia syndrome. *Semin Arthritis Rheum* 1996;26:605-611.

197. Buskila D, Neumann L. Fibromyalgia syndrome (FM) and nonarticular tenderness in relatives of patients with FM. *J Rheumatol* 1997;24:941-944.

198. Burda CD, Cox FR, Osborne P. Histocompatibility antigens in fibrositis (fibromyalgia) syndrome. *Clin Exp Rheumatol* 1986;4:355-358.

199. Bondy B, Spaeth M, Offenbaecher M, et al. The T102C polymorphism of the 5–HT2A-receptor gene in fibromyalgia. *Neurobiol Dis* 1999;6:433-439.

200. Yunus MB, Kahn MA, Rawlings KK, Green JR, Olson JM, Shah S. Genetic linkage analysis of multicase families with fibromyalgia syndrome. *J Rheumatol* 1999;26:408-412.

201. Gursoy S, Erdal E, Herken H, Madenci E, Alashirli B, Erdai N. Significance of catechol-O-methyltransferase gene polymorphism in fibromylgia syndrome. *Rheumatol Int* 2003;23:104-107.

202. Gursoy S, Erdal E, Herken H, Madenci E, Alasehirli B, Erdal N. Significance of catechol-O-methyltransferase gene polymorphism in fibromyalgia syndrome. *Rheumatol Int* 2002;23:104-107.

203. Karaaslan Y, Haznedaroglu S, Ozturk M. Joint hypermobility and primary fibromyalgia: a clinical enigma. *J Rheumatol* 2000;27:1774-1776.

204. Haley RW, Billecke S, La Du BN. Association of low PON1 type Q (type A) aryl esterase activity with neurologic symptom complexes in Gulf War veterans. *Toxicol Appl Pharmacol* 1999;157:227-233.

205. Binkley K, King N, Poonai N, Seeman P, Ulpian C, Kennedy J. Idiopathic environmental intolerance: increased prevalence of panic disorder associated with cholecystokin B receptor allele. *J Allergy Clin Immunol* 2001;107:887-890.

206. McKeown-Eyssen G, Baines C, Cole DE, et al. Case-control study of genotypes in multiple chemical sensitivity: CYP2D6, NAT1, NAT2, PON1, PON2, MTHFR. *Int J Epidemiol* in press 2004.

207. Koenen KC, Lyons MJ, Goldberg J, et al. A high risk twin study of combat-related PTSD. *Twin Res* 2003;6:218-226.

208. Stein MB, Jang KL, Taylor S, Vernon PA, Livesley WJ. Genetic and environmental influences on trauma exposure and posttraumatic stress disorder symptoms. *Am J Psychiatry* 2002;159:1675-1681.

209. Segman RH, Cooper-Kazaz R, Macciardi F, et al. Association between the dopamine transporter gene and posttraumatic stress disoder. *Mol Psychiatry* 2002; 7:903-907.

210. Radant A, Tsuang D, Peskind ER, McFall M, Raskind W. Biological markers and diagnostic accuracy in the genetics of posttraumatic stress disorder. *Psychiatry Res* 2001;102:203-215.

211. Hukkanen V, Broberg E, Salmi A, Eralinna JP. Cytokines in experimental herpes simplex virus infection. *Int Rev Immunol* 2002;21:355-371.

212. Imanishi J. Expression of cytokines in bacterial and viral infections and their biochemical targets. *J Biochem* 2000;127:525-530.

213. Skoldenberg B. Herpes simplex encephalitis. *Scand J Infect Dis Suppl* 1996;100:8-13.

214. Cals-Grierson MM, Ormerod AD. Nitric oxide function in the skin. *Nitric Oxide* 2004;10:179-193.

215. Novick A, Weiner M. Enzyme induction as an all-or-none phenomenon. *Proc Natl Acad Sci USA* 1957;43:553-566.

216. Guilherme L, Kalil J. Rheumatic fever: the T cell response leading to autoimmune aggression in the heart. *Autoimmun Rev* 2002;1:261-266.

217. Quinn A, Kosanke S, Fischetti VA, Factor SM, Cunningham MW. Induction of autoimmune valvular heart disease by recombinant streptococcal M protein. *Infect Immun* 2001;69:4072-4078.

218. Veasy LG, Hill HR. Immunologic and clinical correlations in rheumatic fever and rheumatic heart disease. *Pediatr Infect Dis* 1997;16:400-407.

219. Anonymous. Sydney Brenner to keynote digital biology symposium. *ASBMB Today.* Aug 2003:16.

220. Pilgeram L. A crisis developing in biology. *ASBMB Today.* Nov 2003:2.

Chapter 2

1. Nathan C, Xie QW. Nitric oxide synthases: roles, tolls and controls. *Cell* 1994; 78:915-918.

2. Knowles RG, Moncada S. Nitric oxide synthases in mammals. *Biochem J* 1994;298:249-258.

3. Bredt DS, Snyder SH, Nitric oxide: a physiologic messenger molecule. *Ann Rev Biochem* 1994;63:175-195.

4. Murad F. Regulation of cytosolic guanylyl cyclase by nitric oxide: the NO-cyclic GMP signal transduction system. *Adv Pharmacol* 1994;26:19-33.

5. Beckman JS, Koppenol WH. Nitric oxide, superoxide and peroxynitrite: the good, the bad and the ugly. *Am J Physiol* 1996;271:C1424-C1437.

6. Pryor WA, Squadrito GL. The chemistry of peroxynitrite: a product from the reaction of nitric oxide and superoxide. *Am J Physiol* 1995;268:L699-L722.

7. Szabo C. Multiple pathways of peroxynitrite cytotoxicity. *Toxicol Lett* 2003; 140-141:105-112.

8. Hogg N. The biochemistry and physiology of S-nitrosothiols. *Ann Rev Pharmacol Toxicol* 2002;42:585-600.

9. Aleryani S, Milo E, Rose Y, Kostka P. Superoxide-mediated decomposition of biological S-nitrosothiols. *J Biol Chem* 1998;273:6041-6045.

10. Rauhala P, Lin AM, Chiueh CC. Neuroprotection by S-nitrosoglutathione on the brain dopamine neurons from oxidative stress. *FASEB J* 1998;12:165-173.

11. Fridovich I. Superoxide radical and superoxide dismutases. *Ann Rev Biochem* 1995;64:97-112.

12. Lebovitz RM, Zhang H, Vogel H, et al. Neurodegeneration, myocardial injury and perinatal death in mitochondrial superoxide dismutase-deficient mice. *Proc Natl Acad Sci USA* 1996;93:9782-9787.

13. Pall ML. Elevated, sustained peroxynitrite levels as the cause of chronic fatigue syndrome. *Med Hypoth* 2000;54:115-125.

14. Radi R, Cassina A, Hodara R, Quijano C, Castro L. Peroxynitrite reactions and formation in mitochondria. *Free Radic Biol Med* 2002;33:1451-1464.

15. Szabo C, Dawson VL. Role of poly (ADP-ribose) synthetase inflammation and ischaemia–reperfusion. *Trends in Pharmacol Sci* 1998;19:287-298.

16. Pieper AA, Verma A, Zhang J, Snyder SH. Poly (ADP-ribose) polymerase, nitric oxide and cell death. *Trends in Pharmacol Sci* 1999;20:171-181.

17. Ellithorpe RR, Settinery RA, Nicolson GL. Pilot study: reduction of fatigue by use of a supplement containing dietary glycophospholipids. *J Am Neutraceutical Assoc* 2003;6:23-28.

18. Nathan C. Nitric oxide as a secretory product of mammalian cells. *FASEB J* 1992;6:3051-3064.

19. Moncada S, Higgs A. The L-arginine-nitric oxide pathway. *New Eng J Med* 1993;329:2002-2012.

20. Brunori M, Giuffre A, Forte E, Mastronicola D, Barone MC, Sarti P. Control of cytochrome C oxidase activity by nitric oxide. *Biochim Biophys Acta* 2004; 1655:365-371.

21. Gardner PR, Costantino G, Szabo C, Salzman AL. Nitric oxide sensitivity of the aconitases. *J Biol Chem* 1997;272:25071-25076.

22. Gardner PR. Superoxide-driven aconitase FE-S center cycling. *Biosci Rep* 1997;17:33-42.

23. Castro L, Rodriguez M, Radi M. Aconitase is readily inactivated by peroxynitrite, but not its precursor nitric oxide. *J Biol Chem* 1994;269:29409-29415.

24. Keller JN, Kindy MS, Holtsberg FW. Mitochondrial manganese superoxide dismutase prevents neural apoptosis and reduces ischemic brain injury: suppression of peroxynitrite production, lipid peroxidation, and mitochondrial dysfunction. *J Neurosci* 1998;18:687-697.

25. Kim PK, Zamora R, Petrosko P, Billiar TR. The regulatory role of nitric oxide in apoptosis. *Int Immunopharmacol* 2001;1:1421-1441.

26. Vojdani A, Ghoneum M, Choppa PC, Magtoto L, Lapp CW. Elevated apoptotic cell populations in patients with chronic fatigue syndrome: the pivotal role of protein kinase RNA. *J Intern Med* 1997;242:409-410.

27. Krueger GR, Koch B, Hoffman A, et al. Dynamics of chronic active herpesvirus-6 infection in patients with chronic fatigue syndrome: data acquisition for computer modeling. *In Vivo* 2001 Nov-Dec. 2001;461-465.

28. Kennedy G, Spence V, Underwood C, Belch JJ. Increased neutrophil apoptosis in chronic fatigue syndrome. *J Clin Pathol* 2004;57:891-893.

29. Baschetti R. Cortisol deficiency may account for elevated apoptotic cell population in patients with chronic fatigue syndrome. *J Int Med* 1999;245:409-410.

30. Vojdani A, Mordechai E, Brautbar N. Abnormal apoptosis and cell cycle progression in humans exposed to methyl tertiary-butyl ether and benzene contaminated water. *Human Expt Toxicol* 1997;16:485-494.

31. Fremont M, D'Haese AD, Roelens S, et al. In Englebienne P. de Meirlier K, eds. *Chronic Fatigue Syndrome: A Biological Approach.* Boca Raton: CRC Press; 2002:131-174.

32. Vojdani A, Ghoneum M, Choppa PC, Magtoto K, Lapp CW. Elevated apopootic cell population in patients with chronic fatigue syndrome: the pivotal role of protein kinase RNA. *J Intern Med* 1997;242:465-478.

33. Hassan IS, Bannister BA, Akbar A, Weir W, Bofill M. A study of immunology of the chronic fatigue syndrome: correlation of immunological parameters to health dysfunction. *Clin Immunol Immunopathol* 1998;87:60-67.

34. Swanink CM, Vercoulen JH, Galama JM, et al. Lymphocyte subsets, apoptosis and cytokines in patients with chronic fatigue syndrome. *J Infect Dis* 1996; 173:460-463.

35. Kozikowski AP, ed. *Neurobiology of the NMDA Receptor: From Chemistry to the Clinic.* New York: VCH Publishers;1991.

36. Mori H, Mishina M. Structure and function of the NMDA receptor channel. *Neuropharmacology* 1995;34:1219-1237.

37. Mody I, MacDonald JF. NMDA receptor-dependent excitotoxicity: the role of intracellular Ca^{2+} release. *Trends Pharmacol Sci* 1995;16:356-359.

38. Kosenko E, Montoliu C, Giordano G, et al. Acute ammonia intoxication induces an NMDA receptor-mediated increase in poly(ADP-ribose) polymerase level and NAD metabolism in nuclei of rat brain cells. *J Neurochem* 2004;89:1101-1110.

39. Pall ML. NMDA sensitization and stimulation by peroxynitrite, nitric oxide and organic solvents as the mechanism of chemical sensitivity in multiple chemical sensitivity. *FASEB J* 2002;16:1407-1417.

40. Iravani MM, Liu L, Rose S, Jenner P. Role of inducible nitric oxide synthase in N-methyl-d-aspartic acid-induced strio-nigral degeneration. *Brain Res* 2004; 1029:103-113.

41. Acarin L, Peluffo H, Gonzalez B, Castellano B. Expression of inducible nitric oxide synthase and cyclooxygenase-2 after excitotoxic damage to the immature rat brain. *J Neurosci Res* 2002;68:745-754.

42. Cardenas A, Moro MA, Hurtado O, et al. Implication of glutamate in the expression of inducible nitric oxide synthase after oxygen and glucose deprivation in rat forebrain slices. *J Neurochem* 2000;74:2041-2048.

43. Yoneda K, Yamamoto T, Ueta E, Osaka T. Suppression by azelastine hydrochloride of NF-kappa B activation involved in generation of cytokines and nitric oxide. *Jpn J Pharmacol* 1997;73:145-153.

44. McInnis J, Wang C, Anastasio N, et al. The role of superoxide and nuclear factor-kappa B signaling in N-methyl-D-aspartate-induced necrosis and apoptosis. *J Pharmacol Exp Ther* 2002;301:478-487.

45. Lafon-Cazal M, Pietri S, Culcasi M, Bockaert J. NMDA-dependent superoxide production and neurotoxicity. *Nature* 1993;364:535-537.

46. Borg J, London J. Copper/zinc superoxide dismutase overexpression promotes survival of cortical neurons exposed to neurotoxins in vitro. *J Neurosci Res* 2002;70:180-189.

47. Hongpaisan J, Winters CA, Andrews SB. Calcium-dependent mitochondrial superoxide modulates nuclear CREB phosphorylation in hippocampal neurons. *Mol Cell Neurosci* 2003;24:1103-1115.

48. Radenovic L, Selakovic V, Kartelija G, Todorovid N, Nedeljkovic M. Differential effects of NMDA and AMPA/kainite receptor antagonists on superoxide production and MnSOD activity in rat brain following intrahippocampal injection. *Brain Res Bull* 2004;64:85-93.

49. Muscoli C, Mollace V, Wheatley J, et al. Superoxide-mediated nitration of spinal manganese superoxide dismutase: a novel pathway in N-methyl-D-aspartate-mediated hyperalgesia. *Pain* 2004;111:96-103.

50. Atlante A, Gagliardi S, Minervini GM, et al. Glutamate neurotoxicity in rat cerebellar granule cells: a major role for xanthine oxidase. *J Neurochem* 1997; 68:2038-2045.

51. Atlante A, Valenti D, Gagliardi S, Passarella S. A sensitive method to assay the xanthine oxidase activity in primary cultures of cerebellar granule cells. *Brain Res Brain Res Protoc* 2000;6:1-5.

52. Pall ML, Anderson JH. The Vanilloid Receptor as a Putative Target of Diverse Chemicals in Multiple Chemical Sensitivity. *Arch Environ Health* 2004;59:363-375.

53. Nielsen GD. Mechanisms of activation of the sensory irritant receptor by airborne chemicals. *CRC Crit Revs Toxicol* 1991;21:183-208.

54. Szallasi A, Blumberg PM. Vanilloid (capsaicin) receptors and mechanisms. *Pharmacol Rev* 1999;51:159-211.

55. Cortright DN, Szallasi A. Biochemical pharmacology of the vanilloid receptor TRPV1: an update. *Eur J Biochem* 2004;271:1814-1819.

56. FerrerMontiel A, Garcia-Martinez C, Morenilla-Palao C, et al. Molecular architecture of the vanilloid receptor: insights for drug design. *Eur J Biochem* 2004; 217:1820-1826.

57. Mery PF, Abi-Gerges N, Vandecasteele G, Jurevicius J, Eschenhagen T, Fischmeister R. Muscarinic regulation of the L-type calcium current in isolated cardiac myocytes. *Life Sci* 1997;60:1113-1120.

58. Ashford NA, Miller CS. *Chemical Exposures: Low Levels and High Stakes.* 2nd ed. New York: John Wiley and Sons;1998.

59. Sorg BA. Multiple chemical sensitivity: potential role for neural sensitization. *Crit Rev Neurobiol* 1999;13:283-316.

60. Patarca-Montero, R. *The Concise Encyclopedia of Fibromyalgia and Myofascial Pain.* Binghamton, NY: Haworth Medical Press;2002.

61. Bell DS. *The Doctor's Guide to Chronic Fatigue Syndrome.* Reading, MA: Addison-Wesley;1995.

62. Yunus MB. Central sensitivity syndromes: a unified concept for fibromyalgia and other maladies. *J Indian Rheumatism Assoc* 2001;8:27-33.

63. Neumann I, Buskila D. Epidemiology of fibromyalgia. *Curr Pain Headache Rep* 2003;7:362-368.

64. Nicolodi M, Sicuteri F. Fibromyalgia and migraine, two faces of the same mechanism. *Adv Exp Med Biol* 1996;398:373-379.

Chapter 3

1. Pall, ML. Elevated, sustained peroxynitrite levels as the cause of chronic fatigue syndrome. *Med Hypoth* 2000;54:115-125.

2. Farquhar WB, Hunt BE, Taylor JA, Darling SE, Freeman R. Blood volume and its relation to peak O(2) consumption and physical activity in patients with chronic fatigue syndrome. *Am J Physiol Heart Circ Physiol* 2002;282:H66-H71.

3. McCully KK, Smith S, Rajaei S, Leigh Jr JS, Natelson BH. Blood flow and muscle metabolism in chronic fatigue syndrome. *Clin Sci (Lond).* 2003;104:641-647.

4. Chazotte B. Mitochondrial dysfunction in chronic fatigue syndrome. In Lemasters, Nieminen, eds. *Mitochondria in Pathogenesis.* New York: Kluwer Academic/Plenum Publishers;2001:393-410.

5. Park JH, Niermann KJ, Olsen N. Evidence for metabolic abnormalities in the muscles of patients with fibromyalgia. *Curr Rheumatol Rep* 2000;2:131-140.

6. Yunus MB, Kalyan Raman UP, Kalyan Raman K. Primary fibromyalgia syndrome and myofascial pain syndrome: clinical features and muscle pathology. *Arch Phys Med Rehabil* 1988;69:451-454.

7. Yunus MB, Kalyan-Raman UP, Kalyan-Raman K, Masi AT. Pathologic changes in muscle in primary fibromyalgia. *Am J Med* 1986;81(3A):38-42.

8. Pongratz DE, Späth M. Morphologic aspects of fibromyalgia. *Z Rheumatol* 1998;57:47-51.

9. Kalyan Raman UP, Kalyan Raman K, Yunus MB, Masi AT. Muscle pathology in primary fibromyalgia syndrome: a light microscopic, histochemical and ultrastructural study. *J Rheumatol* 1984;11:808-813.

10. Lindman R, Hagberg M, Bengtsson A, et al. Capillary structure and mitochondrial volume density in the trapezius muscle of chronic trapezius myalgia, fibromyalgia and healthy subjects. *J Musculoskeletal Pain* 1995;3:5-22.

11. Drewes AM, Andreasen A, Schroder HD, Hogsaa B, Jennum P. Pathology of skeletal muscle fibromyalgia: a histo-immuno-chemical and ultrastructural study. *Br J Rheumatol* 1993;32:479-483.

12. Fassbender HG, Wegner K. Morphologie und Pathogenese des Weichteil-rheumatismus. *Z Rheumaforsch* 1973;33:355-374.

13. Park JH, Phothimat P, Oates CT, Hernanz Schulman M, Olsen NJ. Use of P-31 magnetic resonanace spectroscopy to detect metabolic abnormalities in muscles in patients with fibromylagia. *Arthritis Rheum* 1998;41:406-413.

14. Sprott H, Salemi S, Gay RE, et al. Increased DNA fragmentation and ultrastructural changes in fibromyalgia muscle fibers. *Ann Rheum Dis* 2004;63:245-251.

15. Sheng WS, Lin JC, Apple F, Hu S, Peterson PK, Chao CC. Brain energy stores in C57BL/6 mice after C. parvum injection. *Neuroreport* 1999;10:177-181.

16. Fulle S, Mecocci P, Fano G, et al. Specific oxidative alterations in vastus lateralis muscle in patients with the diagnosis of chronic fatigue syndrome. *Free Radic Biol Med* 2000;29:1252-1259.

17. Richards RS, Roberts TK, McGregor NR, Butt HL. Blood parameters indicative of oxidative stress are associated with symptom expression in chronic fatigue syndrome. *Redox Rep* 2000;5:35-41.

18. Richards RS, Roberts TK, Dunstan RH, McGregor NR, Butt HL. Free radicals in chronic fatigue syndrome: cause or effect? *Redox Rep* 2000;5:146-147.

19. Keenoy BM, Moorkens G, Vertommen J, DeLeeuw I. Antioxidant status and lipoprotein oxidation in chronic fatigue syndrome. *Life Sci* 2001;68:2037-2049.

20. Logan AC, Wong C. Chronic fatigue syndrome: oxidative stress and dietary modifications. *Altern Med Rev* 2001;6:450-459.

21. Smirnova IV, Pall ML. Elevated levels of protein carbonyls in sera of chronic fatigue syndrome patients. *Mol Cell Biochem* 2003;248:93-95.

22. Kurup RK, Kurp PA. Hypothalamic digoxin, cerebral chemical dominance and myalgic encephalomyelitis. *Intern J Neuroscience* 2003;113:445-457.

23. Vecchiet J, Cipollone F, Falasca K, et al. Relationship between musculoskeletal symptoms and blood markers of oxidative stress in patients with chronic fatigue syndrome. *Neurosci Lett* 2003;335:151-154.

24. Ionescu G, Merck M, Bradford R. Simple chemiluminescence assays for free radicals in venous blood and serum samples: results in atopic dermatitis, psoriasis, MCS and cancer patients. *Forsch Komplementarmed* 1999;6:294-300.

25. Eisinger J, Gandolfo C, Zakarian H, Ayavou T. Reactive oxygen species, antioxidant status and fibromyalgia. *J Musculoskeletal Pain* 5(4):5-15.

26. Eisinger J, Zakarian H, Pouly F, Plantamura A, Ayavou T. Protein peroxidation, magnesium deficiency and fibromyalgia. *Magnes Res* 1996;9:313-316.

27. Hein G, Franke S. Are advanced glycation end-product-modified proteins of pathogenetic importance in fibromylagia? *Rheumatology* 2002;41:1163-1176.

28. Bagis S, Tamer L, Sahin G, et al. Free radicals and antioxidants in primary fibromyalgia: an oxidative stress disorder? *Rheumatol Int* 2005;25:188-190.

29. Tezcan E, Atmaca M, Kuloglu M, Ustundag B. Free radicals in patients with post–traumatic stress disorder. *Neuroreport* 2003;23:913-916.

30. Alptekin N, Seckin S, Dogru Abbasoglu S, et al. Lipid peroxides, glutathione, γ-glutamylocysteine synthetase and γ-glutamyltranspeptidase activities in several tissues of rats following water-immersion stress. eliminary findings. *Int J Biosocial Res* 1996;3:44-47.

31. Seckin S, Alptekin N, Dogru Abbasoglu S, et al. The effect of chronic stress on hepatic and gastric peroxidation in long-term depletion of glutathione in rats. *Pharmacol Res* 1997;36:55-57.

32. Martinez-Augustin O, de Medina FS. Effect of psychogenic stress on gastrointestinal function. *J Physiol Biochem* 2000;56:259-273.

33. Singh A, Garg V, Gupta S, Kulkarni SK. Role of antioxidants in chronic fatigue syndrome in mice. *Indian J Exp Biol* 2002;40:1240-1244.

34. Tirelli U, Chierichetti F, Tavio M, et al. Brain positron emission tomography (PET) in chronic fatigue syndrome: preliminary data. *Am J Med* 1998;105(3A): 54S-58S.

35. MacHale SM, Lawrie SM, Cavanagh JT, et al. Cerebral perfusion in chronic fatigue syndrome and depression. *Br J Psychiatry* 2000;176:550-556.

36. Seissmeier T, Nix WA, Hardt J, et al. Observer independent analysis of cerebral glucose metabolism in patients with chronic fatigue syndrome. *J Neurol Neurosurg Psychiatry* 2003;74:922-928.

37. Lekander M, Frederikson M, Wik G. Neuroimmune relations in patients with fibromyalgia: a positron emission tomography study. *Neurosci Lett* 2000;282:193-196.

38. Heuser G, Wu JC. Deep subcortical (including limbic) hypermetabolism in patients with chemical intolerance: human PET studies. *Ann NY Acad Sci* 2001; 933:319-322.

39. Bell IR, Miller CS, Schwartz GE, Peterson JM, Amend D. Neuropsychiatric and somatic characteristics of young adults with and without self-reported chemical odor intolerance and chemical sensitivity. *Arch Environ Health* 1996;51:9-21.

40. Lekander M, Frederikson M, Wik G. Neuroimmune relations in patients with fibromyalgia: a positron emission tomography study. *Neurosci Lett* 2000;282:193-196.

41. Yunus MB, Young CS, Saeed SA, Mountz JM, Aldag JC. Positron emission tomography in patients with fibromyalgia syndrome and healthy controls. *Arthritis Rheum.* 2004;51:513-518.

42. Bremner JD, Vythilingam M, Vermetten E, et al. MRI and PET study of deficits in hippocampal structure and function in women with childhood sexual abuse and posttraumatic stress disorder. *Am J Psychiatry* 2003;160:924-932.

43. Shin LM, Orr SP, Carson MA, et al. Regional blood flow in the amygdala and medial prefrontal cortex during traumatic imagery in male and female Vietnam veterans with PTSD. *Arch Gen Psychiatry* 2004;61:168-176.

44. Bonne O, Gilboa A, Louzoun Y, et al. Resting regional perfusion in recent posttraumatic stress disorder. *Biol Psychiatry* 54:1077-1086.

45. Bremner JD, Vythilingham M, Vermetten E, et al. MRI and PET study of deficits in hippocampal structure and function in women with childhood sexual abuse and posttraumatic stress disorder. *Am J Psychiatry* 2003;160:924-932.

46. Ichise M, Salit IE, Abbey SE, et al. Assessment of regional cerebral perfusion by 99Tcm-HMPAO SPECT in chronic fatigue syndrome. *Nucl Med Commun* 1992;13:767-772.

47. Schwartz RB, Komaroff AL, Garada BM, et al. SPECT imaging of the brain: comparison of findings in patients with chronic fatigue syndrome, AIDS dementia complex and major unipolar depression. *Am J Roentgenol* 1994;162:943-951.

48. Dickinson CJ. Chronic fatigue syndrome—aetiological aspects. *Eur J Clin Invest* 1997;27:257-267.

49. Fischler B, D'Haenen H, Cluydts R, et al. Comparison of 99m Tc HMPAO SPECT scan between chronic fatigue syndrome, major depression and healthy controls: an exploratory study of clinical correlates of regional cerebral blood flow. *Neuropsychobiology* 1996;34:175-183.

50. Simon T, Hickey D, Fincher C, Johnson A, Ross G, Rea W. Single photon emission computed tomography of the brain in patients with chemical sensitivities. *Toxicol Ind Health* 1994;10:573-577.

51. Heuser G, Mena I, Alamos F. Neurospect findings in patients exposed to neurotoxic chemicals. *Toxicol Ind Health* 1994;10:561-572.

52. Ross GH, Rea WJ, Johnson AR, Hickey DC, Simon TR. Neurotoxicity in single photon emission computed tomography brain scans of patients reporting chemical sensitivities. *Toxicol Ind Health* 1999;15:415-420.

53. Kwiatek R, Barnden L, Tedman R, et al. Regional blood flow in fibromyalgia: single-photon-emission computed tomography evidence of reduction of the pontine tegmentum and thalami. *Arthritis Rheum* 2000;43:2823-2833.

54. Pitman RK, Shin LM, Rauch SL. Investigating the pathogenesis of post-traumatic stresss disorder with neuroimaging. *J Clin Psychiatry* 2001;62(Suppl) 17:47-54.

55. Villarreal G, King CY. Brain imaging in posttraumatic stress disorder. *Semin Clin Neuropsychiatry* 2001;6:131-145.

56. Van Der Kolk BA. The psychobiology and psychopharmacology of PTSD. *Hum Psychopharmacol* 2001;16(S1):S49-S64.

57. Mirzaei S, Knoll P, Keck A, et al. Regional cerebral blood flow in patients suffering from post-traumatic stress disorder. *Neuropsychobiology* 2001;43:260-264.

58. Zubieta JK, Chinitz JA, Lombardi U, et al. Medial frontal cortex involvement in PTSD symptoms: a SPECT study. *J Psychiatr Res* 1999;33:259-264.

59. Aoki T, Miyakoshi H, Usuda Y, Heberman RB. Low NK syndrome and its relationship to chronic fatigue syndrome. *Clin Immunol Immunopath* 1993;69:253-265.

60. Natelson BH, Haghighi MH, Ponzio NM. Evidence for the presence of immune dysfunction in chronic fatigue syndrome. *Clin Diagnostic Lab Immunol* 2002;9:747-752.

61. Komaroff AL, Buchwald DS. Chronic fatigue syndrome: an update. *Ann Rev Med* 1998;49:1-13.

62. Pall ML. Elevated peroxynitrite as the caused of chronic fatigue syndrome. *Medical Hypoth* 2000;54:115-125.

63. Patarca R. Cytokines and chronic fatigue syndrome. *Ann NY Acad Sci* 2001; 933:185-200.

64. Ashford NA, Miller C. *Chemical Exposures: Low Levels and High Stakes.* New York: John Wiley and Sons;1998.

65. Sorg BA. Multiple chemical sensitivity: potential role for neural sensitization. *Crit Rev Neurobiol* 1999;13:283-316.

66. Landis CA, Lentz MJ, Tsuji J, Buchwald D, Shaver JL. Pain, psychological variables, sleep quality, and natural killer cell activity in midlife women with and without fibromyalgia. *Brain Behav Immun* 2004;18:304-313.

67. Patarca-Montero R. *The Concise Encyclopedia of Fibromyalgia and Myofascial Pain.* Binghamton, NY: Haworth Medical Press;2002.

68. Mosnaim AD, Wolf ME, Maturana P, et al. In vitro studies of natural killer cell activity in posttraumatic stress disorder patients. *Immunopharmacology* 1993; 25:107-116.

69. Ironson G, Wynings C, Schneiderman N, et al. Posttraumatic stress symptoms, intrusive thoughts, loss and immune function after Hurricane Andrew. *Psychsom Med* 1997;59:142-243.

70. Inoue-Sakurai C, Maruyama S, Morimoto K. Posttraumatic stress and lifestyles are associated with natural killer cell activity in victims of the Hanshin-Awaji earthquake in Japan. *Prev Med* 2000;31:467-473.

71. Kawamura N, Kim Y, Asukai N. Suppression of cellular immunity in men with a past history of posttraumatic stress disorder. *Am J Psychiatry* 2001;158: 484-486.

72. Skowera A, Cleare A, Blair D, Bevis L, Wessely SC, Peakman M. High levels of type 2 cytokine-producing cells in chronic fatigue syndrome. *Clin Exp Immunol.* 2004;135:294-302.

73. Pall ML. The nitric oxide synthase product, citrulline is elevated in the sera of chronic fatigue syndrome patients. *J Chronic Fatigue Syndr* 2002;10(3/4):37-42.

74. Patarca-Montero R. *Chronic Fatigue Syndrome and the Body's Immune Defense System.* Binghamton, NY: Haworth Medical Press;2002.

75. Gur A, Karakoc M, Erdogan S, Nas K, Cevik R, Sarac AJ. Regional cerebral blood flow and cytokines in young females with fibromyalgia. *Clin Exp Rheumatol* 2002;20:753-760.

76. Salemi S, Rethage J, Wollina U, et al. Detection of interleukin 1beta (IL-1beta), IL-6, and tumor necrosis factor-alpha in skin of patients with fibromyalgia. *J Rheumatol* 2003;30:146-150.

77. Maes M, Lin AH, Delmeire L, et al. Elevated serum interleukin-6 (IL-6) and IL-6 receptor concentrations in posttraumatic stress disorder following accidental man-made traumatic events. *Biol Psychiatry* 1999;45:833-839.

78. Spivak B, Shohat B, Mester R, et al. Elevated levels of serum interleukin-1β in combat related posttraumatic stress disorder. *Biol Psychiatry* 1997;42:345-348.

79. Baker DG, Ekhator NN, Kasckow JW, et al. Plasma and cerebrospinal fluid interleukin-6 concentrations in posttraumatic stress disorder. *Neuroimmunomodulation* 2001;9:209-217.

80. Aurer A, Aurer-Kozelj J, Stavljenic-Rukavina A, Kalenic S, Ivic-Kardum M, Haban V. Inflammatory mediators in saliva of patients with rapidly progressive periodontitis during war stress induced incidence increase. *Coll Antropol* 1999; 23:117-124.

81. Ushio H, Nohara K, Fujimaki H. Effects of environmental pollutants on the production of inflammatory cytokines by normal human dermal keratinocytes. *Toxicol Lett* 1999;105:17-24.

82. Watkins LR, Martin D, Ulrich P, Tracey KJ, Maier SF. Evidence for involvement of spinal cord glia in subcutaneous formalin induced hyperalgesia in the rat. *Pain* 1997;71:225-235.

83. Demitrack MA, Dale JK, Straus SE, et al. Evidence for impaired activation of the hypothalamic-pituitary-adrenal axis in patients with chronic fatigue syndrome. *J Clin Endocrinol Metab* 1991;73:1224-1234.

84. Demitrack MA. Neuroendocrine correlates of chronic fatigue syndrome: a brief review. *J Psychiat Res* 1997;31:69-82.

85. Appels A. Exhausted subjects, exhausted systems. *Acta Physiol Scand Suppl* 1997;640:153-154.

86. Cleare AJ. The HPA axis and the genesis of chronic fatigue syndrome. *Trends Endocrinol Metab* 2004;15:55-59.

87. Thompson D, Lettich L, Takeshita J. Fibromyalgia: an overview. *Curr Psychiatry* 2003;5:211-217.

88. Okifuji A, Turk DC. Stress and psychophysiology dysregulation in patients with fibromyalgia syndrome. *Appl Psychophysiol Biofeedback* 2002;27:129-141.

89. Adler GK, Manfredsdottir VF, Creskoff KW. Neuroendocrine abnormalities in fibromyalgia. *Curr Pain Headache Rep* 2002;6:289-298.

90. Crofford LJ. The hypothalamic-pituitary-adrenal axis in pathogenesis of rheumatic diseases. *Endocrinol Metab Clin North Am* 2002;31:1-13.

91. Clauw DJ. Potential mechanisms in chemical intolerance and related conditions. *Ann NY Acad Sci* 2001;933:235-253.

92. Nawab SS, Miller CS, Dale JK, et al. Self-reported sensitivity to chemical exposures in five clinical populations and healthy controls. *Psychiatry Res* 2000; 95:67-74.

93. Yehuda R, Giller EL, Southwick SM, Lowy MT, Mason JW. Hypothalamic-pituitary-adrenal dysfunction in post-traumatic stress disorder. *Biol Psych* 1991; 30:1031-1048.

94. Yehuda R, Boisoneau D, Lowy MT, Giller EL, Jr. Dose-response changes in plasma cortisol and lymphocyte glucocorticoid receptors following dexamethasone administration in combat veterans with and without posttraumatic stress disorder. *Arch Gen Psych* 1996;52:583-593.

95. Grossman R, Yehuda R, New A, et al. Dexamethasone suppression of test findings in subjects with personality disorders: association with posttraumatic stress disorder and major depression. *Am J Psychiatry* 2003;160:1291-1298.

96. Thaller V, Vrkljan M, Hotujac L, Thakore J. The potential role of hypercortisolism in the pathophysiology of PTSD and psoriasis. *Collegium Anthropologicum* 1999;23:611-619.

97. Kellner M, Yassouridis A, Hubner R, Baker DG, Wiedemann K. Endocrine and cardiovascular responses to corticotropin-releasing hormone in patients with posttraumatic stress disorder: a role for atrial natriuretic peptide? *Neuropsychobiology* 2003;47:102-108.

98. Yehuda R, Golier JA, Kaufman S. Circadian rhythm of salivary cortisol in holocaust survivors with and without PTSD. *Am J Psychiatry* 2005;162:998-1000.

99. Sorg BA, Bailie TM, Tschirigi ML, Li N, Wu WR. Exposure to repeated low-level-formaldehyde in rats increases basal corticosterone levels and enhances the corticosterone response to subsequent formaldehyde. *Brain Res* 2001;898:314-320.

100. Bell DS. *The Doctor's Guide to Chronic Fatigue Syndrome.* Reading, MA: Addison-Wesley;1995.

101. Fukuda K, Strauss SE, Hickie I, Sharpe MC, Dobbin JG, Komaroff A. The chronic fatigue syndrome: A comprehensive approach to definition and study. International Chronic Fatigue Syndrome Group. *Ann Intern Med* 1994;121:953-959.

102. Goldenberg DL. Fibromyalgia syndrome a decade later: What have we learned? *Arch Intern Med* 1999;159:777-785.

103. Larson AA, Kovacs KJ. Nociceptive aspects of fibromyalgia. *Curr Pain Headache Rep* 2001;5338-346.

104. Adamec R. Modelling anxiety disorders following chemical exposures. *Toxicol Ind Health* 1994;10:391-420.

105. Bell IR, Peterson JM, Schwartz GE. Medical histories and psychological profiles of middle-aged women with and without self-reported illness from environmental chemicals. *J Clin Psychiatry* 1995;56:151-160.

106. Moore LJ, Boehnlein JK. Posttraumatic stress disorder, depression and somatic symptoms in U.S. Mein patients. *J Nerv Ment Dis* 1991;179:728-733.

107. Jones F, Vermaas RH, McCartney H, et al. Flashbacks and post-traumatic stress disorder: the genesis of a 20th century diagnosis. *Br J Psychiatry* 2003; 182:158-163.

108. Bennett A. A view of violence contained in chronic fatigue syndrome. *J Anal Psychol* 1997;42:237-251.

109. Bell IR, Baldwin CM, Fenandez M, Schwartz GE. Neural sensitization model of multiple chemical sensitivity. *Toxicol Indust Health* 1999.

110. Chemtob CM, Novaco RW, Hamada RS, Gross DM, Smith G. Anger regulation deficits in combat-related posttraumatic stress disorder. *J Trauma Stress* 1998;10:17-36.

111. Sandman CA, Barron JL, Nackoul K, Goldstein J, Fidler F. Memory deficits associated with chronic fatigue immune dysfunction syndrome. *Biol Psychiatry* 1993;33:618-123.

112. Michiels V, Cluydts R, Fischler B. Attention and verbal learning in patients with chronic fatigue syndrome. *J Int Neuropsychol Soc* 1998;4:456-466.

113. Servatius RJ, Tapp WN, Bergen MT, et al. Impaired associative learning in chronic fatigue syndrome. *Neuroreport* 1998;9:1153-1157.

114. Busichio K, Tiersky LA, DeLuca J, Natelson BH. Neuropsychological deficits in patients with chronic fatigue syndrome. *J Int Neuropsych Soc* 2004; 10:278-285.

115. Pall, ML. Elevated peroxynitrite as the cause of chronic fatigue syndrome: Other inducers and mechanisms of symptom generation. *J Chronic Fatigue Syndr* 2000;7(4):39-44.

116. Okifuji A, Ashburn MA. Fibromyalgia syndrome: toward an integration of the literature. *Crit Revs Physical Rehab Med* 2001;13:27-54.

117. Lipschitz EL. Chronic fatigue syndrome and posttraumatic stress disorder. *JAMA* 2001;286:916-917.

118. Brandes D, Ben-Schachar G, Gilboa A, Bonne O, Freedman S, Shalev AY. PTSD symptoms and cognitive performance in recent trauma survivors. *Psychiatry Res* 2002;110:102-110.

119. Horner MD, Hamner MB. Neurocognitive functioning in posttraumatic stress disorder. *Neuropsychol Rev* 2002;12:15-30.

120. Burloux G, Forestier P, Dalery J, Guyotat J. Chronic pain and posttraumatic stress disorders. *Psychother Psychosom* 1989;52:119-124.

121. Beckham JC, Crawford AL, Feldman ME, et al. Chronic posttraumatic stress disorder and chronic pain in Vietnam combat veterans. *J Psychosom Res* 1997;43:379-389.

122. Dagan Y, Zinger Y, Lavic P. Actigraphic sleep monitoring in posttraumatic stress disorder (PTSD) patients. *J Psychosom Res* 1997;42:577-581.

123. Mellman TA, Bustamante V, Fins AI, Pigeon WR, Nolan B. REM sleep and the early development of posttraumatic stress disorder. *Am J Psychiatry* 2002; 159:1696-1701.

124. Rowe PC, Bou Holaigah I, Kan J, Calkins H. Is neurally mediated hypotension an unrecognized cause of chronic fatigue? *Lancet* 1995;345:623-624.

125. Stewart JM, Gewitz MH, Weldon A, et al. Patterns of delayed orthostatic intolerance: the orthostatic tachycardia syndrome and adolescent chronic fatigue syndrome. *J Pediatr* 1999;135:218-225.

126. Bell IR, Baldwin CM, Russek LG, Schwartz GE, Hardin EE. Early life stress, negative paternal relationships, and chemical intolerance in middle-aged women: support for a neural sensitization model. *J Women's Health* 1998;7:1135-1147.

127. Orr SP, Meyerhoff JL, Edwards JV, Pitman RK. Heart rate and blood pressure resting levels and responses to generic stressors in Vietnam veterans with posttraumatic stress disorder. *J Trauma Stress* 1998;11:155-164.

128. Hinton D, Ba P, Peou S, Um K. Panic disorder among Cambodian refugees attending a psychiatric clinic. Prevalence and subtypes. *Gen Hosp Psychiatry* 2000; 22:437-444.

129. Pietrini P, Teipel SJ, Bartenstein P, et al. PET and the effects of aging and neurodegeneration on brain function: basic principles. *Drug News Perspect* 1998;11: 161-165.

130. Holthoff VA, Beuthien-Baumann B, Zundorf G, et al. Changes in brain metabolism associated with remission in unipolar major depression. *Acta Psychiatr Scand* 2004;110:184-194.

131. Silverman DH, Small KA, Chang CY, et al. Positron emission tomography in evaluation of dementia: regional brain metabolism and long-term outcome. *JAMA* 2001;286:2120-2127.

132. Jacquier-Sarlin MR, Polla BS, Slosman DO. Oxido-reductive state: the major determinant for cellular retention of technetium-99m-HMPAO. *J Nucl Med* 1996;37:1413-1416.

133. Suess E, Malessa K, Ungersbock K, et al. Techetium-99m-D,L-hexamethl-propyleneamine oxime (HMPAO) uptake and glutathione content of brain tumors.

134. Meydani SN, Wu D, Santos MS, Hayek MG. Antioxidants and immune response in aged persons: overview of present evidence. *Am J Clin Nutr* 1995; 62(Suppl):1462S-1476S.

135. Nakamura K, Matsunaga K. Susceptibility of natural killer (NK) cells to reactive oxygen species (ROS) and their restoration by the mimics of superoxide dismutase (SOD). *Cancer Biothe Radiopharm* 1998;13:275-2090.

136. Hansson M, Asea A, Ersson U, Hermodsson S, Hellstrand K. Induction of apoptosis in NK cells by monocyte-derived reactive oxygen metabolites. *J Immunol* 1996;156:42-47.

137. Takeuchi M, Nagai S, Nakajima A, et al. Inhibition of lung natural killer cell activity by smoking: the role of alveolar macrophages. *Respiration* 2001; 168:262-267.

138. Heuser G, Vojdani A. Enhancement of natural killer cell activity and T and B cell function by buffered vitamin C in patients exposed to toxic chemicals: the role of protein kinase C. *Immunopharmacol Immuntoxicol* 1997;19:291-312.

139. Ogawa M, Nishiura T, Yoshimura M, et al. Decreased nitric oxide-mediated natural killer cell activation in chronic fatigue syndrome. *Eur J Clin Invest* 1998; 28:937-943.

140. Riedel WS. Role of nitric oxide in the control of the hypothalamic-pituitary-adrenal axis. *Z Rheumatol* 2000;59(Suppl 2):36-42.

141. Chikanza IC. Neuroendocrine immune features of pediatric inflammatory rheumatic diseases. *Ann NY Acad Sci* 1999;876:71-80.

142. Bomholt SF, Harbuz MS, Blackburn-Munro G, Blackburn-Munro RE. Involvement and role of the hypothalamo-pituitary-adrenal (HPA) stress axis in animal models of chronic pain and inflammation. *Stress* 2004;7:1-14.

143. Buske-Kirschbaum A, Hellhammer DH. Endocrine and immune responses to stress in chronic inflammatory skin disorders. *Ann NY Acad Sci* 2003;992:231-240.

144. Huitinga I, Erkut ZA, van Beurden D, Swaab DF. The hypothalamo-pituitary-adrenal axis in multiple sclerosis. *Ann NY Acad Sci.* 2003;992:118-128.

145. Bornstein SR, Rutkowski H. The adrenal hormone metabolism in the immune/inflammatory reaction. *Endocr Res* 2002;28:719-728.

146. Adamec RE. Evidence that NMDA-dependent limbic neural plasticity in the right hemisphere medicated pharmacological stressor (FG-7142)-induced lasting increased in anxiety-like behavior. *J Psychopharmacol* 1998;12:122-128.

147. Davis M. Neurobiology of fear responses: the role of the amygdala. *J Neuropsychiatry Clin Neurosci* 1997;9:382-402.

148. Adamec RE, Burton P, Shallow T, Budgell J. Unilateral block of NMDA receptors in the amygdala prevents predator stress-induced lasting increases in anxiety-like behavior and unconditioned startle—effective hemisphere depends on behavior. *Physiol Behav* 1999;65:739-751.

149. Shekhar A, Sajdyk TJ, Gehlert DR, Rainnie DG. The amygdala, panic disorder, and cardiovascular responses. *Ann NY Acad Sci* 2003;985:308-325.

150. Volke V, Koks S, Vasar E, et al. Inhibition of nitric oxide synthase causes anxiolytic-like behavior in an elevated plus-maze. *Neuroreport* 6:1413-1416.

151. Faria MS, Muscara MN, Moreno Junior H, et al. Acute inhibition of nitric oxide synthesis induces anxiolysis in the plus maze test. *Eur J Pharmacol* 1997; 323:37-43.

152. Monzon ME, Varas MM, De Barioglio SR. Anxiogenesis induced by nitric oxide synthase inhibition and anxiolytic effect of melanin-concentrating hormone (MCH) in rat brain. *Peptides* 2001;22:1043-1047.

153. Werner C, Raivich G, Cowen M, et al. Importance of NO/cGMP signaling via cGMP-dependent protein kinase II for controlling emotionality and neurobehavioural effects of alcohol. *Eur J Neurosci* 2004;20:3498-3506.

154. Volke V, Wegener G, Vasar E. Augmentation of the NO–cGMP cascade induces anxiolytic-like effect in mice. *J Physiol Pharmacol* 2003;54:653-660.

155. Kurt M, Bilge SS, Aksoz E, et al. Effect of sidenafil on anxiety in the plus-maze test in mice. *Pol J Pharmacol* 2004;56:55-59.

156. Papageiorgioua C, Grapsab NG, Chritodoulouc NG, et al. Association of serum nitric oxide with depressive symptoms: a study with end-stage renal failure patients. *Psychother Psychosomatics* 2001;70:216-220.

157. Suzuki E, Yagi G, Nakaki T, Kanba S, Asai M. Elevated plasma nitrate levels in depressive states. *J Affect Disord* 2001;63:221-224.

158. McLeod TM, Lopez-Figueroa AL, Lopez-Figueroa MO. Nitric oxide, stress and depression. *Psychopharmacol Bull* 2001;35:24-41.

159. Paul IA, Skolnik P. Glutamate and depression: clinical and preclinical studies. *Ann N Y Acad Sci* 2003;1003:250-272.

160. Finkel MS, Laghrissi-Thode F, Pollock BG, Rong J. Paroxetine is a novel nitric oxide synthase inhibitor. *Psychopharmacol Bull* 1996;32:653-658.

161. Angulo J, Peiro C, Sanchez-Ferrer CF, et al. Differential effects of serotonin reuptake inhibitors on erective responses, NO-production, and neuronal NO synthase expression in rat corpus cavernosum tissue. *Br J Pharmacol* 2001;134:1190-1194.

162. Capuron L, Dantzer R. Cytokines and depression: the need for a new paradigm. *Brain Behav Immun* 2003;17(Suppl 1):S119-S124.

163. Anisman H, Merali Z. Cytokines, stress and depressive illness: brain-immune interactions. *Ann Med* 2003;35:2-11.

164. O'Brien SM, Scott LV, Dinan TG. Cytokines: abnormalities in major depression and implications for pharmacological treatment. *Hum Psychopharmacol* 2003;19:397-403.

165. Bandler R. Induction of 'rage' following microinjections of glutamate into midbrain but not hypothalamus of cats. *Neurosci Lett* 1982;30:183-188.

166. Schubert K, Shaik MB, Siegel A. NMDA receptors in the midbrain of periacqueductal gray mediate hypothalamically evoked hissing behavior in cat. *Brain Res* 1996;726:80-90.

167. Greg TR, Siegel A. Brain structures and neurotransmitters regulating aggression in cats: implications for human aggression. *Prog Neuropsychopharmacol Biol Psychiatry* 2001;25:91-140.

168. Gammie SC, Nelson RJ. Maternal aggression is reduced in neuronal nitric oxide synthase-deficient mice. *J Neurosci* 1999;19:8027-8035.

169. Albensi BC. Models of brain injury and alterations and alterations in synaptic plasticity. *J Neurosci Res* 2001;65:279-283.

170. Bliss TV, Collingridge GL. A synaptic model of memory: long-term potentiation in the hippocampus. *Nature* 1993;361:31-39.

171. Bennett MR. The concept of long term potentiation of transmission at synapses. *Prog Neurobiol* 2000;60:109-137.

172. Platenik J, Kuramoto N, Yoneda Y. Molecular mechanisms associated with long-term consolidation of the NMDA signals. *Life Sci* 2000;67:231-253.

173. Prast H, Philippu A. Nitric oxide as a modulator of neuronal function. *Prog Neurobiol* 2001;64:51-68.

174. Cotman CW, Monaghan DT, Ganong AH. Excitatory amino acid neurotransmission: NMDA receptors and Hebb-type synaptic plasticity. *Ann Rev Neurosci* 1988;11:61-80.

175. Bliss TV, Douglas RM, Errington ML, Lynch MA. Correlation between long-term potentiation and release of endogenous amino acids from dentate gyrus of anesthetized rats. *J Physiol* 1986;377:391-408.

176. Kuriyama K, Ohkuma S. Role of nitric oxide in central synaptic transmission: effects on neurotransmitter release. *Jpn J Pharmacol* 1995;34:347-350.

177. Zhang J, Snyder SH. Nitric oxide in the nervous system. *Annu Rev Phamacol Toxicol* 1995;35:213-233.

178. Williams JH. Retrograde messengers and long-term potentiation: a progress report. *J Lipid Mediat Cell Signal* 1996;14:331-339.

179. Hawkins RD, Son H, Arancio O. Nitric oxide as a retrograde messenger during long-term potentiation in hippocampus. *Prog Brain Res* 1998;118:155-172.

180. Tegeder I, Del Turco D, Schmidtko A, et al. Reduced inflammatory hyperalgesia with preservation of acute thermal nociception in mice lacking cGMP-dependent protein kinase I. *Proc Natl Acad Sci USA* 2004;101:3253-3257.

181. Brune Kay, Handwerker Hermann, eds. *Hyperalgesia: Molecular Mechanisms and Clinical Implications.* Seattle: IASP Press;2004.

182. Turkoski BB. Tired blood. Part I. *Orthop Nurs* 2003;22:222-227; Sobrero A, Puglisi F, Guglielmi A, et al. Fatigue: a main component of anemia symptomatology. *Semin Oncol* 2001;28(Suppl 8):15-18.

183. Annibele B, Marignani M, Monarca B, et al. Reversal of iron deficiency anemia after Helicobacter pylori eradicatgion in patients with asymptomatic gastritis. *Ann Intern Med* 1999;131:668-672.

184. Kaltwasser JP, Kessler U, Gottschalk R, Stucki G, Moller B. Effect of recombinant human erythropoietin and intravenous iron on anemia and disease activity in rheumatoid arthritis. *J Rheumatol* 2001;28:2430-2436.

185. Littlewood TJ, Bajetta E, Nortier JWR, et al. Effects of Epoetin Alfa on hematologic parameters and quality of life in cancer patients receiving nonplatinum chemotherapy: results of a randomized, double blind, placebo-controlled trial. *J Clin Oncol* 2001;19:2865-2874.

186. Nybo L. CNS fatigue and prolonged exercise: effect of glucose supplementation. *Med Sci Sports Exerc* 2003;35:589-594.

187. Brouns F. Nutritional aspects of health and performance at lowland and altitude. *Int J Sports Med* 1993;13(suppl 1):S100-S106.

188. Costill DL, Hargreaves M. Carbohydrate nutrition and fatigue. *Sports Med* 1992;13:86-92.

189. Griggs RC, Karpati G. Muscle pain, fatigue and mitochondriopathies. *New Eng J Med* 1999;341:1077-1078.

190. Kabbouche MA, Powers SW, Vockell AL, LeCates SL, Hershey AD. Carnitine palmityltransferase II (CPT2) deficiency and migraine headaches: two case reports. *Headache* 2003;43:490-495.

191. Hooper RG, Thomas AR, Kearl RA. Mitochondrial enzyme deficiency causing exercise limitation in normal-appearing adults. *Chest* 1995;107:317-322.

192. Wouters BG, Delahoussaye YM, Evans JW, et al. Mitochondrial dysfunction after aerobic exposure to the hypoxic cytotoxin tirapazamine. *Cancer Res* 2001;61:145-152.

193. Neri S, Pistone GF, Saraceno B, et al. L-carnitine decreases severity and type of fatigue induced by interferon-α in the treatment of patients with hepatitis C. *Neuropsychobiology* 2003;47:94-97.

194. Brass EP, Adler S, Sietsema KE, Hiatt WR, Orlando AM, Amato A. Intravenous L-carnitine increases plasma carnitine, reduces fatigue, and may preserve exercise capacity in hemodialysis patients. *Am J Kidney Dis* 2001;37:1018-1028.

195. Plioplys AV, Plioplys S. Amantadine and L-carnitine treatment of chronic fatigue. *Neuropsychobiology* 1997;35:16-23.

196. Ellithorpe RR, Settinery RA, Nicolson GL. Pilot study: reduction of fatigue by use of a supplement containing dietary glycophospholipids. *J Am Neutraceutical Assoc* 2003;6:23-28.

197. Agadjanyan M, Vasilevko V, Ghochikyan A, et al. Nutritional supplement (NT Factor) restores mitochondrial function and reduces moderately severe fatigue in aged subjects. *J Chronic Fatigue Syndr* 2003;11(4):1-12.

198. Singh RB, Neki NS, Kartikey K, et al. Effect of coenzyme Q10 on risk of atherosclerosis in patients with recent myocardial infarction. *Mol Cell Biochem* 2003;246:75-82.

199. Sahlin K. Metabolic factors in fatigue. *Sports Med* 1992;13:99-107; Green HJ. Mechanisms of muscle fatigue in intense exercise. *J Sports Sci* 1997; 15:247-256.

200. McLester JR, Jr. Muscle contraction and fatigue. The role of adenosine 5'-diphosphate and inorganic phosphate. *Sports Med* 1997;23:287-305.

201. Dengler R, Wohlfarth K, Zierz S, Jobges M, Schubert M. Muscle fatigue, lactate and pyruvate in mitochondrial myopathy with progressive external ophthalmoplegia. *Muscle Nerve* 1996;19:456-462.

202. Roussel M, Bendahan D, Mattei JP, Le Fur Y, Cozzone PJ. P-31 magnetic resonance spectroscopy study of phosphocreatine recovery kinetics by skeletal muscle: the issue of intersubject variability. *Biochim Biophys Acta* 2000;1457:18-26.

203. Benington JH, Heller HC. Restoration of brain energy metabolism as the function of sleep. *Prog Neurobiol* 1995;45:347-360.

204. Kreuger JM, Obal FJ, Fang J, Kubota T, Taishi P. The role of cytokines in physiological sleep regulation. *Ann NY Acad Sci* 2001;933:211-221.

205. Liew FY. Interactions between cytokines and nitric oxide. *Adv Neuroimmunol* 1995;5:201-209.

206. Burlet S, Leger L, Cespuglio R. Nitric oxide and sleep in the rat: a puzzling relationship. *Neuroscience* 1999;92:627-639.

207. Nijs J, De Meirleir K, Meeus M, McGregor NR, Englebienne P. Chronic fatigue syndrome: intracellular immune deregulations as a possible etiology for abnormal exercise response. *Med Hypoth* 2004;62:759-765.

208. Garland EM, Winker R, Williams SM, et al. Endothelial NO synthase polymorphisms and postural tachycardia syndrome. *Hypertension* 2005;46:1103-1110.

209. Krukoff TL. Central control of autonomic function: no brakes? *Clin Exp Pharmacol Physiol* 1998;25:474-478.

210. Chowdhary S, Townsend JN. Nitric oxide and hypertension: not just and endothelium derived relaxing factor. *J Hum Hypertens* 2001;15:219-227.

211. Hirooka Y, Kishi T, Sakai K, Shimokawa H, Takeshita A. Effect of overproduction of nitric oxide in the brain stem on the cardiovascular response in conscious rats. *J Cardiovasc Pharmacol* 2003;41(Suppl 1):S119-S126.

212. Akaike T, Suga M, Maeda, H. Free radicals in viral pathogenesis: molecular mechanisms involving superoxide and NO. *Proc Soc Exp Biol Med* 1998;217:64-73.

213. Kawashima H, Watanabe Y, Ichiyama T, et al. High concentrations of serum nitrite/nitrate obtained from patients with influenza-associated encephalopathy. *Pediatr Int* 2002;44:705-707.

214. Akaike T, Maeda H. Nitric oxide and virus infection. *Immunology* 2000; 101:300-308.

215. Suliman HB, Ryan LK, Bishop L, Folz RJ. Prevention of influenza-induced long injury in mice overexpressing extracellular superoxide dismutase. *Am J Physiol Lung Cell Mol Physiol* 2001;280:L69-L78.

216. Mori I, Liu B, Hossain MJ, et al. Successful protection by amantadine hydrochloride agains lethal encephalitis caused by highly virulent recombinant influenza A virus in mice. *Virology* 2002;303:287-296.

217. Rigden S, Barrager E, Bland JS. Evaluation of the effect of a modified enteropathic resuscitation program in chronic fatigue syndrome patients. *J Adv Med* 1998;11:247-262.

218. Logan AC, Rao AV, Irani D. Chronic fatigue syndrome: lactic acid bacteria may be of therapeutic value. *Med Hypoth* 2003;60:915-923.

219. Gomborone JE, Gorard DA, Dewsnap PA, et al. Prevalence of irritable bowel syndrome in chronic fatigue syndrome. *J R Coll Physicians Lond* 1996;30:512-513.

220. Aaron LA, Burke MM, Buchwald D. Overlapping conditions among patients with chronic fatigue syndrome, fibromyalgia and temperomandibular disorder. *Arch Intern Med* 2000;160:221-227.

221. Chang L. The association of functional gastrointestinal disorders and fibromyalgia. *Eur J Surg* 1998;(Suppl 583):32-36.

222. Barton A, Pal B, Whorwell PJ, Marshall D. Increased prevalence of sicca comples and fibromyalgia in patients with irritable bowel syndrome. *Am J Gastroenterol* 1999;94:1898-1901.

223. Sperber AD, Carmel S, Neumann L, et al. Fibromyalgia in the irritable bowel syndrome: studies of prevalence and clinical implications. *Am J Gastroenterol* 1999;94:3541-3546.

224. Irwin C, Falsetti SA, Lydiard RB, et al. Comorbidity of posttraumatic stress disorder and irritable bowel syndrome. *J Clin Psychiatry* 1996;57:576-578.

225. Kendall-Tackett KA. Physiological correlates of childhood abuse: chronic hyperarousal in PTSD, depression and irritable bowel syndrome. *Child Abuse Negl* 2000;24:799-810.

226. Mayer EA, Craske M, Naliboff BD. Depression, anxiety and the gastrointestinal system. *J Clin Psychiatry* 2001;62(Suppl 8):28-36.

227. Azpiroz F, Dapoigny M, Pace F, et al. Nongastrointestinal disorders in irritable bowel syndrome. *Digestion* 2000;62:66-72.

228. Crissinger KD, Kvietys PR, Granger DN. Pathophysiology of gastrointestinal mucosal permeability. *J Intern Med Suppl* 1990;732;145-154.

229. Peters TJ, Bjarnason I. Uses and abuses of intestinal permeability measurements. *Can J Gastroenterol* 1988;2:127-132.

230. Rooney PJ, Jenkins RT, Buchanan WW. A short review of the relationship between intestinal permeability and inflammatory joint disease. *Clin Exp Rheumatol* 1990;8:75-83.

231. Walker WA. Antigen absorption from the small intestine and gastrointestinal disease. *Pediatr Clin North Am* 1975;22:731-746.

232. Jacobson P, Baker R, Lessof M. Intestinal permeability in patients with eczema and food allergy. *Lancet* 1981;1(8233):1285-1286.

233. Vojdani A. A single blood test for the detection of food allergy, candidiasis, microflora imbalance, intestinal barrier dysfunction, and humoral immunodeficiencies. *Biomed Ther* 1999;XVII:129-135.

234. Manu P, Matthews DA, Lane TJ. Food intolerances in patients with chronic fatigue syndrome. *In J Eat Disord* 1993;13:203-209.

235. Miller CS, Prihoda TJ. A controlled comparison of symptoms and chemical intolerances reported in Gulf War veterans, implant recipients and persons with multiple chemical sensitivity. *Toxicol Indust Health* 1999;15:386-397.

236. Ross GH. Clinical characteristics of chemical sensitivity: an illustrative case history of asthma and MCS. *Environ Health Perspect* 1997;105(Suppl 2):437-441.

237. Bell IR. Multiple chemical sensitivities. *Psychiatric Times* 2003;XX(1): January.

238. Becherel PA, Chosidow O, Le Goff L, et al. Inducible nitric oxide synthase and proinflammatory cytokine expression by human keratinocytes during acute urticaria. *Mol Med* 1997;3:686-694.

239. Bayon Y, Alonso A, Sanchez Crespo M. Immunoglobulin-E/dinitrophenyl complexes induce nitric oxide synthesis in rat peritoneal macrophages by a mechanism involving CD23 and NF-kappa B activation. *Biochem Biophys Res Commun* 242:570-574.

240. van Straaten EA, Koster-Kamphuis L, Bovee-Oudenhoven IM, van der Meer R, Forget PP. Increase urinary nitric oxidation products in children with active coeliac disease. *Acta Paediatr* 1999;88:528-531.

241. Fargeas MJ, Theodorou V, Weirich B, Fioramonte J, Bueno L. Decrease in sensitization rate and intestinal anaphylactic response after nitric oxide synthase inhibition in a food hypersensitivity model. *Gut* 1996;38:598-602.

242. Barau E, Dupont C. Modifications of intestinal permeability during food provocation procedures in pediatric irritable bowel syndrome. *J Pediatr Gastroenterol Nutr* 1990;11:72-77.

243. Goyal RK, Hirano I. The enteric nervous system. *N Engl J Med* 1996; 334:1106-1115.

244. Dawson TM, Bredt DS, Fotuhi PM, Hwang PM, Snyder SH. Nitric oxide synthase and neuronal NADPH diaphorase are identical in brain and peripheral tissues. *Proc Natl Acad Sci USA* 1991;88:7797-7801.

245. Xue L, Farrugia G, Miller SM, et al. Carbon monoxide and nitric oxide as coneurotransmitters in the enteric nervous system: evidence from genomic deletion of biosynthetic enzymes. *Proc Natl Acad Sci USA* 2000;97:1851-1855.

246. Burns GA, Stephens KE. Expression of mRNA for the N-methyl-D-aspartate (NMDAR1) receptor and vasoactive intestinal polypeptide (VIP) co-exist in enteric neurons of the rat. *J Auton Nerv Syst* 1995;55:207-210.

247. Izzo AA, Capasso R, Pinto L, et al. Effect of vanilloid drugs on gastrointestinal transit in mice. *Br J Pharmacol* 2001;132:1411-1416.

248. Fiocchi C. Intestinal inflammation: a complex interplay of immune and nonimmune cell interactions. *Am J Physiol* 1997;273:G769-G775.

249. Holzer P. Sensory neurone responses to mucosal noxae in the upper gut: relevance to mucosal integrity and gastrointestinal pain. *Neurogastroenterol Motil* 2002;14:459-475.

250. Cortright DN, Szallasi A. Biochemical pharmacology of the vanilloid receptor TRPV1. An update. *Eur J Biochem* 2004;271:1814-1819.

251. Robinson DR, McNaughton PA, Evans ML, Hicks GA. 2004 *Characterization of the primary afferent innervation of the mouse colon using retrograde labeling.*

252. Stanghellini V, De Ponti F, De Georgio R, et al. New developments in the treatment of functional dyspepsia. *Drugs* 2003;63:869-892.

253. Fritz E, Hammer J, Schmidt B, Eherer AJ, Hammer HF. Stimulation of the nitric oxide-guanosine 3',5'-cyclic monophosphate pathway by sildenafil: effect on rectal muscle tone, distensibility, and perception of health and irritable bowel syndrome. *Am J Gastroenterol* 2003;98:2253-2260.

254. Evans R. *Nitric oxide and IBD. Inflammation 2003-Sixth World Congress,* Canada: Vancouver;2003:August 2-6.

255. Casellas F, Mourelle M, Papo M, et al. Bile acid induced colonic irritation stimulates introcolonic nitric oxide release in humans. *Gut* 1996;38:719-723.

256. Ritchie J. Mechanisms of pain in the irritable bowel syndrome. In: Read N Ed. *Irritable Bowel Syndrome.* Philadelphia: Grune and Stratton;1985:163-170.

257. Kolhekar R, Gebhart GF. Modulation of spinal visceral nociceptive transmission by NMDA receptor activation in the rat. *Brain Res* 1996;651:215-226.

258. Rice AS, McMahon SB. Pre-emptive intrathecal administration of an NMDA receptor antagonist (AP-5) prevents hyper-reflexia in a model of persistent visceral pain. *Pain* 1994;57:335-340.

259. Robinson DR, McNaughton PA, Evans ML, Hicks GA. Characterization of the primary spinal afferent innervation of the mouse colon using retrograde labelling. *Neurogastroenterol Motil* 2004;16:113-124.

260. Verne GN, Price DD. Irritable bowel syndrome as a common precipitant of central sensitization. *Curr Rheumatol Rep* 2002;4:322-328.

261. Xu DZ, Lu Q, Deitch EA. Nitric oxide directly impairs intestinal barrier function. *Shock* 2002;17:139-145.

262. Fink MP. Intestinal epithelial hyperpermeability: update on the pathogenesis of gut mucosal barrier dysfunction in critical illness. *Curr Opin Crit Care* 2003;9:143-151.

263. Chavez AM, Menconi MJ, Hodin RA, Fink MP. Cytokine–induced intestinal hyperpermeability: role of nitric oxide. *Crit Care Med* 1999;27:2246-2251.

264. Han X, Uchiyama I, Sappington PL, et al. NAD$^+$ ameliorates inflammation-induced epithelial barrier dysfunction in cultured enterocytes and mouse ileal mucosa. *J Pharmacol Exp Ther* 2003;307:443-449.

265. Chavez AM, Menconi MJ, Hodin RA, Fink MP. Cytokine-induced intestinal hyperpermeability: role of nitric oxide. *Crit Care Med* 1999;27:2246-2251.

266. Banan A, Fields JZ, Zhang Y, Keshavarzian A. iNOS upregulation mediates oxidant-induced disruption of F-actin and barrier of intestinal monolayers. *Am J Physiol Gastrointest Liver Physiol* 2001;280:G1234-1246.

267. Jagtap P, Soriano FG, Virag L, et al. Novel phenanthridinone inhibitors of poly (adenosine 5'-diphosphate-ribose) synthetase: potent cytoprotective and anti-shock agents. *Crit Care Med* 2002;30:1071-1082.

268. Kennedy M, Denenberg AG, Szabo C, Salzman AL. Poly(ADP-ribose) synthetase activation mediates increased permeability induced by peroxynitrite in Caco-2BBe cells. *Gastroenterology* 1998;114:510-518.

269. Cuzzocrea S, Mazzon E, De Sarro A, Caputi AP. Role of free radicals and poly(ADP-ribose) synthetase in intestinal tight junction permeability. *Mol Med* 2000;6:766-778.

270. Sappington PL, Yang R, Yang H, et al. HMGB1 box increases permeability of Caco-2 enterocyte monolayers and impairs intestinal barrier function in mice. *Gastroenterology* 2002;123:790-802.

271. Banan A, Fields JZ, Zhang Y, Keshavarzian A. iNOS upregulation mediates oxidant-induced disruption of F-actin and barrier intestinal monolayers. *Am J Physiol Gastrointest Liver Physiol* 2001;280:G1234-G1246.

Chapter 4

1. Chen B, Deen WM. Analysis of the effects of cell spacing and liquid depth on nitric oxide and its oxidation products in cell culture. *Chem Res Toxicol* 2001; 14:135-147.

2. Lancaster JR. Simulation of the diffusion and reaction of endogenously produced nitric oxide. *Proc Natl Acad Sci USA* 1994;91:8137-8141.

3. Wood J, Garthwaite J. Models of diffusional spread of nitric oxide: implications for neural signaling and its pharmacological properties. *Neuropharmacology* 1994;33:1235-1244.

4. Lebovitz RM, Zhang H, Vogel H, et al. Neurodegeneration, myocardial injury, and perinatal death in mitochondrial superoxide dismutase-deficient mice. *Proc Natl Acad Sci USA* 1996;93:9782-9787.

5. Copin S, Gasche Y, Chan PH. Overexpression of copper/zinc superoxide dismutase does not prevent neonatal lethality in mutant mice that lack manganese superoxide dismutase. *Free Radic Biol Med* 2000;28:1571-1576.

6. Taylor RR, Friedberg F, Jason LA. *A Clinician's Guide to Controversial Illness: Chronic Fatigue Syndrome, Fibromyalgia, Multiple Chemical Sensitivities.* Sarasota, FL: Professional Resource Press;2001.

7. Sorg BA. Multiple chemical sensitivity: potential role for neural sensitization. *Crit Rev Neurobiol* 1999;13:283-316.

8. Fukuda K, Stauss SE, Hickie I, et al. The chronic fatigue syndrome: a comprehensive approach to its definition and study. International Chronic Fatigue Syndrome Group. *Ann Intern Med* 1994;121:953-959.

9. Pawloski JR, Hess DT, Stamler JS. Export by red blood cells of nitric oxide bioactivity. *Nature* 2001;409:622-626.

10. Pall ML. Elevated peroxynitrite as the caused of chronic fatigue syndrome. *Medical Hypoth* 2000;54:115-125.

11. American Psychiatric Association, *Diagnostic and Statistical Manual of Mental Disorders.* 4th ed. DSM-IV. Washington, DC: American Psychiatric Press;1994. Reprinted with permission from APA.

Chapter 5

1. Mowbray JF, Yousef GE. Immunology of postviral fatigue syndrome. *Br Med Bull* 1991;47:886-894.

2. Behan PO, Bakheit AMO. Clinical spectrum of postviral fatigue syndrome. *Br Med Bull* 1991;47:793-808.

3. White PD, Thomas JM, Amess J, et al. The existence of a fatigue syndrome after glandular fever. *Psychol Med* 1995;25:907-916.

4. Gow JW, Behan WM, Simpsom K, et al. Studies of enterovirus in patients with chronic fatigue syndrome. *Clin Infect Dis* 1994;18(Suppl 1):S126-S129.

5. Lloyd A. Postinfectious fatigue. In: Jason LA, Fennell PA, Taylor RR, eds. *Handbook of Chronic Fatigue Syndrome.* New Jersey: John Wiley and Sons;2003: 108-123.

6. Kerr JR, Bracewell J, Laing I, et al. Chronic fatigue syndrome and arthralgia following parvovirus B19 infection. *J Rheumatol* 2002;29:595-602.

7. Selden SM, Cameron AS. Changing epidemiology of Ross River virus disease in South Australia. *Med J Aust* 1996;165:313-317.

8. Richardson J. Myalgic encephalomyelitis. *J Chron Fatigue Syndr* 2002; 10(1):65-80.

9. Shadick NA, Phillips CB, Sangha O, et al. Musculoskeletal and neurologic outcomes in patients with previously treated Lyme disease. *Ann Intern Med* 1999; 131:919-926.

10. Sigal LH. Summary of the first 100 patients seen at a Lyme disease referral center. *Am J Med* 1990;88:577-581.

11. Wildman MJ, Smith EG, Groves J, et al. Chronic fatigue following infection by Coxiella burnetii (Q fever): ten-year follow-up of the 1989 UK outbreak cohort. *QJM* 2002;95:527-538.

12. Natelson BH, Lange G. A status report on chronic fatigue syndrome. *Environ Health Perspect* 2002;110(Suppl 4):673-677.

13. Pall ML. Elevated, sustained peroxynitrite levels as the cause of chronic fatigue syndrome. *Med Hypoth* 2000;54:115-125.

14. Donnay A. On the recognition of multiple chemical sensitivity in medical literature and government policy. *Int J Toxicol* 1999;18:383-392.

15. Donnay A. Carbon monoxide as an unrecognized cause of neurasthenia: a history. In: Penney D, ed. *Carbon Monoxide Toxicity*. Boca Raton, Florida: CRC; 2000:231-260.

16. Pall ML. Common etiology of posttraumatic stress disorder, fibromyalgia, chronic fatigue syndrome and multiple chemical sensitivity via elevated nitric oxide/ peroxynitrite. *Med Hypoth* 2001;57:139-145.

17. Thom SR, Fisher D, Zhang J, et al. Neuronal nitric oxide synthase and N-methyl-D-aspartate neurons in experimental carbon monoxide poisoning. *Toxicol Appl Pharmacol* 2004;194:280-295.

18. Tahmaz N, Soutar A, Cherrie JW. Chronic fatigue and organophosphate pesticides in sheep farming: a retrospective study amongst people reporting to a UK pharmacovigilance scheme. *Ann Occup Hyg* 2003;47:261-267.

19. Kennedy G, Abbot NC, Spence V, Underwood C, Belch JJ. The specificity of the CDC-1994 criteria for chronic fatigue syndrome: comparison of health status in three groups of patients who fulfill the criteria. *Ann Epidemiol* 2004;14:95-100.

20. Pall ML, Satterlee Elevated nitric oxide/peroxynitrite mechanism for the common etiology of multiple chemical sensitivity, chronic fatigue syndrome and posttraumatic stress disorder. *Ann NY Acad Sci* 2001;933:323-329.

21. Pearn JH. Chronic fatigue syndrome: chronic ciguatera toxin poisoning as a differential diagnosis. *Med J Aust* 1979;166:309-310.

22. Racciatti D, Vecchiet J, Ceccomancini A. Ricci F, Pizzigallo E. Chronic fatigue syndrome following toxic exposure. *Sci Total Environ* 2001;270:27-31.

23. Lewis RJ. Ion channels and therapeutics: from cone snail venoms to ciguatera. *Ther Drug Monit* 2000;22:61-64.

24. Yu XM, Salter MW. Gain control of NMDA-receptor currents by intracellular sodium. *Nature* 1998;396:469-474.

25. Li WI, Berman FW, Okino T, et al. Antillatoxin is a marine cyanobacterial toxin that potently activates voltage-gated sodium channels. *Proc Natl Acad Sci USA* 2001;98:7599-7604.

26. Parada CA, Vivancos GG, Tambeli CH, et al. Activation of presynaptic NMDA receptors coupled to NaV 1.8-resistant sodium channel C-fibers causes retrograde mechanical nociceptor sensitization. *Proc Natl Acad Sci USA* 2003;100: 2923-2928.

27. Verleye M, Andre N, Heulard I, Gillardin JM. Nefopam blocks voltage-sensitive sodium channels and modulates glutamatergic transmission in rodents. *Brain Res* 2004;1013:249-255.

28. Dravid SM, Baden DG, Murray TF. Brevetoxin augments NMDA receptor signaling in murine neocortical neurons. *Brain Res* 2005;1031:30-38.

29. Berman FW, Murray TF. Brevetoxins cause acute excitotoxicity in primary cultures of rat cerebellar granule neurons. *J Pharmacol Exp Ther* 1999;290:439-444.

30. De Meirleir K, De Becker P, Nijs J, et al. CFS etiology, the immune system, and infection. In: Englebienne P, De Meirleir K, eds, *Chronic Fatigue Syndrome, A Biological Approach.* Boca Raton: CRC Press;2002.

31. Brunet LR. Nitric oxide and parasitic infections. *Int Immunopharmacol* 2001;1:1457-1467.

32. Khan IA, Schwartzman JD, Matsuura T, Kasper LH. Dichotomous role for nitric oxide during acute Toxoplasma gondii infection in mice. *Proc Natl Acad Sci USA* 1997;94:13955-13960.

33. Scharton-Kersten TM, Yap G, Magram J, Sher A. Inducible nitric oxide is essential for host control of persistent but not acute infection with the intracellular pathogen Toxoplasma gondii. *J Exp Med* 1997;185:1261-1273.

34. Bell DS. *The Doctor's Guide to Chronic Fatigue Syndrome.* Addison Wesley Reading, Massachusetts: Publishing Co.;1995.

35. Fukuda K, Strauss SE, Hickie I, et al. The chronic fatigue syndrome: a comprehensive approach to its definition and study. *Ann Intern Med* 1994;121:953-959.

36. Carruthers BM, Jain AK, De Meirleir KL, et al. Myalgic encephalomyelitis/ chronic fatigue sydnrome: clinical working case definition, diagnostic and treatment protocols. *J Chronic Fatigue Syndr* 2003;11(1):7-115.

37. Sharpe M, Archard LC, Banatvala JE, et al. A report—chronic fatigue syndrome: guidelines for research. *J R Soc Med* 1991;84:118-121.

38. Komaroff AL, Buchwald DS. Chronic fatigue syndrome: an update. *Ann Rev Med* 1998;49:1-13.

39. Jason LA, Richman JA, Rademaker AW, et al. A community based study of chronic fatigue syndrome. *Arch Intern Med* 1999;159:2129-2137.

40. Pall ML. Elevated peroxynitrite as the cause of chronic fatigue syndrome: other inducers and mechanisms of symptom generation. *J Chronic Fatigue Syndr* 2000;7(4):45-58.

41. Pall ML. Levels of nitric oxide synthase product citrulline are elevated in sera of chronic fatigue syndrome patients. *J Chronic Fatigue Syndr* 2002;10(3/4): 37-41.

42. Pall ML. Cobalamin used in chronic fatigue syndrome therapy is a nitric oxide scavenger. *J Chronic Fatigue Syndr* 2001;8(2):39-44.

43. Smirnova IV, Pall ML. Elevated levels of protein carbonyls in sera of chronic fatigue syndrome patients. *Mol Cell Biochem* 2003;248:93-95.

44. Pall ML. Nitric oxide and the etiology of chronic fatigue syndrome: Giving credit where credit is due. *Med Hypotheses* 2005:Jun2.

45. Chao CC, De La Hunt M, Hu S, Close K, Peterson PK. Immunologically mediated fatigue: a murine model. *Clin Immunol Immunopathol* 1992;64:161-165.

46. Sheng WS, Hu S, Lamkin A, Peterson PK, Chao CC. Susceptibility to immunologically mediated fatigue in C57BL/6 versus Balb/C mice. *Clin Immunol Immunopathol* 1996;81:161-167.

47. Sheng WS, Lin JC, Apple F, Hu S, Peterson PK, Chao CC. Brain energy stores in C57BL/6 mice after C. parvum injection. *Neuroreport* 1999;10:177-81.

48. Sheng WS, Hu S, Ding JM, Chao CC, Peterson PK. Cytokine expression in the mouse brain in response to immune activation by Corynebacterium parvum. *Clin Diagn Lab Immunol* 2001;8:446-448.

49. Ambs S, Ogunfusika MO, Merriam WG, Bennett WP, Billiar TR, Harris CC. Up-regulation of inducible nitric oxide synthase expression in cancer–prone p53 knockout mice. *Proc Natl Acad Sci USA* 1998;95:8823-8828.

50. Cook HT, Bune AJ, Jansen AS, Taylor GM, Loi RK, Cattell V. Cellular localization of inducible nitric oxide synthase in experimental endotoxic shock in the rat. *Clin Sci (Lond).* 1994;87:179-186.

51. Kurup RK, Kurup PA. Hypothalamic digoxin, cerebral chemical dominance and myalgic encephalomyelitis. *Int J Neurosci* 2003;113:445-457.

52. Patarca R. Cytokines and chronic fatigue syndrome. *Ann NY Acad Sci USA* 2001;933:185-200.

53. Vernon SD, Unger ER, Dimulescu IM, Rajeevan M, Reeves WC. Utility of the blood for gene expression profiling and biomarker discovery in chronic fatigue. *Dis Markers* 2002;18:193-199.

54. Buskila D. Fibromyalgia, chronic fatigue syndrome and myofascial pain syndrome. *Curr Opin Rheumatol* 2001;13:117-127.

55. Cannon JG, Angel JB, Ball RW, et al. Acute phase responses and cytokine secretion in chronic fatigue syndrome. *J Clin Immunol* 1999;19:414-421.

56. Droge W, Holm E. Role of cysteine and glutathione in HIV infection and other diseases associated with muscle wasting and immunological dysfunction. *FASEB J* 1997;11:1077-1089.

57. Bounos G, Molson J. Competition for glutathione precursors between the immune system and the skeletal muscle: pathogenesis of chronic fatigue syndrome. *Med Hypoth* 1999;53:347-349.

58. McGregor NR, Dunstan RH, Zerbes M, et al. Preliminary determination of the association between symptom expression with urinary metabolites in subjects with chronic fatigue syndrome. *Biochem Mol Med* 1996;58:85-92.

59. Young A. 1999 *Hypercitricemia in chronic fatigue syndrome.* Presentation at the 1999 Sydney ME/CFS Conference.

60. Carpman V. CFIDS treatment: the Cheney clinic's strategic approach. *CFIDS Chronicle Spring* 1995:38-45.

61. Hoh D. Treatment at the Cheney clinic. *CFIDS Chronicle* 1998;11(4):13-14.

62. Goldstein JA. *Tuning the Brain: Principles and Practice of Neurosomatic Medicine.* Binghamton, NY: Haworth Medical Press;2004.

63. Manuel y Keenoy B, Moorkens G et al. Magnesium status and parameters of the oxidant-antioxidant balance in patients with chronic fatigue: effects of supplementation with magnesium. *J Am Coll Nutr* 2000;19:374-382.

64. Werbach MR. Nutritional strategies for treating chronic fatigue syndrome. *Altern Med Rev* 2000;5:93-108.

65. Tarello W. Chronic Fatigue Syndrome (CFS) in 15 dogs and cats with specific biochemical and microbiological. *Comp Immunol Microbiol Infect Dis* 2001; 24:165-185.

66. Tarello W. Chronic fatigue and immune dysfunction syndrome associated with Staphylococcus spp. bacteraemia responsive to thiacetarsamide sodium in eight birds of prey. *J Vet Med B Infect Dis Vet Public Health*·2001;48:267-281.

67. Fulle S, Mecocci P, Fano G, et al. Specific oxidative alterations in vastus lateralis muscle of patients with the diagnosis of chronic fatigue syndrome. *Free Radic Biol Med* 2000;15:1252-1259.

68. Richards RS, Roberts TK, Mathers MB, Dunstan RH, McGregor NR, Butt HL. Investigation of erythrocyte oxidative damage in rheumatoid arthritis and chronic fatigue syndrome. *J Chronic Fatigue Syndr* 2000;6(1):37-46.

69. Richards RS, Roberts TK, McGregor NR, Dunstan RH, Butt HL. Blood parameters indicative of oxidative stress are associated with symptom expression in chronic fatigue syndrome. *Redox Rep* 2000;5:35-41.

70. Richards RS, Roberts TK, Dunstan RH, McGregor NR, Butt HL. Free radicals in chronic fatigue syndrome: cause or effect? *Redox Rep* 2000;5:146-147.

71. Keenoy BM, Moorkens G, Vertommen J, DeLeeuw I. Antioxidant status and lipoprotein oxidation in chronic fatigue syndrome. *Life Sciences* 2001;68: 2037-2049.

72. Manuel y Keenoy B, Moorkens G, Vertommen J, et al. Magnesium status and parameters of the oxidant-antioxidant balance in patients with chronic fatigue: effects of supplementation with magnesium. *J Am Coll Nutr* 19:374-382.

73. Vecchiet J, Cipollone F, Falasca K, et al. Relationship between musculo-skeletal symptoms and blood markers of oxidative stress in patients with chronic fatigue syndrome. *Neurosci Lett* 2003;335:151-154.

74. Jammes Y, Steinberg JG, Mambrini O, et al. Chronic fatigue syndrome: assessment of increased oxidative stress and altered muscle excitability in response to incremental exercise. *J Intern Med* 2005;257:299-310.

75. Kennedy G, Spence VA, McLaren M, et al. Oxidative stress levels are raised in chronic fatigue syndrome and are associated with clinical symptoms. *Free Radic Biol Med* 2005;39:584-589.

76. Singh A, Garg V, Gupta S, Kulkarni SK. Role of antioxidants in chronic fatigue syndrome in mice. *Indian J Exp Biol* 2002;40:1240-1244.

77. Logan AC, Wong C. Chronic fatigue syndrome: oxidative stress and dietary modifications. *Altern Med Rev* 2001;6:450-459.

78. Rigden S, Barrager E, Bland JS. Evaluation of the effect of a modified entero-hepatic resuscitation program in chronic fatigue syndrome patients. *J Adv Med* 1998;11:247-262.

79. Majib A. Ascorbic acid reverses abnormal erythrocyte morphology in chronic fatigue syndrome. *Am J Clin Pathol* 1991;94:515.

80. Behan WM, More IA, Behan PO. Mitochondrial abnormalities in the postviral fatigue syndrome. *Acta Neuropathol* 1991;83:61-65.

81. Plioplys AV, Plioplys S. Serum levels of carnitine in chronic fatigue syndrome: clinical correlates. *Neuropsychobiology* 1995;32:132-138.

82. Kuratsune H, Yamaguti K, Lindh G, et al. Low levels of serum acylcarnitine in chronic fatigue syndrome and chronic hepatitis type C but not seen in other diseases. *Int J Mol Med* 1998;2:51-56.

83. Wong R, Lopaschuk G, Zhu G, et al. Skeletal muscle metabolism in the chronic fatigue syndrome. In vivo assessment by 31P nuclear magnetic resonance. *Chest* 1992;102:1716-1722.

84. Barnes PR, Taylor DJ, Kemp GJ, Radda GK. Skeletal muscle bioenergetics in the chronic fatigue syndrome. *J Neurol Neurosurg Psychiatry* 1993;56:679-683.

85. McCully KK, Natelson BH, Iotti S, Sisto S, Leigh JS Jr. Reduced oxidative muscle metabolism in chronic fatigue syndrome. *Muscle Nerve* 1997;19:621-625.

86. Vecchiet L, Monanari G, Pizzigally E, et al. Sensory characterization of somatic parietal tissues in humans with chronic fatigue syndrome. *Neurosci Lett* 1996; 208:117-120.

87. Hayakawa M, Hattori K, Sugiyama S, Ozawa T. Age-related oxygen damage and mutations in mitochondrial DNA in human hearts. *Biochem Biophys Res Commun* 1992;189:979-985.

88. Farquhar WB, Hunt BE, Tayler JA, Darling SE, Freeman R. Blood volume and its relation to peak O(2) consumption and physical activity in patients with chronic fatigue. *Am J Physiol Heart Circ Physiol* 2002;282:H66-H71.

89. McCully KK, Smith S, Rajaei S, Leigh JS, Natelson BH. Muscle metabolism with blood flow restriction in chronic fatigue syndrome. *J Appl Physiol* 2004; 96:871-878.

90. Kaushik N, Fear D, Richards SC, et al. Gene expression in peripheral blood mononuclear cells from patients with chronic fatigue syndrome. *J Clin Pathol* 2005; 58:826-832.

91. Plioplys AV, Plioplys S. Amantadine and L-carnitine treatment of chronic fatigue. *Neuropsychobiology* 1997;35:16-23.

92. Vermeulen RC, Scholte HR. Exploratory open label, randomized study of acetyl- and proprionylcarnitine in chronic fatigue syndrome. *Psychosom Med* 2004; 66:276-282.

93. Ellithorpe RR, Settinery RA, Nicolson GL. Pilot study: reduction of fatigue by use of a supplement containing dietary glycophospholipids. *J Am Neutraceutical Assoc* 2003;6:23-28.

94. Agadjanyan M, Vasilevko V, Ghochikyan A, et al. Nutritional supplement (NT Factor[TM]) restores mitochondrial function and reduces moderately severe fatigue in aged subjects. *J Chronic Fatigue Syndr* 2003;11(4):1-12.

95. Aaron LA, Herrell R, Ashton S, et al. Comorbid clinical conditions in chronic fatigue: a co-twin study. *J Gen Intern Med* 2001;16:24-31.

96. Buchwald D, Herrell R, Ashton S, et al. A twin study of chronic fatigue. *Psychosom Med* 2001;63:936-943.

97. Keller RH, Lane JL, Klimas N, et al. Association between HLA class II antigens and the chronic fatigue immune dysfunction syndrome. *Clin Infect Dis* 1994; 18(Suppl 1):S154-S156.

98. Torpy DJ, Bachmann AW, Grice JE, et al. Familial corticosteroid-binding globulin deficiency due to a novel null mutation: association with fatigue and relative hypotension. *J Clin Endocrinol Metab* 2001;86:3692-3700.

99. Torpy DJ, Bachmann AW, Gartside M, et al. Association between chronic fatigue syndrome and the corticosteroid-binding globulin geen ALA SER224 polymorphism. *Endocrine Res* 2004;30:417-429.

100. Narita M, Nishigami N, Narita N, et al. Association between serotonin transported gene polymorphism and chronic fatigue syndrome. *Biochem Biophys Res Commun* 2003;311:264-266.

101. Vladutiu GD, Natelson BH. Association of medically unexplained fatigue with ACE insertion/deletion polymorphism in Gulf War veterans. *Muscle Nerve* 2004;30:38-43.

102. Das UN. Long-chain polyunsaturated fatty acids interact with nitric oxide, superoxide anion, and transforming growth factor-beta to prevent essential human hypertension. *Eur J Clin Nutr* 2004;58:195-203.

103. Wolf G. Free radical production and angiotensin. *Curr Hypertens Rep* 2000;2:167-173.

104. Rowe PC, Barron DF, Calkins H, Maumenee IH, Tong PY, Geraghty MT. Orthostatic intolerance and chronic fatigue associated with Ehlers-Danlos syndrome. *J Pediatr* 1999;135:494-499.

105. Yeowell HN, Pinnell SR. The Ehlers-Danlos syndromes. *Semin Dermatol* 1993;12:229-240.

106. de Paepe A. The Ehlers-Danlos syndrome: a heritable collagen disorder as a cause of bleeding. *Thromb Haemost* 1996;75:379-386.

107. Kuivaniemi H, Tromp G, Prockop DJ. Mutations in fibrillar collagens (types I, II, II, and XI) fibril-associated collagen (type IX), and network-forming collagen (type X) cause a spectrum of diseases of bone, cartilage, and blood vessels. *Hum Mutat* 1997;9:300-315.

108. McGregor NR, Dunstan RH, Butt HL, et al. A preliminary assessment of the association of SCL-90-R psychological inventory responses with changes in urinary metabolites in patients with chronic fatigue syndrome. *J Chronic Fatigue Syndr* 1997;3(1):17-37.

109. Jones MG, Cooper E, Amjad S, Goodwin SC, Barron JL, Chambers RA. Urinary and plasma organic acids and amino acids in chronic fatigue syndrome. *Clin Chim Acta* 2005;361:150-158.

110. Hokama Y, Uto GA, Palafox NA, et al. Chronic phase lipids in sera of chronic fatigue syndrome (CFS), chronic ciguatera fish poisoning (CCFP), hepatitis B, and cancer with antigenic epitope resembling ciguatoxin, as assesses with MAb-CTX. *J Clin Lab Anal* 2003;17:132-139.

111. Buchwald D, Wener MH, Pearlman T, Kith P. Markers of inflammation and immune activation in chronic fatigue and chronic fatigue syndrome. *J Rheumatol* 1997;24:372-376.

112. Fehsel K, Plewe D, Kolb-Bachofen. Nitric oxide induced expression of C-reactive protein islet cells is a very early marker for islet stess in the rat pancreas. *Nitric Oxide* 1997;1:254-262.

113. Ford ES, Liu S, Mannino DM, et al. C-reactive protein concentrations and concentrations of blood vitamins, carotenoids and selenium among United State adults. *Eur J Clin Nutr* 2003;57:1157-1163.

114. Horrobin DF. Post-viral fatigue syndrome, viral infections in atopic eczema, and essential fatty acids. *Med Hypoth* 1990;32:211-217.

115. Liu Z, Wang D, Xue Q, et al. Determination of fatty acid levels in erythrocyte membranes in patients with chronic fatigue syndrome. *Nutr Neurosci* 2004; 6:389-392.

116. Berg D, Berg LH, Couvaras J, Harrison H. Chronic fatigue syndrome and/or fibromyalgia as a variation of antiphospholipid antibody syndrome: an explanatory model and approach to laboratory diagnosis. *Blood Coagul Fibrinolysis* 2004;10: 435-438.

117. Hannan KL, Berg DE, Baumzweiger W, et al. Activation of the coagulation system in Gulf War Illness: a potential pathophysiologic link with chronic fatigue syndrome. A laboratory approach to diagnosis. *Blood Coagul Fibrinolysis* 2000; 11:673-678.

118. Horkko S, Miller E, Dudl E, et al. Antiphospholipid antibodies are directed against epitopes of oxidized phospholipids. Recognition of cardiolipin by monoclonal antibodies to epitopes of oxidized low density lipoproteins. *J Clin Invest* 1996;98:815-825.

119. Iuliano L, Practico D, Ferro D, et al. Enhanced lipid peroxidation in patients positive for antiphospholipid antibodies. *Blood* 1997;90:3931-3935.

120. Pawlak K, Borawski J, Naumnik B, Mysliwiec M. Relationship between oxidative stress and extrinsic coagulation pathway in haemodialized patients. *Throm Res* 2003;109:247-251.

121. Tomiyama K, Kushiro T, Okazaki R, et al. Influences of increased oxidative stress on endothelial function, and fibrinolysis in hypertension associated with glucose intolerance. *Hypertens Res* 2003;26:295-300.

122. Chaudhuri A, Watson WS, Pearn J, Behan PO. The symptoms of chronic fatigue syndrome are related to abnormal ion channel function. *Med Hypoth* 2000; 54:59-63.

123. Zhang C, Imam SZ, Ali SF, Mayeux PR. Peroxynitrite and the regulation of Na^+, K^+-ATPase activity by angiotensin II in the rat proximal tubule. *Nitric Oxide* 2002;7:30-35.

124. Muriel P, Casteneda G, Ortega M, Noel F. Insights into the mechanism of erythrocyte Na^+/K^+-ATPase inhibition by nitric oxide and peroxynitrite anion. *J Appl Toxicol* 2003;23:275-278.

125. http://phoenix-cfs.org/Cardio%20IVa%20Superoxide.htm

126. Dulhunty A, Haarman C, Green D, Hart J. How many cysteine residues regulate ryanodine receptor channel activity? *Antioxid Redox Signal* 2000;2:27-34.

127. Suhadolnik RJ, Reichenbach NL, Hitzges P, et al. Upregulation of the 2-5A synthetase/RNase L pathway associated with chronic fatigue syndrome. *Clin Infect Dis* 1994;18(Suppl 1):S96-S104.

128. Suhadolnik RJ, Peterson DL, O'Brien K, et al. Biochemical evidence for a novel low molecular weight 2-5A-dependent RNase L in chronic fatigue syndrome. *J Inteferon Cytokine Res* 1997;17:377-385.

129. Shetzline SE, Suhadolnik RJ. Characterization of a 2',5'-oligoadenylate (2-5A)–dependent 35 kDa RNase: azido photoaffinity labeling and 2-5A-dependent activation. *J Biol Chem* 2001;276:23707-23711.

130. Shetzline SE, Martinand-Mari C, Reichenbach NL, et al. Structural and functional features of the 37-kDa 2-5A-dependent RNase L in chronic fatigue syndrome. *J Interferon Cytokine Res* 2002;22:443-456.

131. De Meirleir K, Bisbal C, Campine I, et al. A 37 kDa 2-5A binding protein as a potential biochemical marker for chronic fatigue syndrome. *Am J Med* 2000; 108:99-105.

132. Suhadolnik RJ, Peterson DL, Reichenbach BS, et al. Clinical and biochemical characteristics differentiation chronic fatigue syndrome from major depression and healthy control populations: relation to dysfunction of he RNase L pathway. *J Chronic Fatigue Syndr* 2004;12(1):5-35.

133. Fremont M, El Bakkouri K, Vaeyens F, et al. 2',5'-Oligoadenylate size is critical to protect RNase L against proteolytic cleavage in chronic fatigue syndrome. *Exp Mol Pathol* 2005;78:239-246.

134. Choppa PC, Vojdani A, Tagle C, Andrin R, Magtoto L. Multiplex PCR for detection of Micoplasma fermentans, M. hominia and M. penetrans in cell cultures and blood samples of patients with chronic fatigue syndrome. *Mol Cell Probes* 1998;12:301-308.

135. Nicolson GL, Gan R, Haier J. Evidence for Brucella spp. and Mycoplasma spp. co-infections in blood of chronic fatigue syndrome patients. *J Chronic Fatigue Syndr* 2004;12(2):5-17.

136. Nasralla M, Haier J, Nicolson GL. Multiple mycoplasmal infections detected in blood of chronic fatigue syndrome and fibromyalgia patients. *Eur J Clin Microbiol Infect Dis* 1999;18:859-865.

137. Nicolson GL, Gan R, Haier J. Multiple co-infections(Mycoplasma, Chlamydia, human herpes virus-6) in blood of chronic fatigue syndrome patient: association of signs and symptoms. *APMIS* 2003;111:557-566.

138. Nijs J, Nicolson GL, de Becker P, Coomans D, De Meirleir K. High prevalence o mycoplasmal infections among European chronic fatigue syndrome patients. Examination of four mycoplasmal species in chronic fatigue syndrome patients. *FEMS Immunol Med Microbiol* 2002;34:209-214.

139. Lane RJ, Soteriou BA, Zhang H, Archard LC. Entervirus related metabolic myopathy: a postviral fatigue syndrome. *J Neurol Neurosurg Psychiatry* 2003; 74:1382-1386.

140. Douche-Aourik F, Berlier W, Feasson L, et al. Detection of enterovirus in human skeletal muscle from patients with chronic inflammatory muscle disease or fibromyalgia and healthy subjects. *J Med Virol* 2003;71:540-547.

141. Lane RJM, Soteriou BA, Zhang H, Archard LC. Enterovirus related metabolic myopathy: a postviral fatigue syndrome. *J Neurol Neurosurg Psychiatry* 2003; 74:1382-1286.

142. Dunstan RH, McGregor NR, Butt HL, Roberts TK. Biochemical and microbiological anomalies in chronic fatigue syndrome: the development of laboratory based tests and possible role of toxic chemicals. *J Nutr Environ Med* 1999;9:97-108.

143. Jason LA, Taylor RR. Applying cluster analysis to define typology of chronic fatigue in medically-evaluated, random community sample. *Psychol Health* 2002;17:323-337.

144. Natelson BH, Weaver SA, Tseng CL, Ottenweller JE. Spinal fluid abnormalities in patients with chronic fatigue syndrome. *Clin Diagn Lab Immunol* 2005; 12:52-55.

145. Ramsay MA. *Myalgic Encephalomyelitis and Postviral Fatigue State: The Saga of Royal Free Disease.* 2nd ed. London: Gower;1988.

146. Demitrack MA, Crofford LJ. Evidence for and pathophysiologic implications of the hypothalamic-pituitary-adrenal axis dysregulation in fibromyalgia and chronic fatigue syndrome. *Ann NY Acad Sci* 1998;840:684-697.

147. Adler GK, Manfredsdottir VF, Rackow RM. Hypothalamic-pituitary-adrenal axis function in fibromyalgia and chronic fatigue sydrome. *The Endocrinologist* 2002;12:513-524.

148. Ottenweller JE, Sisto SA, McCarty RC, Natelson BH. Hormonal responses to exercise in chronic fatigue syndrome. *Neuropsychobiology* 2001;43:34-41.

149. Scott LV, The J, Reznek R, Martin A, Sohaib A, Dinan TG. Small adrenal glands in chronic fatigue syndrome: a preliminary computer tomography study. *Endocrinology* 1999;24:759-768.

150. Neeck G, Crofford LJ. Neuroendocrine perturbations in fibromyalgia and chronic fatigue syndrome. *Rheum Dis Clin North Am* 2000;26:989-1002.

151. Torpy DJ. Neuroendocrinology, genetics and chronic fatigue syndrome. *CFS Res Rev* 2001;2(4):1-3.

152. Baschetti R. Chronic fatigue syndrome, exercise, cortisol and lymphoadenopathy. *J Intern Med* 2005;258:291-292.

153. Segal TY, Hindmarsh PC, Viner RM. Disturbed adrenal function in adolescents with chronic fatigue syndrome. *J Pediatr Endocrinol Metab* 2005;18:295-301.

154. LaManca JJ, Sisto SA, DeLuca J, et al. Influence of exhaustive treadmill exercise on cognitive functioning in chronic fatigue syndrome. *Am J Med* 1998; 105(3A):59S-65S.

155. Peckerman A, LaManca JJ, Dahl KA, et al. Abnormal impedance cardiography predicts symptom severity in chronic fatigue syndrome. *Am J Med* 2003; 326:55-60.

156. Peckerman A, LaManca JJ, Qureshi B, et al. Baroreceptive reflex and integrative stress responses in chronic fatigue syndrome. *Psychosom Med* 2003;65: 889-895.

157. Aoyama T, Matsui T, Novikov M, et al. Serum and glucocorticoid-responsive kinase-1 regulates cardiomyocyte survival and hypertrophic response. *Circulation* 2005;111:1653-1659.

158. Narayanan N, Yang C, Xur A. Dexamethasone treatment improves sarcoplasmic reticulum function and contractile performance in aged myocardium. *Mol Cell Biochem* 2004;266:31-36.

159. Chiu CZ, Nakatani S, Zhang G, et al. Prevention of left ventricular remodeling by long-term corticosteroid therapy in patients with cardiac sarcoidosis. *Am J Cardiol* 2005;95:143-146.

160. Iga K, Hori K, Gen H. Deep negative T waves associated with reversible left ventricular dysfunction in acute adrenal crisis. *Heart Vessels* 1992;7:107-111.

161. Allolio B, Ehses W, Steffen HM, Muller R. Reduced lymphocyte beta 2-adreoreceptor density and impaired diastolic left ventricular function in patients with glucocorticoid deficiency. *Clin Endocrinol* 1994;40:769-775.

162. Boachour G, Tirot P, Varache N, et al. Hemodynamic changes in acute adrenal insufficiency. *Intensive Care Med* 1994;20:138-141.

163. Emir M, Ozisik K, Cagli K, et al. Beneficial effect of methylprednisone on cardiac myocytes in a rat model of severe brain injury. *Tohoku J Exp Med* 2005;207:119-124.

164. Shojaiefard M, Christie DL, Lang F. Stimulation of the creatine transporter SLC6A8 by the protein kinases SGK1 and SGK3. *Biochem Biophys Res Commun* 2005;334:742-746.

165. Boehmer C, Wilhelm V, Palmada M, et al. Serum and glucocorticoid inducible kinases in the regulation of the cardiac sodium channel SCN5A. *Cardiovasc Res* 2003;57:1079-1084.

166. Conwell LS, Gray LM, Delbridge RG, Thomsett MJ, Batch JA. Reversible cardiomyopathy in paediatric Addison's disease—a cautionary tale. *J Pediatr Endocrinol Metab* 2003;16:1191-1195.

167. Hyde BM, ed. *The Clinical and Scientific Basis of Myalgic Encephalomyelitis/Chronic Fatigue Syndrome.* Ottawa, Canada: The Nightingale Research Foundation; 1992.

Chapter 6

1. Ellis FR, Nasser S. A pilot study of vitamin B_{12} in the treatment of tiredness. *Br J Nutr* 1973;30:277-283.

2. Bjorkegren K. Vitamin B_{12}, chronic fatigue and injection therapy. *Lakartidningen* 1999;96:5610.

3. Wiebe E. N of 1 trials. Managing patients with chronic fatigue syndrome: two case reports. *Can Fam Physician* 1996;42:2214-2217.

4. http://www.drmyhill.co.uk/article.cfm?id=341

5. Lapp CW. Using vitamin B-12 for the management of CFS. *The CFIDS Chronicle* 1999;12(6):14-16.

6. Hoh D. Treatment at the Cheney clinic. *The CFIDS Chronicle* 1998;1(4):13-14.

7. Pall ML. Cobalamin used in chronic fatigue syndrome therapy is a nitric oxide scavenger. *J Chronic Fatigue Syndr* 2001;8(2):39-44.

8. Gaby AR. Intravenous nutrient therapy: the "Myers' cocktail". *Altern Med Rev* 2002;7:389-403.

9. Gaby AR. Literature review & commentary. *Townsend Letter for Doctors & Patients* 1997;Feb/Mar.

10. http://utopia.knoware.nl/

11. http://www.wholehealthmd.com/news/viewarticle/1,1513,1045,00.html

12. Leroy J, Haney Davis I, Jason LA. Data derived from "Treatment Efficacy: A survey of 305 MCS patients" *The CFIDS Chronicle*1996;Winter:52-53.

13. Lawhorne L, Rindgahl D. Cyanocobalamin injections for patients without documented deficiency. *JAMA* 1989;261:1920-1923.

14. Mellman I, Willard HF, Youngdahl-Turner P, Rosenberg LE. Cobalamin coenzyme synthesis in normal and mutant human fibroblasts. Evidence for a processing enzyme activity deficient in cblC cells. *J Biol Chem.* 1979;254:11847-11853.

15. Rochelle LG, Morana SJ, Kruszyna H, et al. Interactions between hydroxocobalamin and nitric oxide (NO): Evidence for a redox reaction between NO and reduced cobalamin and reversible NO binding to oxidized cobalamin. *J Pharmacol Expt Therapeut* 1995;275:48-52.

16. Ellis A, Lu H, Li CG, Rand MJ. Effects of agents that inactivate free radical NO(NO•) released from the nitroxyl anion donor Angeli's salt. *Br J Pharmacol* 2001;134:521-528.

17. Zheng D, Yan L, Birke RL. Electrochemical and spectral studies of the reaction of aquocobalamin with nitric oxide and nitric ion. *Inorg Chem* 2002;41: 2548-2555.

18. Rajanayagam MAS, Li CG, Rand MJ. Differential effects of hydroxocobalamin in NO-mediated relaxations of rat aorta and anococcygeus muscle. *Br J Pharmacol* 1993;108:3-5.

19. Greenberg SS, Xie J, Zatarain JM, Kapusta DR, Miller MJ. Hydroxocobalamin (vitamin B12a) prevents and reverses endotoxin-induced hypotension in rodents: role of nitric oxide. *J Pharmacol Exp Therapeut* 1995;273:257-265.

20. Wanstall JC, Jeffery TK, Gambino A, et al. Vascular smooth muscle relaxation mediated by nitric oxide donors: a comparison with acetylcholine, nitric oxide and nitroxyl ion. *Br J Pharmacol* 2001;134:463-472.

21. Tracey A, Bunton D, Irvine J, MacDonald A, Shaw AM. Relaxation of bradykinin in bovine pulmonary supernumerary arteries can be mediated by both a nitric oxide-dependent and -independent mechanism. *Br J Pharmacol* 2002;137:538-544.

22. Nabeyrat E, Jones GE, Fenwick PS, et al. Mitogen-activated protein kinases mediate peroxynitrite-induced cell death in human bronchial epithelial cells. *Am J Physiol Lung Cell Mol Biol* 2003;284:L1112-L1120.

23. Schubert R, Kein U, Wulfsen I, et al. Nitric oxide donor sodium nitroprusside dilates rat small arteries by activation of inward rectifies potassium channels. *Hypertension* 2004;43:891-896.

24. Weinberg JB, Sauls DL, Misukonis MA, Shugars DC. Inhibition of productive human immunodeficiency virus-1 infection by cobalamins. *Blood* 1995;86: 1281-1287.

25. Weinberg JB, Misukonis MA, Shami PJ et al. Human mononuclear phagocyte inducible nitric oxide synthase (iNOS): analysis of iNOS mRNA, iNOS protein, biopterin, and nitric oxide production by blood monocytes and peritoneal macrophages. *Blood* 1995;86:1184-1195.

26. van der Kuy PH, Merkus FW, Lohman JJ, ter Berg JW, Hooymans PM. Hydroxocobalamin, a nitric oxide scavenger, in the prophylaxis of migraine: an open pilot study. *Cephalagia* 2002;22:513-519.

27. Simpson LO, Murdoch JC, Herbison GP. Red cell shape changes following trigger finger fatigue in subjects with chronic tiredness [CFS] and healthy controls. *New Zealand Medical Journal* 1993;106:104-107.

28. http://listserv.nodak.edu/scripts/wa.exe.?A2=ind9905D&L=co-cure&P= R356

29. Deliconstatinos G, Villiotou V, Stavrides JC, Salemes N, Gogas J. Nitric oxide and peroxynitrite production by human erythrocytes: a causative factor of toxic anemia in breast cancer patients. *Anticancer Res* 1995;15:1435-1446.

30. Kaslow JE, Rucker L, Onishi R. Liver extract-folic acid-cyanocobalamin vs placebo for chronic fatigue syndrome. *Arch Intern Med* 1989;149:2501-2503.

31. Regland B, Andersson M, Abrahamsson L, Bagby J, Dyrehag LE, Gottfries CG. Increased concentrations of homocysteine in the cerebrospinal fluid in patients with fibromyalgia and chronic fatigue syndrome. *Scand J Rheumatol* 1997; 26:301-307.

32. Newbold HL. Vitamin B-12: a placebo or neglected therapeutic tool. *Med Hypoth* 1989;28:155-164.

33. Akyol O, Zoroglu SS, Armutcu F, Sahin S, Gurel A. Nitric oxide as a pathophysiological factor in neuropsychatric disorders. *In Vivo* 2004;18:377-390.

34. Finkel MS, Laghrissi-Thode F, Pollock BG, Rong J. Paroxetine is a novel nitric oxide synthase inhibitor. *Psychopharmacol Bull* 1996;32:653-658.

35. Angulo J, Peiro C, Sanchez-Ferrer CF, et al. Differential effects of serotonin reuptake inhibitors on erectile responses, NO-production, and neuronal NO synthase expression in rat corpus cavernosum tissue. *Brit J Pharmacol* 2001;134: 1190-1194.

36. Wegener G, Volke V, Harvey BH, Rosenberg R. Local, but not systemic, administration of serotonergic antidepressants decreases hippocampal nitric oxide synthase activity. *Brain Res* 2003;959:128-134.

37. Altschuler EL, Kast RE. Paroxetine for hepatopulmonary syndrome? *Med Hypoth* 2004;62:446-44733.

38. Davidson JR. Treatment of posttraumatic stress disorder: the impact of paroxetine. *Psychopharmacol Bull* 2003;37(suppl 1):76-88.

39. Asnis GM, Kohn SR, Henderson M, Brown NL. SSRIs versus non-SSRIs in post-traumatic stress disorder: an update with recommendations. *Drugs* 2004; 64:3 83-404.

40. Bourin M, Chue P, Guillon Y. Paroxetine: a review. *CNS Drug Rev* 2001; 7:25-47.

41. Black DW. Paroxetine for multiple chemical sensitivity. *Am J Psychiatry* 2002;159:1436-1437.

42. Stenn P, Binkley K. Successful outcome in a patient with chemical sensitivity: treatment with psychological desensitization and selective serotonin reuptake inhibitor. *Psychosomatics* 1998;39:547-550.

43. Andine P, Ronnback L, Jarvholm B. Successful use of a selective serotonin reuptake inhibitor in a patient with multiple chemical sensitivities. *Acta Psychiatr Scand* 1997;96:82-83.

Chapter 7

1. Pall ML, Satterlee JD Elevated nitric oxide/peroxynitrite mechanism for the common etiology of multiple chemical sensitivity, chronic fatigue syndrome and posttraumatic stress disorder. *Ann NY Acad Sci* 2001;933:323-329.

2. Pall ML. NMDA sensitization and stimulation by peroxynitrite, nitric oxide and organic solvents as the mechanism of chemical sensitivity in multiple chemical sensitivity. *FASEB J* 2002;16:1407-1417.

3. Pall ML. Elevated nitric oxide/peroxynitrite theory of multiple chemical sensitivity: central role on N-methyl-D-aspartate receptors in the sensitivity mechanism. *Environ Health Perspect* 2003;111:1461-1464.

4. Pall ML. The simple truth about multiple chemical sensitivity. *Environ Health Perspect* 2004;112:A266-A267.

5. Pall ML, Anderson JH. The vanilloid receptor as a putative target of diverse chemicals in multiple chemical sensitivity. *Arch Environ Health* 2004;59:363-375.

6. Pall ML. Elevated nitric oxide/peroxynitrite neurochemical mechanism of multiple chemical sensitivity. In: Kohji Fukunaga ed. *Neurochemistry*, in press.

7. Rosenthal N. Multiple chemical sensitivity: lessons from seasonal affective disorder. *Toxicol Ind Health* 1994;10:623-632.

8. Ashford NA, Miller CS. *Chemical Exposures: Low Levels and High Stakes.* 2nd ed. New York: John Wiley & Sons, Inc;1998.

9. Sorg BA. Multiple chemical sensitivity: potential role for neural sensitization. *Crit Rev Neurobiol* 1999;13:283-316.

10. Straus DC, Cooley JD, Wong WC, Jumper CA. Studies on the role of fungi in sick building syndrome. *Arch Environ Health* 2003;58:475-478.

11. Meggs WJ. RADS and RUDS—The toxic induction of asthma and rhinitis. *Clin Toxicol* 1994;32:487-501.

12. Meggs WJ. Multiple chemical sensitivities—Chemical sensitivity as a symptom of airway inflammation. *Clin Toxicol* 1995;33:107-110.

13. Meggs WJ, Elsheik T, Metzger WJ, Albernaz M, Bloch RM. Nasal pathology and ultrastructure in patients with chronic airways inflammation(RADS and RUDS) following irritant exposure. *Clin Toxicol* 1996;34:383-396.

14. Meggs WJ. Mechanisms of allergy and chemical sensitivity. *Toxicol Ind Health* 1999;15:331-338.

15. Lieberman AD, Craven MR. Reactive intestinal dysfunction syndrome (RIDS) caused by chemical exposure. *Arch Environ Health* 1998;53:354-358.

16. Miller CS. Are we on the threshold of a new theory of disease? Toxicant-induced loss of tolerance and its relationship in addiction and abdiction. *Toxicol Ind Health* 1999;15:284-294.

17. Ionescu G, Merck M, Bradford R. Simple chemiluminescence assays for free radicals in venous blood and serum samples: results in atopic dermatitis, psoriasis, MCS and cancer patients. *Forsch Komplementarmed* 1999;6:294-300.

18. Levine SA, Parker J. Selenium and human chemical hypersensitivities: preliminary findings. *Int J Biosocial Res* 1982;3:44-47.

19. Levine SA. Oxidants/anti-oxidants and chemical hypersensitivities (Part one). *Int J Biosocial Res* 1983;4:51-54.

20. Levine SA. Oxidants/anti-oxidants and chemical hypersensitivities (Part two). *Int J Biosocial Res* 1983;4:102-105.

21. Kuklinski B, Scheifer R, and Bleyer H. Hirnschrankenprotein S-100 und Xenobiotica-Susceptibilitat. *Umwelt Medizin Gesellschaft* 2003;16:112-120.

22. Corrigan FM, MacDonald S, Brown A, Armstrong K, Armstrong EM. Neurasthenic fatigue, chemical sensitivity and GABA a receptor toxins. *Med Hypoth* 1994;43:195-200.

23. Narahashi T. Neuronal ion channels as the target of insecticides. *Pharmacol Toxicol* 1996;79:1-14.

24. Sunol C, Vale C, Rodriguez-Farre E. Polychlorocycloalkane insecticide action on GABA- and glycine-dependent chloride flux. *Neurotoxicology* 1998;19: 573-580.

25. Adamec R. Modelling anxiety disorders following chemical exposures. *Toxicol Indust Health* 1994;10:391-420.

26. Gupta RC, Milatovic D, Dettbarn WD. Nitric oxide modulates high-energy phosphates in brain regions of rat intoxicated with diisopropylphosphofluoridate or carbofuran: prevention by N-tert-butyl-alpha-phenylnitrone or vitamin E. *Arch Toxicol* 2001;75:346-356.

27. Wu A, Liu Y. Effects of deltamethrin on nitric oxide synthase and poly(ADP-ribose) polymerase in rat brain. *Brain Res* 1999;850:249-252.

28. El-Gohary M, Awara WM, Nassar S, Hawas S. Deltamethin-induced testicular apoptosis in rats: the protective effect of nitric oxide synthase inhibitor. *Toxicology* 1999;132:1-8.

29. Dhouib M, Lugnier A. Induction of nitric oxide synthase by chlorinated pesticides (p,p'-DDT, chlordane, endosulfan) in rat liver. *Cent Eur J Public Health* 1996;4(suppl 48).

30. Bell IR, Baldwin CM, Schwartz GE. Illness from low levels of environmental chemicals: relevance to chronic fatigue syndrome and fibromyalgia. *Am J Med* 1998;105:74S-82S.

31. Bell IR, Miller CS, Schwartz GE. An olfactory-limbic model of multiple chemical sensitivity: possible relationships to kindling and effective spectrum disorders. *Biol Psychiatry* 1992;32:218-242.

32. Bell IR, Schwartz GE, Baldwin CM, Hardin EE. Neural sensitization and physiological markers in multiple chemical sensitivity. *Regul Toxicol Pharmacol* 1996;24:S39-S47.

33. Bell IR, Szarek MJ, Dicensor DR, Baldwin CM, Schwartz GE, Bootzin RR. Patterns of waking EEG spectral power in chemical intolerant individuals during repeated chemical exposures. *Int J Neurosci* 1999;97:41-59.

34. Sorg BA, Bell IR, eds. The role of neural plasticity in chemical intolerance. *Ann NY Acad Sci* Vol 933. New York: The New York Academy of Sciences;2001.

35. Gadea A, Lopez-Colome AM. Glial transporters for glutamate, glycine and GABA I. Glutamate transporters. *J Neurosci Res* 2001;63:456-460.

36. Bliss TM, Ip M, Cheng E, et al. Dual-gene, dual-cell therapy against excitotoxic insult by bolstering neuroenergetics. *J Neurosci* 2004;24:6202-6208.

37. Izquierdo I, Medina JH. Correlation between the pharmacology of long-term potentiation and the pharmacology of memory. *Neurobiol Learn Mem* 1995; 63:19-32.

38. Jerusalinsky D, Kornisiuk E, Izquierdo I. Cholinergic neurotransmission and synaptic plasticity concerning memory processing. *Neurochem Res* 1997;22: 507-515.

39. Ustinova EE, Schultz HD. Activation of cardiac gagal afferents by oxygen-derived free radicals in rats. *Circ Res* 1994;74:895-903.

40. Schultz HD, Ustinova EE. Capsaicin receptors mediate free radical-induced activation of cardiac afferent endings. *Cardiovascular Res* 1998;38:348-355.

41. Cerutti PA. Mechanisms of action of oxidant carcinogens. *Cancer Detect Prev* 1989;14:281-284.

42. Chakraborti T, Ghosh SK, Michael JR, Batabyal SK, Chakraborti S. Targets of oxidative stress in cardiovascular system. *Mol Cell Biochem* 1998;187:1-10.

43. Gopalakrishna R, Jaken S. Protein kinase C signaling and oxidative stress. *Free Radic Biol Med* 2000;28:1349-1361.

44. Vellani V, Mapplebeck S, Morionda A, Davis JB, McNaughton PA. Protein kinase C activation potentiates gating of the vanilloid receptor VR1 by capsaicin, protons, head and anandamide. *J Physiol* 2001;534:813-825.

45. Zhou Y, Li GD, Zhao ZQ. State-dependent phosphorylation of epsilon-isozyme of protein kinase C in adult rat dorsal root ganglia after inflammation and nerve injury. *J Neurochem* 2003;85:571-580.

46. Abou-Donia MB, Goldstein LB, Dechovskaia A, Bullman S, Jones KH, Herrick EA, Abdel-Rahman AA, Khan WA. Effects of daily dermal application of DEET and permethrin alone and in combination, on sensorimotor performance, blood-brain barrier, and blood-testis barrier in rats. *J Toxicol Environ Health* A 2001;62:523-541.

47. Miller C, Mitzel H. Chemical sensitivity attributed to pesticide exposure versus remodeling. *Arch Environ Health* 1995;50:119-129.

48. Rea WJ. *Chemical Sensitivity,* Vol. 1, Boca Raton: Lewis Publishers;1992.

49. Binkley K, King N, Poonai N, Seeman P, Ulpian C, Kennedy J. Idiopathic environmental intolerance: increased prevalence of panic disorder associated cholecy-stokinin B receptor allele 7. *J Allergy Clin Immunol* 2001;107:887-890.

50. Haley RW, Billecke S, La Du BN. Association of the low PON1 type Q (type A) arylesterase activity with neurological symptom complexes in Gulf War veterans. *Toxicol Appl Pharmacol* 1999;157:227-233.

51. McKeown-Eyssen G, Baines C, Cole DE, et al. Case-control study of genotypes in multiple chemical sensitivity: CYP2D6, NAT1, NAT2, PON1, PON2 and MTHFR. *Int J Epidemiol* 2004;33:971-978.

52. Coderre TJ, Melzack R. The role of NMDA receptor-operated calcium channels in persistent nociception after formalin-induced tissue injury. *J Neurosci* 1992; 12:3671-3675.

53. Elliott KJ, Brodsky M, Hynansky AD, Foley KM, Inturrisi CE. Dextromethorphan suppresses both formalin-induced nociceptive behavior and the formalin-induced increase in spinal cord c-fos mRNA. *Pain* 1995;61:401-409.

54. Davis AM, Inturrisi CE. Attenuation of hyperalgesia by LY235959, a competitive N-methyl-D-aspartate receptor antagonist. *Brain Res* 2001;894:150-153.

55. Haxhiu MA, Erokwu B, Dreshaz IA. The role of excitatory amino acids in airway reflex responses in anesthetized dogs. *J Auton Nervous Syst* 1997;67:192-199.

56. Silverman RA, Osborn H, Runge J, et al. IV magnesium sulfate in the treatment of acute severe asthma: a multicenter randomized controlled trial. *Chest* 2002; 122:396-398.

57. Bessmertny O, DiGregorio RV, Cohen H, et al. A randomized clinical trial of nebulized magnesium sulfate in addition to albuterol in the treatment of acute mild-to-moderate asthma exacerbations in adults. *Ann Emerg Med* 2002;39:585-591.

58. Becherel PA, Chosidow O, Le Goff L, et al. Inducible nitric oxide synthase and proinflammatory cytokine expression by human keratinocytes during acute urticaria. *Mol Med* 1997;3:686-694.

59. Bayon Y, Alonso A, Sanchez Crespo M. Immunoglobulin-E/dinitrophenyl complexes induce nitric oxide synthesis in rat peritoneal macrophages by a mechanism involving CD23 and NF-kappa B activation. *Biochem Biophys Res Commun* 242:570-574.

60. van Straaten EA, Koster-Kamphuis L, Bovee-Oudenhoven IM, van der Meer R, Forget PP. Increase urinary nitric oxidation products in children with active coeliac disease. *Acta Paediatr* 1999;88:528-531.

61. Fargeas MJ, Theodorou V, Weirich B, Fioramonte J, Bueno L. Decrease in sensitization rate and intestinal anaphylactic response after nitric oxide synthase inhibition in a food hypersensitivity model. *Gut* 1996;38:598-602.

62. Barau E, Dupont C. Modifications of intestinal permeability during food provocation procedures in pediatric irritable bowel syndrome. *J Pediatr Gastroenterol Nutr* 1990;11:72-77.

63. McKemy DD, Neuhausser WM, Julius D. Identification of a cold receptor reveals a general role for TRP channels in thermosensation. *Nature* 2002;416:52-58.

64. Story GM, Peier AM, Reeve AJ, et al. ANKTM1, a TRP-like channel expressed in nociceptive neurons is activated by cold temperatures. *Cell* 2003;112:819-129.

65. Levallois P, Neutra R, Lee G, Hristova L. Study of self-reported hypersensitivity to electromagnetic fields in California. *Environ Health Perspect* 2002;110 (Suppl 4):619-623.

66. McKay BE, Koren SA, Persinger MA. Behavioral effects of combined perinatal L-NAME and 0.5 Hz magnetic field treatments. *Int J Neurosci* 2003; 113:119-139.

67. Irmak MK, Fadillioglu E, Gulec M, et al. Effects of electromagnetic radiation from cellular telephone on the oxidant and antioxidant levels in rabbits. *Cell Biochem Funct* 2002;20:279-283.

68. Kim SS, Shin HJ, Eom DW, et al. Enhanced expression of neuronal nitric oxide synthase and phospholipase C-γ in regenerating murine neuronal cells by pulsed electromagnetic fields. *Exp Mol Med* 2002;34:53-59.

69. Yoshikawa T, Tanagawa M, Tanigawa T, et al. Enhancement of nitric oxide generation by low frequency electromagnetic field. *Pathophysiology* 2000;7:131-135.

70. Miura M, Takayama K, Okada J. Increase in nitric oxide and cyclic GMP in rat cerebellum by radio frequency burst-type electromagnetic field radiation. *J Physiol* 1993;461:513-524.

71. Graham-Bermann SA, Seng J. Violence exposure and traumatic stress symptoms as additional predictors of health problems in high-risk children. *J Pediatr* 2005;146:349-354.

72. Dobie DJ, Kivliahan DR, Maynard C, et al. Posttraumatic stress disorder in female veterans: association with self-reported health problems and functional impairment. *Arch Intern Med* 2004;164:394-400.

73. Fagan J, Galea S, Ahern J, Bonner S, Vlahov D. Relationship of self-reported asthma severity and urgent health care utilization to psychological sequelae of the September 11, 2001 terrorist attack on the World Trade Center among New York City area residents. *Psychosom Med* 2003;65:993-996.

74. Weisberg RB, Bruce SE, Machan JT, et al. Nonpsychiatric illness among primary care patients with trauma histories and posttraumatic stress disorder. *Psychiatr Serv* 53:848-854.

75. Wamboldt MZ, Weintraub P, Krafchick D, Wamboldt FS. Psychiatric family history in adolescents with severe asthma. *J Am Acad Adolesc Psychiatry* 1996; 35:1042-1049.

76. Massaro AF, Gaston D, Kita C, et al. Expired nitric oxide levels during treatment of acute asthma. *Am J Respir Crit Care Med* 1995;152:800-803.

77. Kharitonov SA, Chung KF, Evans D, O'Connor BJ, Barnes PJ. Increased exhaled nitric oxide in asthma is mainly derived from the lower respiratory tract. *Am J Respir Crit Care Med* 1996;153:1773-1780.

78. Deykin A, Halpern O, Massaro AF, Drazen JM, Israel E. Expired nitric oxide after bronchoprovocation and repeated spirometry in patients with asthma. *Am J Respir Crit Care Med* 1998;157:769-775.

79. Persson MG, Zetterstrom O, Agrenius V, Ihre E, Gustafsson LE. Single–breath nitric oxide measurements in asthmatic patients and smokers. *Lancet* 1994; 343:146-147.

80. Nelson BV, Sears S, Woods J, et al. Expired nitric oxide as a marker for childhood asthma. *J Pediatr* 130:423-427.

81. Arruda LK, Sole D, Baena-Cagnani CE, Naspitz CK. Risk factors for asthma and atopy. *Curr Opin Allergy Clin Immunol* 2005;5:153-159.

82. Mapp CE. Genetics and the occupational environment. *Curr Opin Allergy Clin Immunol* 2005;5:113-118.

83. Hynes HP, Brugge D, Osgood ND, et al. Investigations into the indoor environment and respiratory health in Boston public housing. *Rev Environ Health* 2004; 19:271-289.

84. Arshad SH, Kurukulaaratchy RJ, Fenn M, Matthews S. Early life risk factors for current wheeze, asthma and bronchial hyperresponsiveness at 10 years of age. *Chest* 2005;127:502-508.

85. Sutherland ER, Brandorff JM, Martin RJ. Atypical bacterial pneumonia and asthma risk. *J Asthma* 2004;41:863-868.

86. Millqvist E, Bengtsson U, Lowhagen O. Provocations with perfume in the eyes induce airway symptoms in patients with sensory hyperreactivity. *Allergy* 1999; 54:495-499.

87. Pall ML. Levels of nitric oxide synthase product citrulline are elevated in sera of chronic fatigue syndrome patients. *J Chronic Fatigue Syndr* 2002;10(3/4): 37-41.

88. Kimata H. Effect of exposure to volatile organic compounds on plasma levels of neuropeptides, nerve growth factor and histamine in patients with self-reported multiple chemical sensitivity. *In J Hyg Environ Health* 2004;207:159-163.

89. Millqvist E, Ternesten-Hasseus E, Stahl A, Bende M. Changes in levels of nerve growth factor in nasal secretions after capsaicin inhalation in patients with airway symptoms from scents and chemicals. *Environ Health Perspect* 2005;113: 849-852.

90. Shinohara N, Mizukoshi A, Yanagisawa Y. Indentification of responsible volatile chemicals that induce hypersensitive reactions to multiple chemical sensitivity patients. *J Expo Anal Environ Epidemiol* 2004;14:84-91.

91. Joffres MR, Sampalli T, Fox RA. Physiologic and symptomatic responses to low-level substances in individuals with and without chemical sensitivities: a randomized controlled blinded pilot booth study. *Environ Health Perspect* 2005;113: 1178-1183.

Chapter 8

1. Wolfe D. Fibromyalgia. *Rheum Dis Clin North Am* 1990;16:681-698.

2. Leventhal LJ, Naides SJ, Freundlich B. Fibromyalgia and parvovirus infection. *Arthritis Rheum* 1991;34:1319-1324.

3. Bujak DI, Weinstein A, Dornbush RL. Clinical and neurocognitive features of the post Lyme syndrome. *J Rheumatol* 1996;23:1392-1397.

4. Buskila D, Shnaider A, Neumann L, et al. Fibromyalgia in hepatitis C infection. Another infectious disease relationship. *Arch Intern Med* 1997;157:2497-2500.

5. Laine M, Luukkainen R, Jalava J, et al. Prolonged arthritis associated with sindbis-related (Pogosta) virus infection. *Rheumatol* 2000;39:1272-1274.

6. Massarotti EM. Lyme arthritis. *Med Clin North Am* 2002;86:297-309.

7. Daoud KF, Barkhuizen A. *Curr Pain Headache Rep* 2002;6:284-288.

8. Waylonis GW, Perkins RH. Post-traumatic fibromyalgia. A long-term follow-up. *Am J Phys Med Rehabil* 1994;73:403-412.

9. Buskila D, Neumann L, Vaisberg G, Alakalay D, Wolfe F. Increased rates of fibromylagia following cervical spine injury. A controlled study of 161 cases of traumatic injury. *Arthritis Rheum* 1997;40:446-452.

10. Greenfield S, Fitzcharles MA, Esdaile JM. Reactive fibromylagia syndrome. *Arthritis Rheum* 1992;35:678-681.

11. Aaron LA, Bradley LA, Alacon GS, Triana Alexander M, Alexander RW, Martin MY, 12. Alberts KR. Perceived physical and emotional trauma as precipitating events in fibromyalgia. Associations with health care seeking and disability status but not pain severity. *Arthritis Rheum* 1997;40:453-460.

13. Al-Allaf AW, Dunbar KL, Hallum NS, et al. A case-control study examining the role of physical trauma in the onset of fibromyalgia syndrome. *Rheumatology* 2002;41:450-453.

14. Gebhard F, Nussler AK, Rosch M, Pfetsch H, Kinzl L, Bruckner UB. Early posttraumatic increase in the production of nitric oxide in humans. *Shock* 1998; 10:237-242.

15. Schwentker A, Billiar TR. Nitric oxide and wound repair. *Surg Clin North Am* 2003;83:521-530.

16. Prasad D. Dhillon MS, Khullar M, Nagi ON. Evaluation of oxidative stress after fractures. A preliminary study. *Acta Oethop Belg* 2003;69:546-551.

17. Sun GB, Huang ZH, Sun YG, Yang WY. Intervention with nitric oxide synthase inhibitors for traumatic shock in rats. *Di Yi Jun Yi Da Xue Xue Bao* 2003; 23:306-309.

18. Feng HM, Huang ZH, Huang XL, et al. Dynamic changes in serum level of nitric oxide and its mechanism in rats with traumatic shock. *Di Yi Jun Yi Da Xue Xue Bao* 2002;22:891-894.

19. Wallis RA, Panizzon KL, Girard JM. Traumatic neuroprotection with inhibitors of nitric oxide and ADP-ribosylation. *Brain Res* 1996;710:169-177.

20. Stoll G, Jander S, Schroeter M. Detrimental and beneficial effects of injury-induced inflammation and cytokine expression in the nervous system. *Adv Exp Med Biol* 2002;513:87-113.

21. Wada K, Chatzipanteli K, Busto R, Dietrich WD. Role of nitric oxide in traumatic brain injury in the rat. *J Neurosurg* 1998;89:807-818.

22. Lewen A, Matz P, Chan PH. Free radical pathways in CNS injury. *J Neurotrauma* 2000;17:871-890.

23. Khaldi A, Chiueh CC, Bullock MR, Woodward JJ. The signficance of nitric oxide production in the brain after injury. *Ann NY Acad Sci* 2002;962:53-59.

24. Obrenovitch TP, Urenjak J. Is extracellular glutamate the key to excitotoxicity after brain injury? *J Neurotrauma* 1997;14:677-698.

25. Alexander RW, Bradley LA, Alarcon GS, et al. Sexual and physical abuse in women with fibromyalgia: association with outpatient health care utilization and pain medication usage. *Arth Care Res* 1998;11:102-115.

26. Anderberg UM, Marteinsdottir I, Theorell T, et al. The impact of life events in female patient with fibromyalgia and femaled health controls. *Eur Psychiatry* 2000;15:295-301.

27. Goldberg RT, Pachas WN, Keith D, et al. Relationship between traumatic events in childhood and chronic pain. *Disability Rehab* 1999;21:23-30.

28. Walker EA, Keegan D, Gardner G, et al. Psychosocial factors in fibromyalgia compared with rheumatoid arthritis: II. Sexual, physical and emotional abuse and neglect. *Psychosom Med* 1997;59:572-577.

29. Winfield JB. Psychological determinants of fibromyalgia and related syndromes. *Curr Rev Pain* 2000;4:276-286.

30. Hench PK, Mitler MM. Fibromyalgia 1. Review of a common rheumatologic syndrome. *Postgrad Med* 1986;80:47-56.

31. Grafe A, Wollina U Tebbe B, et al. Fibromyalgia in lupus erythematosus. *Acta Derm Venereol* 1999;79:62-64.

32. Eisinger J, Gandolfo C, Zakarian H, Ayavou T. Reactive oxygen species, antioxidant status and fibromyalgia. *J Musculoskeletal Pain* 1997;5(4):5-15.

33. Eisinger J, Zakarian H, Pouly F, Plantamura A, Ayavou T. Protein peroxidation, magnesium deficiency and fibromyalgia. *Magnes Res* 1996;9:313-316.

34. Ayavou T. Statut anti-oxydant et fibromyalgia. *Lyon Med Med* 36:12-13.

35. Hein G, Franke S. Are advanced glycation end-product-modified proteins of pathogenic importance in fibromyalgia? *Rheumatology* 2002;41:1163-1167.

36. Eisinger J, Ayavou T, Plantamura A, Lawson K, Danneskold-Samsoe B. Lipid and protein peroxidations in fibromyalgia. *Myalgies Int* 2002;3:37-42.

37. Bagis S, Tamer L, Sahin G, et al. Free radicals and antioxidants in primary fibromyalgia: an oxidative stress disorder? *Rheumatol Int* 2005;25:188-190.

38. Ali M. Respiratory-to-fermentative (RTF) shift in ATP production in chronic energy deficit states. *Townsend Lett Doctors Patients* 2004;Aug/Sept:64-65.

39. Ali M. Fibromyalgia: an oxidative-dysoxygenative disorder (ODD). *J Integrative Med* 1999;3:17-37.

40. Klein R, Berg PA. High incidence of antibodies to 5-hydroxytryptamine, gangliosides and phospholipids in patients with chronic fatigue syndrome and fibromyalgia syndrome and their relatives: evidence for a clinical entity of both disorders. *Eur J Med Res* 1995;1:21-26.

41. Bramwell B, Ferguson S, Scarlett N, Macintosh A. The use of ascorbigen in the treatment of fibromyalgia patients: a preliminary trial. *Alt Medical Revs* 2000; 5:455-462.

42. Merchant RE, Carmack CA, Wise CM. Nutritional supplementation with Chlorella pyrenoidosa for patients with fibromyalgia syndrome A: a pilot study. *Phytotherapy Res* 2000;14:167-173.

43. Edwards AM, Blackburn L, Christie S, et al. Food supplements in the treatment of primary fibromyalgia: a double-blind crossover trial of anthocyanidins and placebo. *J Nutr Environ Med* 2000;10:189-199.

44. Lister RE. An open, pilot study to evaluate the potential benefits of coenzyme Q10 combined with Ginkgo biloba extract in fibromyalgia syndrome. *J Int Med Res* 2002;30:195-199.

45. Wallace D, Linker-Israeli, Hallegua D, et al. Cytokines plan an aetiopathogenetic role in fibromyalgia–a hypothesis and a pilot study. *Rheumatology* 2001; 40:743-749.

46. Patarca-Montero R. *The Concise Encyclopedia of Fibromyalgia and Myofascial Pain.* Binghamton, NY: Haworth Medical Press;2002.

47. Thompson ME, Barkhuizen A. Fibromyalgia, hepatitis C infection and the cytokine connection. *Curr Pain Headache Rep* 2003;7:342-347.

48. Gur A, Karakoc M, Nas, K, et al. Cytokines and depression in cases with fibromyalgia. *J Rheumatol* 2002;29:358-361.

49. Gur A, Karakoc M, Erdogan S, Nas K, Cevik R, Sarac AJ. Regional cerebral blood flow and cytokines in young females with fibromyalgia. *Clin Exp Rheumatol* 2002;20:753-760.

50. Salemi S, Rethage J, Wollina U, et al. Detection of interleukin 1β (IL-1β), IL-6, and tumor necrosis factor-alpha in skin of patients with fibromyalgia. *J Rheumatol* 2003;30:146-150.

51. Larson AA, Giovengo SL, Russell IJ, Michalek JE. *Pain* 2000;87:201-211.

52. Bradley LA, Weigent DA, Sotolongo A, et al. Blood serum levels on nitric oxide (NO) are elevated in women with fibromyalgia (FM): possible contributions to central and peripheral sensitization. *Arthritis Rheum* 2000;43(Suppl 9):S173.

53. Helme RD, Littlejohn GO, Weinstein C. Neurogenic flare responses in chronic rheumatic pain syndromes. *Clin Exp Neurol* 1987;23:91-94.

54. Morris V, Cruwys S, Kidd B. Increased capsaicin-induced secondary hyperalgesia as a marker of abnormal sensory activity in patients with fibromyalgia. *Neurosci Lett* 1998;250:205-207.

55. Staud R, Smitherman ML. Peripheral and central sensitization in fibromyalgia: pathogenetic role. *Curr Pain Headache Rep* 2002;6:259-266.

56. Sorensen J, Bengtsson A, Backman E, et al. Pain analysis in patients with fibromyalgia. Effects of intravenous morphine, lidocaine and ketamine. *Scand J Rheumatol* 1995;24:360-365.

57. Bennett R. Fibromyalgia, chronic fatigue syndrome and myofascial pain. *Curr Opin Rheumatol* 1998;2:95-103.

58. Nicolodi M, Volpe AR, Sicuderi F. Fibromyalgia and headache: failure of serotonergic analgesia and N-methyl-D-aspartate-mediated neuronal plasticity: their common clues. *Cephalalgia* 1998;18(Suppl 21):41-44.

59. Graven-Nielsen T, Aspergren Kendall S, Hensiksson KG, et al. Ketamine reduces muscle pain, temporal summation, and referred pain in fibromyalgia patients. *Pain* 2000;85:483-491.

60. Stoll AL. Fibromyalgia symptoms relieved by flupirtine: an open label case series. *Psychosomatics* 2000;41:371-372.

61. Buskila D. Fibromyalgia, chronic fatigue syndrome and myofascial pain syndrome. *Curr Opin Rheumatol* 2001;13:117-127.

62. Henriksson KG, Sorensen J. The promise of N-methyl-D-aspartate receptor antagonists in fibromyalgia. *Rheum Dis Clin North Am* 2002;28:343-351.

63. Hocking G, Cousins MJ. Ketamine in chronic pain management: an evidence-based review. *Anesth Analg* 2003;97:1730-1739.

64. Staud SR, Vierck CJ, Robinson ME, Price DD. Effects of the N-methyl-D-aspartate receptors antagonist dextromethorphan on temporal summation of pain are similar in fibromyalgia patients and normal control subjects. *J Pain* 2005;6:323-332.

65. Peres MF, Zukerman E, Senne Soares CA, et al. Cerebrospinal fluid glutamate levels in chronic migraine. *Cephalalgia* 2004;24:735-739.

66. Smith JD, Terpening CM, Schmidt SOF, Gums JG. Relief of fibromyalgia symptoms following discontinuation of dietary excitotoxins. *Ann Pharmacother* 2001;35:702-706.

67. Lidbeck J. Central hyperexcitability in chronic musculoskeletal pain: a conceptual breakthrough. *Pain Res Manag* 2002;7:81-92.

68. Clauw DJ, Crofford LJ. Chronic widespread pain and fibromyalgia: what we know, and what we need to know. *Best Pract Res Clin Rheumatol* 2003;17:685-701.

69. Desmeules JA, Cedraschi C, Rapiti E, et al. Neurophysiologic evidence for a central sensitization in patients with fibromyalgia. *Arthritis Rheum* 2003;48: 1420-1429.

70. Staud R. Evidence of involvement of central neural mechanisms in generating fibromyalgia pain. *Curr Rheumatol Rep* 2002;4:299-305.

71. Bradley LA, McKendree-Smith NL, Alarcon GS, Cianfrini LR. Is fibromyalgia a neurologic disease? *Curr Pain Headache Rep* 2002;6:106-114.

72. Staud R, Price DD, Robinson ME, Mauderli AP, Vierck CJ. Maintenance of windup of second pain requires less frequent stimulation in fibromyalgia patients compared with normal controls. *Pain* 2004;110:689-696.

73. Yunus MB. Central sensitivity syndromes: a unified concept for fibromyalgia and other similar maladies. *Fibromyalgia Frontiers* 2001;9(3):3-8.

74. Larson AA, Kovacs KJ. Nociceptive aspects of fibromyalgia. *Curr Pain Headache Rep* 2001;5:338-346.

75. Henriksson KG. Hypersensitivity in muscle pain syndromes. *Curr Pain Headache Rep* 2003;7:426-432.

76. Staud R. Evidence of involvement of central neural mechanisms in generating fibromyalgia pain. *Current Science* 2004;4:299-305.

77. Markenson JA. Mechanisms of chronic pain. *Am J Med* 1996;101:6S-18S.

78. Simone DA, Zhang X, Li J, et al. Comparison of responses of primate spinothalamic tract neurons to pruritic and algogenic stimuli. *J Neurophys* 2004;91: 213-222.

79. Mantyh PW, Hunt SP. Setting the tone: superficial dorsal horn projection neurons regulate pain sensitivity. *Trends Neurosci* 2004;27:582-584.

80. Saab CY, Park YC, Al-Chaer ED. Thalamic modulation of visceral nociceptive processing in adult rats with neonatal colon irritation. *Brain Res* 2004;1008: 186-192.

81. Gauriau C, Bernard JF. A comparative reappraisal of projections from the superficial luminae of the dorsal horn of the rat: the forebrain. *J Comp Neurol* 2004; 468:24-56.

82. Julien N, Goffaux P, Arsenault P, Marchand S. Widespread pain in fibromyalgia is related to a deficit in endogenous pain inhibition. *Pain* 2005; 114:295-302.

83. Mountz JM, Bradley LA, Modell JG, et al. Fibromyagia in women. Abnormalities in regional cerebral blood flow in the thalamus and the caudate nucleus are associated with low pain threshold levels. *Arthritis Rheum* 38:926-938.

84. Wik G, Fischer H, Bragee B, Finer B, Fredrikson M. Functional anatomy of hypnotic analgesia: a PET study of patients with fibromyalgia. *Eur J Pain* 1999;3:7-12.

85. Lekander M, Fredrikson M, Wik G. Neuroimmune relations in patients with fibromyalgia: a positron emission tomography study. *Neurosci Lett* 2000;282: 193-196.

86. Kwiatek R, Barnden L, Tedman R, et al. Regional cerebral blood flow in fibromyalgia: a single-photon-emission computed tomography evidence of reduction in the pontine tegmentum and thalami. *Arthritis Rheum* 2000;43:2823-2833.

87. Anon. *A possible cause of fibromyalgia.* Special Update Edition, The American Fibromyalgia Syndrome Association, Inc;2003:14-18.

88. Zhou M. Canadian Association of Neuroscience review: Cellular and synaptic insights into physiological and pathological pain. *Can J Neurol Sci* 2005;32:27-36.

89. Goettl VM, Huang Y, Hackshaw KV, Stephens RL Jr. Reduced basal release of serotonin from the basolateral thalamus of the rat in a model of neuropathic pain. *Pain* 2002;99:359-366.

90. Bondy B, Spaeth M, Offenbaecher M, et al. The T102C polymorphism of the 5-HT2A-receptor gene in fibromyalgia. *Neurobiol Dis* 1999;6:433-439.

91. Cohen H, Buskila D, Neumann L, Ebstein RP. Confirmation of an association between fibromyalgia and serotonin transporter promoter region (5-HTTLPR) polymorphism, and relationship to anxiety-related personality traits. *Arthritis Rheum* 2002;46:845-847.

92. Neeck G. Neuroendocrine and hormonal perturbations and relations to the serotonergic system in fibromyalgia. *Scand J Rheumatol Suppl* 2000;113:8-12.

93. Miller LJ, Kubes KL. Serotonergic agents in the treatment of fibromyalgia syndrome. *Ann Pharmacother* 2002;36:707-712.

94. Palkar AA, Bilal L, Masand PS. Management of fibromyalgia. *Curr Psychiatry Rep* 2003;5:218-224.

95. Spath M, Stratz T, Farber L, Haus U, Pongratz D. Treatment with fibromyalgia with tropisetron—dose and efficacy correlations. *Scand J Rheumatol Suppl* 2004;119:63-66.

96. Cook DB, Lange G, Ciccone DS, et al. Functional imaging of pain in patients with primary fibromyalgia. *J Rheumatol* 2004;31:364-378.

97. Chang L, Berman S, Mayer EA, et al. Brain responses to visceral and somatic stimuli in patients with irritable bowel syndrome with and without fibromyalgia. *Am J Gastroenterol* 2003;98:1354-1361.

98. Gracely RH, Geisser ME, Giesecke T, et al. Pain catastrophizing and neural responses to pain among persons with fibromyalgia. *Brain* 2004;127:835-843.

Chapter 9

1. American Psychiatric Association, *Diagnostic and Statistical Manual of Mental Disorders.* 4th ed. DSM-IV, Washington, DC: American Psychiatric Press;1994. Reprinted with permission from APA.

2. Miller CS. Are we on the threshold of a new theory of disease? Toxicant-induced loss of tolerance and its relationship in addiction and abdiction. *Toxicol Ind Health* 1999;15:284-294.

3. Lipschitz EL Chronic fatigue syndrome and posttraumatic stress disorder. *JAMA* 2001;286:916-917.

4. Cohen H, Neumann L, Haiman Y, Matar MA, Press J, Buskila D. Prevalence of post-traumatic stress disorder in fibromyalgia patients: overlapping syndromes of post-traumatic fibromyalgia syndrome? *Semin Arthritis Rheum* 2002;32:38-50.

5. Friedman MJ. Neurobiological sensitization models of post-traumatic stress disorder: their possible relevance to multiple chemical sensitivity syndrome. *Toxicol Ind Health* 1994;10:449-462.

6. Gould E, Cameron HA. Early NMDA blockade impairs defensive behavior and increases cell proliferation in the dentate gyrus of developing rats. *Behav Neurosci* 1997;111:49-56.

7. Adamec RE, Burton P, Shallow T, Budgell J. Unilateral block of NMDA receptors in the amygdala prevents predator-induced lasting increases in anxiety-like behavior and unconditioned startle-effective hemisphere depends on behavior. *Physiol Behav* 1999;65:739-751.

8. Shors TJ, Elkabes S, Selcher JC, Black IB. Stress persistently increases NMDA receptor-mediated binding of (3H)PDBu (a marker for protein kinase C) in the amygdala and re-exposure to the stressful context reactivates the increase. *Brain Res* 1997;750:293-300.

9. Miserendino MJ, Sananes CB, Melia KR, Davis M. Blocking of acquisition but not expression of conditioned fear-potentiated startle by NMDA antagonists in the amygdala. *Nature* 1990;345:716-718.

10. Goldstein LE, Rasmusson AM, Bunney BS, Roth RH. The NMDA glycine site antagonist (+)-HA-966 selectively regulates conditioned stress-induced metabolic activation of the mesoprefrontal cortical dopamine but not serotonin systems: a behavioral, neuroendocrine, and neurochemical study in the rat. *J Neurosci* 1994; 14:4937-4950.

11. Charney DS, Deutch AY, Krystal JH, Southwick SM, Davis M. Psychobiology mechanisms in posttraumatic stress disorder. *Arch Gen Psychiatry* 1993;50: 294-302.

12. Chambers RA, Bremner JD, Mogahaddam B, Southwick SM, Charney DS, Krystal JH. Glutamate and post-traumatic stress disorder: toward a psychobiology of dissociation. *Semin Clin Neuropsychiatry* 1999;4:274-281.

13. Antelman SM, Yehuda R. Time-dependent change following acute stress: Relevance to the chronic and delayed aspects of PTSD. In: Murburg MM, ed. *Catecholamine Function in Post-Traumatic Stress Disorder: Emerging Concepts.* Washington, DC: American Psychiatric Press;1994:87-98.

14. Post RM, Weiss SR, Smith M, Li H, McCann U. Kindling vs quenching: Implications for the evolution and treatment of posttraumatic stress disorder. *Ann NY Acad Sci* 1997;821:285-295.

15. Hageman I, Andersen HS, Jorgensen MB. Post-traumatic stress disorder: a review of psychobiology and pharmacotherapy. *Acta Psychiatr Scand* 2001;104: 411-422.

16. Heresco Levy U, Javitt DC. The role of N-methyl-D-aspartate (NMDA) receptor-mediated neurotransmission in the pathophysiology and therapeutics of psychiatric syndromes. *Eur Neuropsychophamacol* 1998;8:141-152.

17. McEwen BS. Possible mechanisms for atrophy in the human hippocampus. *Mol Psychiatr* 1997;2:255-262.

18. Bremner JD. Does stress damage the brain? *Biol Psychiatr* 1999;45:797-805.

19. Birmes P, Senard JM, Escande M, Schmitt L. Facteurs biologiques du stress post-traumatique: neurotransmission et neuromodulation. *Encephale* 2002; 28:241-247.

20. McEwen B. Re-examination of the glucocorticoid hypothesis of stress and aging. *Prog Brain Res* 1992;93:365-378.

21. Sapolsky R. Stress, glucocorticoids and damage to the nervous system. The current state of confusion. *Stress* 1996;1:1-16.

22. Bremner J. Does stress damage the brain? *Biol Psychiatry* 1999;45:797-804.

23. Strijbos PJ, Relton JK, Rothwell NJ. Corticotrophin-releasing factor antagonist inhibits neuronal damage induced by focal ischaemia or activation of NMDA receptors. *Brain Res* 1994;656:405-408.

24. McEwen BS. Possible mechanisms for atrophy of the human hippocampus. *Mol Psychiatry* 1997;2:255-262.

25. Coussens CM, Kerr DS, Abraham WC. Glucocorticoid receptor activation lowers the threshold for NMDA-receptor-dependent homosynaptic long-term depression in the hippocampus through activation of voltage-dependent calcium channels. *J Neurophysiol* 1997;78:2685-2696.

26. Brook SM, Howard SA, Sapolsky RM. Energy dependency of glucocorticoid exacerbation of gp120 neurotoxicity. *J Neurochem* 1998;71:1187-1193.

27. Hergovich N, Singer E, Agneter E, et al. Comparison of the effects of ketamine and memantine on prolactin and cortisol release in men, a randomized, double-blind, placebo-controlled trial. *Neuropsychopharmacology* 2001;24:590-593.

28. Takahashi T, Kimoto T, Tanabe N, Hattori TA, Yasumatsu N, Kawato S. Corticosterone acutely prolonged N-methyl-D-aspartate receptor-mediated Ca^{2+} elevation in cultured rat hippocampal neurons. *J Neurochem* 2002;83:1441-1451.

29. McEwen BS, Magarinos AM. Stress effects on morphology and function of the hippocampus. *Ann NY Acad Sci* 1997;821:271-284.

30. Howard SA, Nakayam AY, Brooke SM, Sapolsky RM. Glucocorticoid modulation of gp120-induced effects on calcium-dependent degenerative events in primary hippocampal and cortical cultures. *Exp Neurol* 1999;158164-170.

31. Harvey AG, Brewin CR, Jones C, Kopelman MD. Coexistence of posttraumatic stress disorder and traumatic brain injury: towards a resolution of the paradox. *J Int Neuropsychological Soc* 2003;9:663-676.

32. Heresco-Levy U, Kremer I, Javitt DC, et al. Pilot-controlled trial of D-cycloserine for the treatment of post-traumatic stress disorder. *Int J Neuropsychopharmacol* 2002;5:301-307.

33. Malek-Ahmadi P. Gabapentin and posttraumatic stress disorder. *Ann Pharmacother* 2003;37:664-666.

34. Zullino DF, Krenz S, Besson J. AMPA blockade may be the mechanism underlying the efficacy of topiramate in PTSD. *J Clin Psychiatry* 2002;64:219-220.

35. Laudanno OM, Cesolari JA, San Miguel P, Bedini OA. Role of inducible nitric oxide synthase in acute gastric mucosal damage in stress, in rats. *Acta Gastroenterol Latinoam* 1996;26:221-224.

36. Martinez-Agustin O, de Medina F. Effect of psychogenic stress on gastrointestinal function. *J Physiol Biochem* 2000;56:259-273.

37. Alptekin N, Seckin S, Dogru Abbasoglu S, et al. Lipid peroxides, glutathione, γ-glutamylocysteine synthetase and γ-glutamyltranspeptidase activities in several tissues of rats following water-immersion stress. *Pharmacol Res* 1996;34:167-169.

38. Seckin S, Alptekin N, Dogru Abbasoglu S, et al. The effect of chronic stress on hepatic and gastric peroxidation in long-term depletion of glutathione in rats. *Pharmacol Res* 1997;36:55-57.

39. Harvey BH, Oosthuizen F, Brand L, Wegener G, Stein DJ. Stress-restress evokes sustained iNOS activity and altered GABA levels and NMDA receptors in rat hippocampus. *Psychopharmacology* 2004;175:494-502.

40. Oosthuizen F, Wegener G, Harvey BH. Role of nitric oxide as inflammatory mediator in post-traumatic stress disorder (PTSD): evidence from an animal model. *Neuropsychiatric Dis Treat* 2005;1:109-124.

41. Harvey BH, Bothma T, Nel A, Wegener G, Stein DJ. Involvement of the NMDA receptor, NO-cyclic GMP and nuclear factor K-β in an animal model of repeated trauma. *Hum Psychopharacol Clin Exp* 2005;20:367-373.

42. Packer MA, Stasiv Y, Benraiss A, et al. Nitric oxide negatively regulates mammalian adult neurogenesis. *Proc Natl Acad Sci USA* 2003;100:9566-9571.

43. Cheng A, Wang S, Cai J, Rao MS, Mattson MP. Nitric oxide acts in a positive feedback loop with BDNF to regulate neural progenitor cell proliferation and differentiation in the mammalian brain. *Dev Biol* 2003;258:319-333.

44. Gibbs SM. Regulation of neuronal proliferation and differentiation by nitric oxide. *Mol Neurobiol* 2003;27:107-120.

45. Cameron HA, McEwen BS, Gould E. Regulation of adult neurogenesis by excitatory input and NMDA receptor activation in the dentate gyrus. *J Neurosci* 1995;15:4687-4692.

46. Gould E, McEwen BS, Tanapat P, Galea LA, Fuchs E. Neurogenesis in the dentate gyrus of the adult tree shrew is regulated by psychosocial stress and NMDA receptor activation. *J Neurosci* 1997;17:2492-2498.

47. McEwen B. Re-examination of the glucocorticoid hypothesis of stress and aging. *Prog Brain Res* 1992;93:365-378.

48. Sapolsky R. Stress, glucocorticoids and damage to the nervous system. The current state of confusion. *Stress* 1996;1:1-16.

49. Bremner J. Does stress damage the brain? *Biol Psychiatry* 1999;45:797-804.

50. Sapolsky RM. Glucocorticoids and hippocampal atrophy in neuropsychiatric disorders. *Arch Gen Psychiatry* 2000;57:925-935.

51. Gilbertson MW, Shenton MF, Ciszewski A, et al. Smaller hippocampal volume predicts pathologic vulnerability to psychological trauma. *Nat Neurosci* 2002; 5:1242-1247.

52. Miserendino MJ, Sananes CB, Melia KR, Davis M. Blocking of acquisition but not expression of conditioned fear-potentiated startle by NMDA antagonists in the amygdala. *Nature* 1990;345:716-718.

53. Falls WA, Miserendino MJ, Davis M. Extinction of fear-potentiated startle: blockade by infusion of an NMDA antagonist into the amygdala. *J Neurosci* 1992; 12:854-863.

54. Bell IR, Miller CS, Schwartz GE, Peterson JM, Amend D. Neuropsychiatric and somatic characteristics of young adults with and without self-reported chemical odor intolerance and chemical sensitivity. *Arch Environ Health* 1996;51:9-21.

55. Sherman JJ, Turk DC, Okifuji A. Prevalence and impact of posttraumatic stress disorder-like symptoms on patients with fibromyalgia. *Clin J Pain* 2000;16: 127-134.

56. Bremer JD. Hypotheses and controversies related to effects of stress on the hippocampus: an argument for stress-induced damage to the hippocampus in patients with posttraumatic stress disorder. *Hippocampus* 2001;11:75-81.

57. Shin LM, Shin PS, Heckers S, et al. Hippocampal function in posttraumatic stress disorder. *Hippocampus* 2004;14:292-300.

58. Friedman A. Pyridostigmine brain penetration under stress enhances neuronal excitability and induces early immediate transcriptional response. *Nat Med* 1996;2:1382-1385.

59. Hanin I. The Gulf War, stress, and a leaky blood-brain barrier. *Nat Med* 1996; 2:1307-1308.

60. Pavolvsky L, Browne RO, Friedman A. Pyridostigmine enhances glutamatergic transmission in hippocampal CA1 neurons. *Expt Neurol* 2003;179:181-187.

61. Abdel-Rahman A, Shetty AK, Abou-Donia MB. Disruption of the blood-brain barrier and neuronal death in cingulated cortex, dentate gyrus, thalamus and hypothalamus in a rat model of Gulf-War syndrome. *Neurobiol Dis* 2002;10: 306-326.

62. Abdel-Rahman A, Abou-Donia SM, El-Masry EM, et al. Stress and combined exposure to low doses of pyridostigmine bromide, DEET and permethrin produce neurochemical and neuropathological alterations in cerebral cortex, hippocampus and cerebellum. *J Toxicol Env Health* 2004;676:163-192.

63. Song X, Tian HL, Bressler J, et al. Acute and repeated restraint have little effect on pyridostigmine toxicity or brain regional cholinesterase inhibition in rats. *Toxicol Sci* 2002;69:157-164.

64. Pall ML. NMDA sensitization and stimulation by peroxynitrite, nitric oxide and organic. *FASEB J* 2002;16:1407-1417.

65. Sapolsky RM. Stress and plasticity in the limbic system. *Neurochem Res* 2003;28:1735-1742.

66. McEwen BS. Plasticity of the hippocampus: adaptation to chronic stress and allostatic load. *Ann NY Acad Sci* 2001;933:265-277.

Chapter 10

1. The Iowa Persian Gulf Study Group. Self-reported illness and health status among Gulf War veterans—a population-based study. *JAMA* 1997;227:238-245.

2. Kipen HM, Hallman W, Kang H, Fiedler N, Natelson BH. Prevalence of chronic fatigue and chemical sensitivities in Gulf Registry Veterans. *Arch Environm Health* 1999;54:313-318.

3. Pollet C, Natelson BH, Lange G, et al. Medical evaluation of Persian Gulf veterans with fatigue and/or chemical sensitivity. *J Med* 1998;29:101-113.

4. Nicolson GL, Nicolson NL. Gulf War illnesses: complex medical, scientific paradox. *Med Confl Surviv* 1998;14:156-165.

5. Hodgson MJ, Kipen HM. Gulf War illnesses: causation and treatment. *J Occup Environ Med* 1999;41:443-452.

6. Baker DG, Mendenhall CL, Simbartl LA, Magan LK, Steinberg JL. Relationship between posttraumatic stress disorder and self-reported physical symptoms in Persian Gulf War veterans. *Arch Intern Med* 1997;157:2076-2078.

7. [no authors listed] Multiple chemical sensitivity: a consensus. *Arch Environ Health* 1999;54:147-149.

8. Kang HK, Mahan CM, Lee KY, Magee CA, Murphy FM. Illnesses among United States veterans of the Gulf War: a population-based survey of 30,000 veterans. *J Occup Environ Med* 2000;42:491-501.

9. Kang HK, Mahan CM, Lee KY, et al. Evidence for deployment-related Gulf War syndrome by factor analysis. *Arch Environ Health* 2002;57:61-68.

10. Steele L. Prevalence and patterns of Gulf War illness in Kansas veterans: associations of symptoms with characteristics of person, place and time of military service. *Am J Epidemiol* 2000;152:992-1002.

11. Proctor SP, Heaton KJ, White RF, Wolfe J. Chemical sensitivity and chronic fatigue in Gulf War veterans: a brief report. *J Occup Environ Med* 2001;43:259-264.

12. Reid S, Hotopf M, Hull L, et al. Multiple chemical sensitivity and chronic fatigue syndrome in British Gulf War veterans. *Am J Epidemiol* 2001;153:604-609.

13. Peckerman A, Dahl K, Chemitiganti R, et al. Effects of posttraumatic stress disorder on cardiovascular stress responses in Gulf War veterans with fatiguing illness. *Auton Neurosci* 2003;108:63-72.

14. Cook DB, Nagelkirk PR, Peckerman A, et al. Perceived exertion in fatiguing illness: Gulf War veterans with chronic fatigue syndrome. *Med Sci Sports Exerc* 2003;35:569-574.

15. McCauley LA, Joos SK, Barkhuzen A, et al. Chronic fatigue in a population–based study of Gulf War veterans. *Arch Environ Health* 2002;57:340-348.

16. Kang HK, Natelson BH, Mahan CM, Lee KY, Murphy FM. Post-traumatic stress disorder and chronic fatigue syndrome-like illness among Gulf War veterans: a population-based survey of 30,000 veterans. *Am J Epidemiol* 2003;157: 141-148.

17. Gray GC, Reed RJ, Kaiser KS, Smith TC, Gastanaga VM. Self-reported symptoms and medical conditions among 11,868 Gulf War-era veterans: the Seabee Health Study. *Am J Epidemiol* 2000;152:992-1002.

18. Eisen SA, Kang HK, Murphy FM, et al. Gulf War veterans' health: medical evaluation of a U.S. cohort. *Ann Intern Med* 2005;142:881-890.

19. Pall ML. Common etiology of posttraumatic stress disorder, fibromyalgia, chronic fatigue syndrome and multiple chemical sensitivity via elevated nitric oxide/peroxynitrite. *Med Hypoth* 2001;57:139-145.

20. Cowan DN, Lange JL, Heller J, Kirkpatrick J, DeBakey S. A case-controlled study of asthma among U.S. Army Gulf War veterans and modeled exposure to oil well fire smoke. *Mil Med* 2002;167:777-782.

21. Lange JL, Schwartz DA, Doebbeling BN, Heller JM, Thorne PS. Exposures to the Kuwait oil fires and their association with asthma and bronchitis among gulf war veterans. *Environ Health Perspect* 2002;110:1141-1146.

22. Unwin C, Blatchley N, Coker W, et al. Health of UK servicemen who served in Persian Gulf War. *Lancet* 1999;353:169-178.

23. Dunphy RC, Bridgewater L, Price DD, et al. Visceral and cutaneous hypersensitivity in Persian Gulf war veterans with chronic gastrointestinal symptoms. *Pain* 2003;102:79-85.

24. Horner RD, Kamins KG, Feussner JR, et al. Occurrence of amyotrophic lateral sclerosis among Gulf War veterans. *Neurology* 2003;61:742-749.

25. Haley RW. Excess incidence of ALS in young Gulf War veterans. *Neurology* 2003;61:750-756.

26. Binns JH, Cherry N, Golomb BA, et al. [Research Advisory Committee on Gulf War Veterans' Illnesses]. 2004 Report and Recommendations.

27. Robbins PJ, Cherniak MG. Review of the biodistribution and toxicity of the insect repellant N,N-diethyl-m-toluamide (DEET). *J Toxicol Environ Health* 1986; 18:503-525.

28. Amichai B, Lazarov A, Halevy S. Contact dermatitis from diethyltoluamide. *Contact Dematitis* 1994;30:188.

29. McKinlay JR, Ross V, Barrett TL. Vesiculobullous reaction to diethyltoluamide revisited. *Cutis* 1998;62:44.

30. Moteiro-Riviere NA, Baynes RE, Riviere JE. Pyridostigmine bromide modulates topical irritant-induced cytokine release from human epidermal keratinocytes and isolated perfused porcine skin. *Toxicology* 2003;183:15-28.

31. Jung M, Dritschilo A. NK-κB signalling pathway as a target for human tumor radiosensitization. *Semin Radiat Oncol* 2001;11:346-351.

32. McBride WH, Pajonk F, Chiang CS, Sun JR. NF-κB, cytokines, proteosomes and low dose radiation exposure. *Mil Med* 2002;167(2 Suppl):66-67.

33. Ibuki Y, Mizuno S, Goto R. γ-Irradiation-induced DNA damage inhances NO production via NF-κB activation in RAW264.7 cells. *Biochim Biophys Acta* 2003; 1593:159-167.

34. Taysi S, Koc M, Buyukokuroglu MF, Altinkaynak K, Sahin YN. Melatonin reduces lipid peroxidation and nitric oxide during irradiation-induced oxidative injury in the rat liver. *J Pineal Res* 2003;34:173-177.

35. Takeda I, Kizu Y, Yoshitaka O, Saito I, Yamane GY. Possible role of nitric oxide in radiation-induced salivary gland dysfunction. *Radiat Res* 2003;159:465-470.

36. Abou-Donia MB, Dechkovskaia AM, Goldstein LB, et al. Uranyl acetate-induced sensorimotor deficit and increased nitric oxide generation in the central nervous system in rats. *Pharmacol Biochem Behav* 2002;72:881-890.

37. Briner W, Murray J. Effectsof short-term and long-term depleted uranium exposure on open-field behavior and brain lipid oxidation in rats. *Neurotoxicol Teratol* 2005;27:135-144.

38. Kengatharan KM, De Kimpe S, Robson C, Foster SJ, Thiemermann C. Mechanism of gram-positive shock: identification of peptidoglycan and lipoteichoic acid moieties essential in the induction of nitric oxide. *J Exp Med* 1998;188:305-315.

39. Tournier JN, Jouan A, Mathieu J, Drouet E. Gulf war syndrome: could it be triggered by biological warfare-vaccines using pertussis as an adjuvant? *Med Hypoth* 2002;58:291-292.

40. Forstermann U, Goppelt-Strube M, Frolich JC, Busse R. Inhibition of acyl-coenzyme A: lysolecithin acyltransferase activated the production of endothelial-derived relaxing factor. *J Pharmacol Exp Therapeutics* 1986;238:252-259.

41. Forstermann U, Goppelt-Strube M, Frolich JC, Busse R. Thimerosal, an inhibitor of endothelial acyl-coenzyme A:lysolecithin acyltransferase, stimulates the production of a nonprostanoid endothelium-derived relaxing factor. *Adv Prostaglandin Thromboxane Leukot Res* 1987;17B:1108-1111.

42. Mulsch A, Bohme E, Busse R. Stimulation of soluble guanylate cyclase by endothelium-derived relaxing factor from cultured endothelial cells. *Eur J Pharmacol* 1987;135:247-250.

43. Beny JL. Thimerosal hyperpolarizes arterial smooth muscles in an endothelium–dependent manner. *Eur J Pharmacol* 1990;185:235-238.

44. Crack P, Cocks T. Thimerosal blocks stimulated but not release of endothelium–derived relaxing factor (EDRF) in dog isolated coronary artery. *Br J Pharmacol* 1992;107:566-572.

45. Chen YJ, Jiang H, Quilley J. The nitric oxide- and prostaglandin independent component of the renal vasodilator effect of thimerosal is mediated by epoxyeicosatienoic acids. *J Pharmacol Exp Ther* 2003;304:1292-1298.

46. Haley RW, Billecke S, La Du BN. Association of the low PON1 type Q (type A) arylesterase activity with neurological symptom complexes in Gulf War veterans. *Toxicol Appl Pharmacol* 1999;157:227-233.

47. Mackness B, Durrington PN, Mackness MI. Low paraoxonase in Persian Gulf War veterans self-reporting Gulf War syndrome. *Biochem Biophys Res Commun* 2000;276:729-733.

48. Lockridge O. Project summary: Butyrylcholinesterase genetic variants in persons with Gulf War illness. Available at: http://www.gulflink.osd.mil.medsearch/GeneticStudies/DoD60.shtml. 1999.

49. Loewenstein-Lichtenstein Y, Schwarz M, Glick D, et al. Genetic predisposition to adverse consequences of anti-cholinesterases in 'atypical' BCHE carriers. *Nat Med* 1995;1:1082-1085.

50. Miller CS, Prihoda TJ. A controlled comparison of symptoms and chemical intolerances reported by Gulf War veterans, implant recipients and persons with multiple chemical sensitivity. *Toxicol Ind Health* 1999;15:386-397.

51. Abu-Qare AW, Abou-Donia MB. Combined exposure to sarin and pyridostigmine bromide increased levels of rat urinary 3-nitrotyrosine and 8-hydroxy-2'-deoxyguanosine, biomarkers of oxidative stress. *Toxicol Lett* 123:51-58.

52. Abu-Qare AW, Suliman HB, Abou-Donia MB. Induction of 3-nitrotyrosine, a marker of oxidative stress, following administration of pyridostigmine bromide, DEET (N,N-diethyl-m-toluamide) and permethrin, along and in combination in rats. *Toxicol Lett* 2001;121:127-134.

53. Abdel-Rahman AA, Shetty AK, Abou-Donia MB. Disruption of the blood-brain barrier and neuronal cell death in cingulate cortex, dentate gyrus, thalamus and hypothalamus in a rat model of Gulf War syndrome. *Neurobiol Dis* 2002;10:306-326.

54. Abu-Qare AW, Abou-Donia MB. Combined exposure to DEET (N,N-dithyl-m-toluamide) and permethrin-induced release of rat brain mitochondrial cytochrome C. *J Toxicol Environ Health A* 2001;63:243-252.

55. Abdel-Rahman AA, Dechkovskaia AM, Goldstein LB, et al. Neurological deficits induced by malathion, DEET, and permethrin, alone and in combination in adult rats. *J Toxicol Environ Health A* 2004;67:331-356.

56. Abou-Donia MB, Suliman HB, Khan WA, Abdel-Rahman AA. Testicular germ cell apoptosis in stressed rats following combined exposure to pyridostigmine bromide, N,N-diethyl-m-toluamide (DEET), and permethrin. *J Toxicol Environ Health A* 2003;66:57-73.

57. Olgun S, Gogal RM Jr., Adeshina F, et al. Pesticide mixtures potentiate the toxicity in murine thymocytes. *Toxicol* 2004;196:181-195.

58. Reaney P. Gulf War illness may never be explained—scientist. Reuters News Service, October 19. http://www.planetark.org/avantgo/dailynewsstory.cfm?newsid=27740. Accessed October 2004.

Chapter 11

1. Cathebras P, Lauwers A, Rousset H. Fibromyalgia. a critical review. *Ann Med Interne* 1998;149:406-414.

2. Neumann L, Buskila D. Epidemiology of fibromyalgia. *Curr Pain Headache Rep* 2003;7:362-368.

3. Shaver JL. Fibromyalgia syndrome in women. *Nurs Clin North Am* 2004;39:195-204.

4. Bennett RM Fibromyalgia: the commonest cause of widespread pain. *Compr Ther* 1995;21:269-275.

5. Wolfe F, Ross K, Anderson J, Russell IJ, Hebert L. The prevalence and characteristics of fibromyalgia in the general population. *Arthritis Rheum* 1995;38:19-28.

6. White KP, Speechley M, Harth M, Ostbye T. The London fibromyalgia epidemiology study: the prevalence of fibromyalgia in London, Ontario. *J Rheumatol* 1999;26:1570-1576.

7. Buskila D. Fibromyalgia, chronic fatigue syndrome and myofascial pain syndrome. *Curr Opin Rheumatol* 2001;13:117-127.

8. Carmona L, Ballina K Gabriel R, Laffon A: EPISER Study Group. The burden of musculoskeletal diseases in the general population of Spain: results from a national survey. *Ann Rheum Dis* 2001;60:1040-1045.

9. Prescott I, Kjoller M, Jacobsen S, et al. Fibromyalgia in the adult Danish population: I. A prevalence study. *Scand J Rheumatol* 1993;22:233-237.

10. Makela M, Heliovaara M. Prevalence of primary fibromyalgia in the Finnish population. *BMJ* 1991;303:216-219.

11. Alvarez Nemegyei J, Nuno Gutierrez BL, Alcocer Sanchez JA. Rheumatic diseases and labor disability in adult rural population. *Rev Med Inst Mex Seguro Soc* 2005;43:287-292.

12. Cardiel MH, Rojas-Serrano J. Community based study to estimate prevalence, burden of illness and help seeking behavior in rheumatic diseases in Mexico City. A COPCORD study. *Clin Exp Rheumatol* 2002;20:617-624.

13. Clark P, Burgos-Vargas R, Medina-Palma C, Lavielle P, Marina FF. Prevalence of fibromyalgia in children: a clinical study of Mexican children. *J Rheumatol* 1998;25:2009-2014.

14. Haq SA, Darmawan J, Islam MN, et al. Prevalence of rheumatic diseases and associated outcomes in rural and urban communities in Bangladesh: a COPCORD study. *J Rheumatol* 2005;32:348-353.

15. Senna ER, De Barros AL, Silva EO, et al. Prevalence of rheumatic diseases in Brazil: a study using the COPCORD approach. *J Rheumatol* 2004;31:594-597.

16. Topbas M, Cakirbay H, Gulec H, et al. The prevalence of fibromyalgia in women aged 20-64 in Turkey. *Scand J Rheumatol* 2005;34:140-144.

17. White KP, Thompson J. Fibromyalgia syndrome in an Amish community: a controlled study to determine disease and symptom prevalence. *J Rheumatol* 2003; 30:1835-1840.

18. Sorg BA. Multiple chemical sensitivity: potential role for neural sensitization. *Crit Rev Neurobiol* 1999;13:283-316.

19. Caress SM, Steinemann AC. National prevalence of asthma and multiple chemical sensitivity: an examination of potential overlap. *J Occup Environ Med* 2005;47:518-522.

20. Caress SM, Steinemann AC. A national population study of the prevalence of multiple chemical sensitivity. *Arch Environ Health* 2004;59:300-305.

21. Caress SM, Steinemann AC. Prevalence of multiple chemical sensitivities: a population-based study in the southeastern United States. *Am J Public Health* 2004; 94:746-747.

22. Caress SM, Steinemann AC. A review of a two-phase population study of multiple chemical sensitivities. *Environ Health Perspect* 2003;111:1490-1497.

23. Kreutzer R, Neutra RR, Lashuay N. Prevalence of people reporting sensitivities to chemicals in a population-based study. *Am J Epidemiol* 1999;150:1-12.

24. Joffres M, Williams T, Sabo B, Rox R. Environmental sensitivities: prevalence of major symptoms in a referral centre: The Nova Scotia Environmental Sensitivities Research Center. *Environ Health Perspect* 2001;109:161-165.

25. Hausteiner C, Bornschein S, Hansen J, Zilker T, Forstl H. Self-reported chemical sensitivity in Germany: a population-based survey. 2005;208:271-278.

26. Yule W. Posttraumatic stress disorder in the general population and in children. *J Clin Psychiatry* 2001;62(Suppl 17):23-28.

27. Breslau N. The epidemiology of posttraumatic stress disorder: what is the extent of the problem? *J Clin Psychiatry* 2001;62(Suppl 17):16-22.

28. Kessler RC. Posttraumatic stress disorder: the burden to the individual and to society. *J Clin Psychiatry* 2001;62(Suppl 17):13-14.

29. Martenyi F. Posttraumatic stress disorder (PTSDS). *Orv Hetil* 2004;145: 2315-2322.

30. Lecrubier Y. Posttraumatic stress disorder in primary care: a hidden diagnosis. *J Clin Psychiatry* 2004;65(Suppl 1):49-54.

31. Kessler RC, Sonnega A, Bromet E, Hughes M, Nelson CB. *Arch Gen Psychiatry* 1995;52:1048-1060.

32. Stein MB, Walker JR, Hazen AL, Forde DR. Full and partial posttraumatic stress disorder: findings from a community survey. *Am J Psychiatry* 1997; 154:1114-1119.

33. Frans O, Rimmo PA, Aberg L, Fredrikson M. Trauma exposure and posttraumatic stress disorder in the general population. *Acta Psychiatr Scand* 2005; 111:291-299.

34. De Albuquerque A, Suares C, De Jesus PM, Alves C. Posttraumatic stress disorder (PTSD). Assessment of its rate of occurrence in the adult population of Portugal. *Acta Med Prot* 2003;16:309-320.

35. Arillo Crespo A, Aguinaga Ontoso I, Guillen Grima F. Prevalence of mental diseases in women of an urban area. *Aten Primaria* 1998;21:265-269.

36. Bleich A, Gelkopf M, Solomon Z. Exposure to terrorism, stress-related mental health symptoms, and coping behavior among a nationally representative sample in Israel. *JAMA* 2003;290:612-620.

37. Afari N, Buchwald D. Chronic fatigue syndrome: a review. *Am J Psychiatry* 2003;160:221-236.

38. Jason LA, Richman JA, Rademaker AW, et al. A community based study of chronic fatigue syndrome. *Arch Intern Med* 1999;159:2129-2137.

39. Huibers MJH, Kant IJ, Swaen GMH, Kasl SV. Prevalence of chronic fatigue syndrome-like caseness in the working population: results from the Maatricht cohort study. *Occup Environ Med* 2004;61:464-466.

40. Evengard B, Jacks A, Pedersen NL, Sullivan PF. The epidemiology of chronic fatigue in the Swedish Twin Registry. *Psychol Med* 2005;35:1317-1326.

41. Aaron LA, Burke MM, Buchwald D. Overlapping conditions among patients with chronic fatigue syndrome, fibromyalgia, and temperomandibular disorder. *Arch Intern Med* 2000;160:221-227.

42. Buchwald D, Garrity D. Comparison of patients with chronic fatigue syndrome, fibromyalgia, and multiple chemical sensitivities. *Arch Intern Med* 1994;154: 2049-2053.

43. Ciccone DS, Natelson BH. Comorbid illness in women with chronic fatigue syndrome: a test of a single syndrome hypothesis. *Psychosom Med* 2003;65:268-275.

44. Aaron LA, Herrell R, Ashton S, et al. Comorbid clinical conditions in chronic fatigue syndrome: a co-twin study. *J Gen Intern Med* 2001;16:24-31.

45. White KP, Speechley M, Harth M, Ostbye T. Co-existence of chronic fatigue syndrome with fibromyalgia syndrome in the general population: a controlled study. *Scand J Rheumatol* 2000;29:44-51.

46. Reynolds KJ, Vernon SD, Bouchery E, Reeves WC. The economic impact of chronic fatigue syndrome. *Cost Eff Resou Alloc* 2004;2:4.

47. Assefi NP, Coy TV, Uslan D, Smith WR, Buchwald D. Financial, occupational, and personal consequences of disability in patients with chronic fatigue syndrome and fibromyalgia compared with other fatiguing conditions. *J Rheumatol* 2003;30:804-808.

48. Wolfe F, Anderson J, Harkness D, et al. Work and disability status of persons with fibromyalgia. *J Rheumatol* 1997;24:1171-1178.

49. Henriksson C, Burckhardt C. Impact of fibromyalgia on everyday life: a study of women in the USA and Sweden. *Disabil Rehabil* 1996;18:241-248.

50. Henriksson C, Liedberg G. Factors of importance for work disability of women with fibromyalgia. *J Rheumatol* 2000;27:1271-1276.

51. Robinson RL, Birnbaum HG, Morley MA, et al. Economic cost and epidemiological characteristics of patients with fibromyalgia pains. *J Rheumatol* 2003; 30:1318-1325. studies reported in a highly selected group of patients, over 2/3 claimed work disability.

52. Terr AI. Environmental Illness: a clinical review of 50 cases. *Arch Intern Med* 1986;146:145-149.

53. Black DW, Rathe A, Goldstein RB. Environmental illness: a controlled study of 26 patients with '20th century disease.' *JAMA* 1990;264:3166-3170.

54. Smith MW, Schnurr PP, Rosenbeck RA. Employment outcomes and PTSD symptom severity. *Ment Health Serv Res* 2005;7:89-101.

55. Matthews LR. Work potential of road accident survivors with posttraumatic stress disorder. *Behav Res Ther* 2005;43:475-483.

56. Mueser KT, Essock SM, Haines M, Wolfe R, Xie H. Posttraumatic stress disorder, supported employment, and outcomes in people with severe mental illness. *CNS Spectr* 2004;9:913-925.

57. MacDonald HA, Colotia V, Flamer S, Karlinsky H. Posttraumatic stress disorder (PTSD) in the workplace: a descriptive study of workers experiencing PTSD resulting from work injury. *J Occup Rehabil* 2003;13:63-77.

58. Prigerson HG, Maciejewski PK, Rosenheck RA. Combat trauma: trauma with highest risk of delayed onset and unresolved posttraumatic stress disorder symptoms, unemployment, and abuse among men. *J Nerv Ment Dis* 2001;189: 99-108.

59. Breslau N, Lucia VC, Davis GC. Partial PTSD versus full PTSD: an empirical examination of associated impairment. *Psychol Med* 2004;34:1205-1214.

Chapter 12

1. Vasquez-Vivar J, Hogg N, Martasek P, et al. Tetrahydrobiopterin-dependent inhibition of superoxide generation from neuronal nitric oxide synthase. *J Biol Chem* 1999;274:26736-26742.

2. Andrew PJ, Mayer B. Enzymatic function of nitric oxide synthases. *Cardiovasc Res* 1999;43:521-531.

3. Gorren AC, Schrammel A, Riethmuller C, et al. Nitric oxide-induced autoinhibition of neuronal nitric oxide synthase in the presence of the autoxidation-resistant pteridine 5-methyltetrahydrobiopterin. *Biochem J* 2000;347(Pt2):475-484.

4. Huisman A, Vos I, van Faasen EE, et al. Anti-inflammatory effects of tetrahydrobiopterin on early rejection in renal allografts: modulation of inducible nitric oxide synthase. *FASEB J* 2002;16:1135-137.

5. Cardounel AJ, Xia Y, Zweier JL. Endogenous methylarginines modulate superoxide as well as nitric oxide generation from neuronal nitric oxide synthase: differences in the effects of monomethyl- and dimethylarginines in the presence and absence of tetrahydrobiopterin. *J Biol Chem* 2005;280:7540-7549.

6. Kuzkaya N, Weissmann N, Harrison DG, Dikalov S. Interactions of peroxynitrite, tetrahydrobiopterin, ascorbic acid, and thiols: implications for uncoupling endothelial nitric oxide synthase. *J Biol Chem* 2003;278:22546-22554.

7. Alp NJ, Channon KM. Regulation of endothelial nitric oxide synthase by tetrahydrobiopterin in vascular disease. *Arteriosler Thromb Vasc Biol* 2004;24:413-420.

8. Kawashima S. Malfunction of vascular control in lifestyle-related diseases: endothelial nitric (NO) synthase/NO system in atherosclerosis. *J Pharmacol Sci* 2004;96(4):411-419.

9. Delgado-Estaban M, Almeida A, Medina JM. Tetrahydrobiopterin deficiency increases neuronal vulnerability to hypoxia. *J Neurochem* 2002;82:1148-1159.

10. Milstien S, Katusic Z. Oxidation of tetrahydrobiopterin by peroxynitrite: implications for vascular endothelial function. *Biochem Biophys Res Commun* 1999; 263:681-684.

11. Kohnen SL, Mouithys-Mickalad AA, Deby-Dupont GP, et al. Oxidation of tetrahydrobiopterin by peroxynitrite or oxoferryl species occurs by a radical pathway. *Free Radic Res* 2001;35:709-721.

12. Kuzkaya N, Weissmann N, Harrison DG, Dikalov S. Interactions of peroxynitrite, tetrahydrobiopterin, ascorbic acid, and thiols: implications for uncoupling endothelial nitric oxide synthase. *J Biol Chem* 2003;278:22546-22554.

13. Kuhn DM, Geddes TJ. Tetrahydrobiopterin prevents nitration of tyrosine hydroxylase by peroxynitrite and nitrogen dioxide. *Mol Pharmacol* 2003;64:946-953.

Chapter 13

1. Davidoff AL, Fogarty L. Methodological flaws of psychogenic MCS studies. *Arch Environ Health* 1994;49:316-324.

2. Davidoff AL, Fogarty LM, Keyl PM. Outpatient inferences from data on psychologic/psychiatric symptoms in multiple chemical sensitivity syndrome. *Arch Environ Health* 2000;55:165-175.

3. Goudsmit E. Response to Renckens. *Psychosom Obster Gynecol* 2001; 22:61-63.

4. Komaroff AL. The biology of chronic fatigue syndrome. *Am J Med* 2000; 108:169-171.

5. www.anapsid.org/cnd/files/mscseige.pdf

6. Radcliffe MJ, Ashurst P, Brostoff J. Unexplained illness: the mind versus the environment. *J R Soc Med* 1995;88:678-679.

7. http://listserv.nodak.edu/cgi-bin/wa.exe?A2=ind0310b&L=co-cure&F=&S= &P=3853

8. Dalen P. Forward. In *Skewed*. London: Slingshot Publications; 2003:ix-xiii.

9. Martin J Walker. *Skewed*. London: Slingshot Publications, 2003.

10. Jason LA, Richman JA, Friedberg F, Wagner L, Taylor R, Jordan KM. Politics, science and the emergence of 'new disease': the case of chronic fatigue syndrome. *Amer Psychol* 1998;52:973-983.

11. Hedrick TE. Response to functional somatic syndromes. *Ann Intern Med* 2000;132:327.

12. Clemenger A. Response to functional somatic syndromes. *Ann Intern Med* 2000;132:327-328.

13. Albrecht F. Response to functional somatic syndromes. *Ann Intern Med* 2000;132:328-329.

14. English TL. Response to functional somatic syndromes. *Ann Intern Med* 2000;132:329.

15. Gots RE. Multiple chemical sensitivities: distinguishing between psychogenic and toxicodynamic. *Reg Toxicol Pharmacol* 1996;24:S8-S15.

16. Barsky AJ, Borus JF. Functional somatic syndromes. *Ann Intern Med* 1999; 130:910-921.

17. Weissmuller GA, Ebel H, Hornberg C, Kwan O, Friel J. Are syndromes in environmental medicine variants of somatoform disorders? *Med Hypoth* 2003;61:419-430.

18. Kellner R. Psychosomatic syndromes, somatization and somatoform disorders. *Psychother Psychosom* 1994;61:4-24.

19. Groopman J. Hurting all over. *New Yorker* 2000;Nov 13:78-92.

20. Staudenmayer H. *Environmental Illness: Myth and Reality.* Boca Raton, FL: Lewis Publishers;1999.

21. Wessely S, Nimnuan C, Sharpe M. Functional somatic syndromes: one or many? *Lancet* 1999;354:936-939.

22. Binder LM, Campbell KA. Medically unexplained symptoms and neuropsychological assessment. *J Clin Exp Neuropsychol* 2004;26:369-392.

23. Staudenmayer H, Binkley KE, Leznoff A, Phillips S. Idiopathic environmental intolerance Part 1: A causation analysis applying Bradford Hill's criteria to the toxicogenic theory. *Toxicol Rev* 2003;22:235-246.

24. Staudenmayer H, Binkley KE, Leznoff A, Phillips S. Idiopathic environmental intolerance Part 2: A causation analysis applying Bradford Hill's criteria to the psychogenic theory. *Toxicol Rev* 2003;22:247-261.

25. Sirois F. Perspectives on epidemic hysteria. In: Ilza Veith, ed. *Hysteria: The History of a Disease,* Chicago: University of Chicago Press;1965:217-236.

26. Smith GR. *Somatization disorder in the medical setting.* U.S. Dept. of Health and Human Services, Public Health Service, Alcohol, Drug Abuse, and Mental Health Administration. Bethesda, MD: National Institute of Mental Health;1990.

27. Janca A. Rethinking somatoform disorders. *Curr Opin Psychiatry* 2005; 18:65-71.

28. Epstein RM, Quill TE, McWhinney IR. Somatization reconsidered: incorporating the patient's experience of illness. *Arch Intern Med* 1999;159:215-222.

29. American Psychiatric Association, *Diagnostic and Statistical Manual of Mental Disorders* 4th ed. DSM-IV, Washington, DC: American Psychiatric Press; 1994. Reprinted with permission of APA.

30. Gervais RO, Russell AS, Green P, et al. Effort testing in patients with fibromyalgia and disability incentives. *J Rheumatol* 2001;28:1892-1899.

31. Mittenberg W, Patton C, Canyock EM, Condit DC. Base rates of malingering and symptom exaggeration. *J Clin Exp Neuropsychol* 2002;24:1094-1102.

32. Khostanteen I, Tunks ER, Goldsmith CH, Ennis J. Fibromyalgia: can one distinguish it from simulation? An observer-blind controlled study. *J Rheumatol* 2000;27:2671-2676.

33. Prins JB, Jongen PJ, van der Meer JW, Bleijenberg. Abnormal neuropsychological findings are not necessarily a sign of cerebral impairment: a matched comparison between chronic fatigue syndreom and multiple sclerosis. *Neuropsychitry Neuropsycholo Behav Neurol* 2000;13:199-203.

34. Porter, Roy. ed. *The Cambridge Illustrated History of Medicine,* UK: Cambridge;1996.

35. Lurie, Hugh James. *Clinical Psychiatry for the Primary Physician.* Nutley, NJ: Roche Laboratories;1976.

36. Stoudemire, Alan. *Human Behavior: An Introduction for Medical Students.* Philadelphia: J.B. Lippincott Co;1994.

37. Deary V. Explaining the unexplained? Overcoming the distortions of a dualist understanding of medically unexplained illness. *J Ment Health* 2005;14: 213-221.

38. Mayou R, Kirmayer LJ, Simon G, Kroenke K, Sharpe M. Somatoform disorders: a time for a new approach in DSM-V. *Am J Psychiatry* 2005;162:847-855.

39. Black DW. Paroxetine for multiple chemical sensitivity. *Am J Psychiatry* 2002;159:1436-1437.

40. Aring CD. Observations of multiple sclerosis and conversion hysteria. *Brain* 1965;88:663-674.

41. Shaskan D, Yarnell H, Alper K. Physical, psychiatric and psychometric studies of post-encephalitic Parkinsonism. *J Nerv Ment Dis* 1942;96:652-662.

42. Booth G. Psychodynamics of Parkinsonism. *Psychosom Med* 1948;10:1-14.

43. Trakas DA. Cutaneous clues to a psychiatric syndrome. *Psychosomatics* 1966;7:221-223.

44. *Campbell's Urology*, 4th ed. Philadelphia, PA: W. B. Saunder's Company; 1979.

45. Martin MJ. Psychogenic factors in headache. *Med Clin North Am* 1978; 62:559-570.

46. Dorfman W. *Closing the Gap between Medicine and Psychiatry*. Springfield, IL: Charles C Thomas, Publisher;1966. Reprinted with permission from the publisher.

47. Haley RW, Billecke S, La Du BN. Association of the low PON1 type Q (type A) arylesterase activity with neurological symptom complexes in Gulf War veterans. *Toxicol Appl Pharmacol* 1999;157:227-233.

48. Furlong CE, Cole TB, Jarvik GP, et al. Role of paraoxonase (PON1) status in pesticide sensitivity: genetic and temportal determinants. *Neurotoxicology* 2005; 26:651-659.

49. McKeown-Eyssen G, Baines C, Cole DE, et al. Case-control study of genotypes in multiple chemical sensitivity: CYP2D6, NAT1, NAT2, PON1, PON2 and MTHFR. *Int J Epidemiol* 2004;33:971-978.

50. Binkley K, King N, Poonai N, Seeman P, Ulpian C, Kennedy K. Idiopathic environmental intolerance: increased prevalence of panic disorder-associated cholecystokinin B receptor allele 7. *J Allergy Clin Immunol* 2001;107:887-890.

51. Pall ML. NMDA sensitization and stimulation by peroxynitrite, nitric oxide and organic solvents as the mechanism of chemical sensitivity in multiple chemical sensitivity. *FASEB J* 2002;16:1407-1417.

52. Stanley I, Salmon P, Peters S. Doctors and social epidemics: the problem of persistent unexplained physical symptoms, including chronic fatigue. *Br J Gen Pract* 2002;52:355-356.

53. Pall ML. Chronic fatigue syndrome/myalgic encepha(lomye) litis. *Br J Gen Pract* 2002;52:762.

54. Stanley I, Salmon P, Peters S. Authors' response. *Br J Gen Pract* 2002; 52:763-764.

55. Bohr TW. Fibromyalgia and myofascial pain syndrome. Do they exist? *Neurol Clin* 1995;13:365-384. Reprinted with permission from Elsevier.

56. Staudenmayer H. Clinical consequences of the EI/MCS "diagnosis": two paths. *Regul Toxicol Pharmacol* 1996;24:S96-S110. Reprinted with permission from Elsevier.

57. Hazemaijer I, Rasker JJ. Fibromylagia and the therapeutic domain. A philosophical study on the origins of fibromyalgia in a specific social setting. *Rheumatol* 2003;42:507-515.

58. Haq SA, Darmawan J, Islam MN, et al. Prevalence of rheumatic diseases and associated outcomes in rural and urban communities in Bangladesh: a COPCORD study. *J Rheumatol* 2005;32:348-353.

59. Cardiel MH, Rojas-Serrano J. Community based study to estimate prevalence, burden of illness and help seeking behavior in rheumatic diseases in Mexico City. A COPCORD study. *Clin Exp Rheumatol* 2002;20:617-624.

60. Topbas M, Cakirbay H, Gulec H, Akgol E, Ak I, Can G. The prevalence of fibromyalgia in women aged 20-64 in Turkey. *Scand J Rheumatol* 2005;34:140-144.

61. White KP, Thompson J. Fibromyalgia syndrome in the Amish community: a controlled study to determine disease and symptom prevalence. *J Rheumatol* 2003; 30:1835-1940.

62. Hill AB. The environment and disease: association or causation. *Proc R Soc Med* 1965;58:295-300.

63. Ashford NA, Miller CS. *Chemical Exposures: Low Levels and High Stakes.* 2nd ed. New York: John Wiley & Sons, Inc;1998.

64. http://www.mcsrr.org/resources/bibliography/allchrono.html

65. Miller CS. Toxicant-induced loss of tolerance—an emerging theory of disease? *Environ Health Perspect* 1997;105(Suppl 2):445-453.

66. Cullen MR, ed. Workers with multiple chemical sensitivities. *Occup Med: State Art Rev* 1987;2:655-806.

67. Cone JE, Sult TA. Acquired intolerance to solvents following pesticide/solvent exposure in a building: a new group of workers at risk for multiple chemical sensitivities? *Toxicol Ind Health* 8:29-39.

68. Miller CS, Mitzel HC. Chemical sensitivity attributed to pesticide exposure versus remodeling. *Arch Environ Health* 1995;50:119-129.

69. Welch LS, Sokas R. Development of multiple chemical sensitivity after an outbreak of sick-building syndrome. *Toxicol Ind Health* 1992;8:47-50.

70. Davidoff AL, Keyl PM. Symptoms and health status in individuals with multiple chemical sensitivities syndrome from four reported sensitizing exposures and a general population comparison group. *Arch Environ Health* 1996;51:201-213.

71. Miller CS, Gammage RB, Jankovic JT. Exacerbation of chemical sensitivity: a case study. *Toxicol Ind Health* 1999;15:398-402.

72. Lee TG. Health symptoms caused by molds in a courthouse. *Arch Environ Health* 2003;58:442-446.

73. Corrigan FM, MacDonald S, Brown A, Armstrong K, Armstrong EM. Neurasthenic fatigue, chemical sensitivity and GABAa receptor toxins. *Med Hypoth* 1994;43:195-200.

74. Cone JE, Harrison R, Reiter R. Patients with multiple chemical sensitivities: clinical diagnostic subsets among an occupational health clinic population. *Occup Med* 1987;2:721-738.

75. Adamec R. Modelling anxiety disorders following chemical exposures. *Toxicol Ind Health* 1994;10:391-420.

76. Ziem G, and McTamney J. Profile of patients with chemical injury and sensitivity *Environ Health Perspect* 1997;105(Suppl 2):417-436.

77. Lohmann K, Prohl A, Schwarz E. Multiple chemical sensitivity disorder in patients with neurotoxic illnesses. *Gesundheitswesen* 1996;58:322-331.

78. Altenkirch H, Hopmann D, Brockmeier B, and Walter G. Neurological investigations in 23 cases of pyrethroid intoxication reported by the German Federal Health Office. *Neurotoxicology* 1996;17:645-651.

79. Terr A. Environmental illness: a review of 50 cases. *Arch Intern Med* 1986; 146:145-149.

80. Terr A. Clinical ecology in the workplace. *J Occup Med* 1989;31:257-261.

81. Lee YL, Pai MC, Chen JH, Guo YL. Central neurological abnormalities and multiple chemical sensitivity caused by chronic toluene exposure. *Occup Med (Lond)* 2003;53:479-482.

82. Caress SM, Steinemann AC. A review of a two-phase population study of multiple chemical sensitivities. *Environ Health Perspect* 2003;111:1490-1497.

83. Simon GE. Epidemic multiple chemical sensitivity in an industrial setting. *Toxicol Ind Health* 1992;8(4):41-46.

84. Henry CJ, Fishbein L, Meggs WJ, et al. Approaches for assessing health risks from complex mixtures in indoor air: a panel overview. *Environ Health Perpect* 1991;95:135-143.

85. Fernandez-Sola, J, Lluis Padierna M, Nogue Xarau S, Munne Mas P. Chronic fatigue syndrome and multiple chemical hypersensitivity after insecticide exposition. *Med Clin (Barc)* 2005;124(12):451-453.

86. Johnson, Alison, ed. *Casualties of Progress: Personal Histories from the Chemically Sensitive*. MCS Information Exchange, Brunswick, ME, 2000.

87. Shinohara N, Y Yanagisawa. Responsible chemicals and behaviors for hypersensitive symptoms in patients with multiple chemical sensitivity. *Jap J Clin Ecol* 2004;13:93-101.

88. Kawamoto MM, Esswein EJ, Wallingford KM, Wothington KA. *Health Hazard Evaluation Report* 96-0012-2652 Brigham and Women's Hospital Boston, MA September 1997. United States Government (NIOSH).

89. Shinohara N, Mizukoshi A, Yanagisawa Y. Identification of responsible volatile chemicals that induce hypersensitive reactions to multiple chemical sensitivity patients. *J Exposure Anal Environ Epidemiol* 2004;14:84-91.

90. Miller CS. Mechanisms of action of addictive stimuli. *Addiction* 2000; 96:115-139.

91. Meggs WJ. Neurogenic inflammation and sensitivity to environmental chemicals. *Environ Health Perspect* 1993;101:234-238.

92. van der Kuy PH, Lohman JJ. The role of nitric oxide in vascular headache. *Pharm World Sci* 2003;25:146-151.

93. Jensen R. Peripheral and central mechanisms in tension-type headache: an update. *Cephalalgia* 2003;23(Suppl 1):49-52.

94. Taylor RR, Friedberg F, Jason LA. *A Clinician's Guide to Controversial Illnesses: Chronic Fatigue Syndrome, Fibromyalgia and Multiple Chemical Sensitivities*. Sarasota, FL: Professional Resource Press;2001.

Chapter 14

1. Miller, C. S. Are we on the threshold of a new theory of disease? Toxicant-induced loss of tolerance and its relationship to addiction and abdiction. *Toxicol Ind Health* 1999;15: 284-294.

2. Kuhn T. *The Structure of Scientific Revolutions*. 3rd ed. Chicago: University of Chicago Press;1966.

3. *Dorland's Illustrated Medical Dictionary*. 24th ed. Philadelphia: W. B. Saunders Company;1965.

4. *Stedman's Medical Dictionary,* 26th ed.; Baltimore: Williams & Wilkins; 1995.

5. Takumida M, Anniko M, Popa R, Zhang DM. Pharmacological models for inner ear therapy with emphasis on nitric oxide. *Acta Otolaryngol* 2001;121:16-20.

6. Shulman A. Neuroprotective drug therapy: a medical and pharmacological treatment for tinnitus control. *Int Tinnitus J* 1997;3:77-93.

7. Denk D-M, Heinzl H, Franz P, Ehrenberger K. Caroverine in tinnitus treatment. *Acta Otolaryngol* 1997;117:825-830.

8. Oestreicher E, Arnold W, Ehrenberger K, Felix D. New approaches for inner ear therapy with glutamate antagonists. *Acta Otolaryngol* 1999;119:174-178.

9. Shulman A, Strashun AM, Goldstein BA. $GABA_A$-Benzodiazepine-chloride receptor-targeted therapy for tinnitus control: preliminary report. *Int Tinnitus J* 2002;8:30-36.

10. Raponi G, Alpini D, Volonte S, Capobianco S, Cesarini A. The role of free radicals and plasmatic antioxidant in Meniere's syndrome. *Int Tinnitus J* 2003; 9:104-108.

11. Takumida M, Anniko M, Ohtani M. Radical scavengers for Meniere's disease after failure of conventional therapy: a pilot study. *Acta Otolaryngol* 2003;123: 697-703.

12. Shulman A. Noise, calpain, calpain inhibitors and neuroprotection: a preliminary report of tinnitus control. *Int Tinnitus J* 1998;4:134-140.

13. Sziklai I. The significance of the calcium signal in the outer hair cells and its possible role in tinnitus of cochlear origin. *Eur Arch Otorhinolaryngol* 2004; 261:517-525.

14. Eybalin M. Neurotransmitters and neuromodulators in the mammalian cochlea. *Physiol Rev* 1993;73:309-373.

15. Johnson KL, Carrasco V, Prazma J, et al. Role of nitric oxide in kainic acid-induced elevation of cochlear compound action potential thresholds. *Acta Otolaryngol (Stockh)* 1998;118:660-665.

16. Kumerova AO, Lece AG, Skesters AP, Orlikov GA, Seleznev JV, Rainsford KD. 2000 Antioxidant defense and trace element imbalance in patients with postradiation syndrome. *Biol Trace Element Res* 77:1-12.

17. Loganovsky KN. Vegetative-vascular dystonia and osteoalgetic syndrome or chronic fatigue syndrome as a characteristic after-effect of radioecological disaster: the Chernobyl accident experience. *J Chronic Fatigue Syndr* 1999;7(3):3-16.

18. Pastel RH. Radiophobia: long-term psychological consequences of Chernobyl. *Mil Med* 2002;167(2 Suppl):134-136.

19. Barnes JG. 'Sensitivity syndromes' related to radiation exposure. *Med Hypoth* 2001;57:453-458.

20. Linard C, Marquette C, Mathieu J, Pennequin A, Clarencon D, Mathe D. Acute induction of inflammatory cytokine expression after γ-irradiation in the rat: effect of an NF-κB inhibitor. *Int J Radia Oncol Biol Phys* 2004; 58:427-434.

21. Li N, Karin M. Ionizing radiation and short wavelength UV activate NF-κB through two distinct mechanisms. *Proc Natl Acad Sci USA* 1998; 95:13012-13017.

22. Prasad AV, Mohan N, Chandrasekar B, Meltz ML. Activation of nuclear factor kappa B in human lymphoblastoid cells by low-dose ionizing radiation. *Radiat Res* 1994;138:367-372.

23. Wang T, Zhang X, Li JJ. The role of NF-κB in the regulation of cell stress responses. *Int Immunopharmacol* 2002;2:1509-1520.

24. Taysi S, Koc M, Muyukokuroglu MF, Altinkaynak K, Sahin YN. Melatonin reduces lipid peroxidation and nitric oxide during irradiation-induced oxidative injury in the rat liver. *J Pineal Res* 2003;34:173-177.

25. Abou-Donia MB, Dechkovskaia AM, Goldstein LB, Shah DU, Bullman SL, Khan WA. Uranyl acetate-induced sensorimotor deficit and increased nitric oxide generation in the central nervous system in rats. *Pharmacol Biochem Behav* 2002; 72:881-890.

26. Takeda I, Kizu Y, Yoshitaka O, Saito I, Yamane GY. Possible role of nitric oxide in radiation-induced salivary gland dysfunction. *Radiat Res* 2003;159:465-470.

27. Ibuki Y, Mizuno S, Goto R. γ-Irradiation-induced DNA damage inhances NO production via NF-κB. *Biochim Biophys Acta* 2003;1593:159-167.

28. Burlakova EB, Antova YS. Mechanism of biological action of low-dose irradiation. In: Bulokova, EB ed. *Consequences of the Chernobyl Catastrophe on Human Health.* Nova Science;1999.

29. Briner W, Murray J. Effects of short-term and long-term depleted uranium exposure on open-field behavior and brain lipid oxidation in rats. *Neurotoxicol Teratol* 2005;27:135-144.

30. Romanenko A, Morimura IK, Wanibuchi H, et al. Increased oxidative stress with gene alteration in urinary bladder urothelium after the Chernobyl accident. *Int J Cancer* 2000;86:790-798.

31. Lykholat EA, Chernaya VI. Parameters of peroxidation and proteolysis in the organism of the liquidators of Chernobyl accident consequences. *Ukr Biokhim Zh* 1999;71:82-85.

32. Chen Y, Rubin P, Williams J, Hernady E, Smudzin T, Okunieff P. Circulating IL-6 as a predictor of radiation pneumonitis. *Int J Radiat Oncol Biol Phys* 2001; 49:641-648.

33. Chiang CS, Hong JH, Stalder A. Sun JR, Withers HR, McBride WH. Delayed molecular responses to brain irradiation. *In J Radiat Biol* 1997;72:45-53.

34. Akiyama M. Late effects of radiation on the human immune system: an overview of immune response among the atomic-bomb survivors. *Int J Radiat Biol* 1995;68:497-508.

35. Vozianov AF, Drannik GN, Petrovskaia IA, Musii MI. Immunity disorders and the increased fatigability syndrome in the residents of the city of Kiev. *Vrach Delo* 1991;(11):14-17.

36. Vyatleva OA, Katargina TA, Puchinskaya LM, Yurkin MM. Electrophysiological characterization of the functional state of the brain in mental disturbances in workers involved in the clean-up following the Chernobyl atomic energy station accident. *Neurosci Behav Physiol* 1997;27:166-172.

37. Rimar VV. Changes in the auditory system related to cerebral circulation in the Ukraine population after the Chernobyl disaster. *Rev Laryngol Otl Rhinol (Bord)* 1999;120:89-92.

38. Loganovsky KN, Yuryev KL. EEG patterns in persons exposed to ionizing radiation as a result of the Chernobyl accident: part 1: conventional EEG analysis. *J Neuropsychiatry Clin Neurosci* 2001;13:441-458.

39. Bruck W, Stadelmann C. Inflammation and degeneration in multiple sclerosis. *Neurol Sci* 2003;24(Suppl 5):S265-S267.

40. Poser CM. Trauma to the central nervous system may result in formation of enlargement of multiple sclerosis plaques. *Arch Neurol* 2000;57:1074-1077.

41. Sobel RA. The pathology of multiple sclerosis. *Neurol Clin* 1995;13:1-21.

42. Gilden DH. Viruses in multiple sclerosis. *JAMA* 2001;286:3127-3129.

43. Steiner I, Wirguin I. Multiple sclerosis—in need of a critical reappraisal. *Med Hypoth* 2000;54:99-106.

44. Barnett MH, Prineas JW. Relapsing and remitting multiple sclerosis: pathology of the newly forming lesion. *Ann Neurol* 2004;55:458-468.

45. Hernan MA, Zhang SM, Lipworth L, Olek MJ, Ascherio A. Multiple sclerosis and age at infection with common viruses. *Epidemiology* 2001;12:301-306.

46. Nielsen NM, Wohlfahrt J, Melbye M, et al. Multiple sclerosis and poliomyelitis. A Danish historical cohort study. *Acta Neurol Scand* 2000;101:384-387.

47. Granieri E. Exogenous factors in aetiology of multiple sclerosis. *J Neurovirol* 2000;6(Suppl 2):S141-S146.

48. Munger KL, Peeling RW, Hernan MA, et al. Infection with Chlamydia pneumoniae and risk of multiple sclerosis. *Epidemiology* 2003;14:141-147.

49. Riise T, Moen BE, Kyvik KR. Organic solvents and the risk of multiple sclerosis. *Epidemiology* 2002;13:718-720.

50. Reis J, Dietermann JL, Warter JM, Poser CM. A case of multiple sclerosis triggered by organic solvents. *Neurol Sci* 2001;22:155-158.

51. Mohr DC, Hart SL, Julian L, Cox D, Pelletier D. Association between stressful life events and exacerbation in multiple sclerosis: a meta-analysis. *BMJ* 2004; 328:731.

52. Buljevac D, Hop WC, Reedeker W, et al. Self reported stressful life events and exacerbations in multiple sclerosis: prospective study. *BMJ* 2003;327:646.

53. Ordonez G, Pineda B, Garcia-Navarrete R, Sotelo J. Brief presence of varicella-zoster viral DNA in mononuclear cells during relapses of multiple sclerosis. *Arch Neurol* 2004;61:529-532.

54. Wallin MT, Page WF, Kurtzke JF. Muliple sclerosis in US veterans of the Vietnam era and later military service: race, sex and geography. *Ann Neurol* 2004; 55:65-71.

55. van der Mei IA, Posonby AL, Dwyer T, et al. Past exposure to sun, skin phenotype, and risk of multiple sclerosis: a case-control study. *BMJ* 2003;327:316.

56. Hayes CE. Vitamin D: a natural inhibitor of multiple sclerosis. *Proc Nutr Soc* 2000;59:531-535.

57. Chang JM, Kuo MC, Kuo HT, et al. 1-alpha,25-Dihydroxyvitamin D3 regulates inducible nitric oxide synthase messenger RNA expression and nitric oxide release in macrophage-like RAW 264.7 cells. *J Lab Clin Med* 2004;143:14-22.

58. Lefebvre d'Hellencourt C, Montero-Menei CN, Bernard R, Couez D. Vitamin D3 inhibits proinflammatory cytokines and nitric oxide production in the EOC13 microglial cell line. *J Neurosci Res* 2003;71:575-582.

59. Smith KJ, Lassmann H. The role of nitric oxide in multiple sclerosis. *Lancet Neurol* 2002;1:232-241.

60. Cross AH, San M, Stern MK, et al. A catalyst of peroxynitrite decomposition inhibits murine experimental autoimmune encephalitis. *J Neuroimmunol* 2000; 107:21-28.

61. Liu JS, Zhao ML, Brosnan CF, Lee SC. Expression of inducible nitric oxide synthase and nitrotyrosine in multiple sclerosis lesions. *Am J Pathol* 2001;158: 2057-2066.

62. Spitsin S, Hooper DC, Leist T, et al. Inactivation of peroxynitrite in multiple sclerosis patients with oral admnistration of inosine may suggest possible approaches to therapy of the disease. *Mult Scler* 2001;7:313-319.

63. Hunter MI, Nlamedim BC, Davidson DL. Lipid peroxidation products and antioxidant proteins in plasma and cerebrospinal fluid from multiple sclerosis patients. *Neurochem Res* 1985;10:1645-1652.

64. Clabrese V, Raffaele R, Cosentino E, Rizza V. *Int J Clin Pharmacol Res* 1994;14:119-123.

65. Vladimirova O, O'Connor J, Cahill A, et al. Oxidative damage to DNA in plaques of MS brains. *Mult Scler* 1998;4:413-418.

66. Greco A, Minghetti L, Sette G, Fieschi C, Levi G. Cerebrospinal fluid isoprostane shows oxidative stress in patients with multiple sclerosis. *Neurology* 1999;53:1876-1879.

67. Gilgun-Sherki Y, Melamed E, Offen D. The role of oxidative stress in the pathogenesis of multiple sclerosis: the need for effective antioxidant therapy. *J Neurol* 2004;251:261-268.

68. Imitola J, Chitnis T, Khouri SJ. Cytokines in multiple sclerosis: from bench to bedside. *Pharmacol Ther* 2005;106:163-177.

69. Biernacki K, Antel JP, Blain M, Narayanan S, Arnold DL, Prat A. Interferon beta promotes nerve growth factor secretion in the course of multiple sclerosis. *Arch Neurol* 2005;62:563-568.

70. Schulte-Herbruggen O, Nassenstein C, Lommatzsch M, et al. Tumor necrosis factor-alpha and interleukin-6 regulate secretion of brain-derived neurotrophic factor in human monocytes. *J Neuroimmunol* 2005;160:204-209.

71. Flachenecker P, Bihler I, Weber F, et al. Cytokine mRNA expression in patients with multiple sclerosis and fatigue. *Mult Scler* 2004;10:165-169.

72. Miterski B, Bohringer S, Klein W, et al. Inhibitors in the NF-kappa B cascade comprise prime candidate genes predisposing to multiple sclerosis, especially in selected combinations. *Genes Immun* 3:211-219.

73. Kaltschmidt B, Sparna T, Kaltschmidt C. Activation of NF-kappa B by reactive oxygen intermediates in the nervous system. *Antioxid Redox Signal* 1999;1:129-144.

74. Bonetti B, Stegagno C, Cannella B, et al. Activation of NF-kappa B and c-jun transcription factors in multiple sclerosis lesions. Implications for oligodendrocyte pathology. *Am J Pathol* 1999;155:1433-1438.

75. Gveric D, Kaltshmidt C, Cuzner ML, Newcombe J. Transcription factor NF-kappa B and inhibitor I kappaB-alpha are localized in macrophages in active multiple sclerosis lesions. *J Neuropathol Exp Neurol* 1998;57:168-178.

76. Paul C, Bolton C. Modulation of blood-brain barrier dysfunction and neurological deficits during acute experimental allergic encephalomyelitis by the N-methyl-D-aspartate receptor antagonist memantine. *J Pharmacol Exp Ther* 2002; 302:50-57.

77. Sarchielli P, Greco L, Floridi A, Floridi A, Gallai V. Excitatory amino acids and multiple sclerosis: evidence from cerebrospinal fluid. *Arch Neurol* 2003;60: 1082-1088.

78. Pitt D, Nagelmeier IE, Wilson HC, Raine CS. Glutamate uptake by oligodendrocytes: Implications for excitotoxicity in multiple sclerosis. *Neurology* 2003;61: 1113-1120.

79. Srinivasan R, Sailsuta N, Hurd R, Nelson S, Pelletier D. Evidence of elevated glutamate in multiple sclerosis using magnetic resonance spectroscopy at 3 T. *Brain* 2005;128:1016-1025.

80. Kent-Braun JA, Sharma KR, Miller RG, Weiner MW. Postexercise phophocreatine resynthesis is slowed in multiple sclerosis. *Muscle Nerve* 1994; 17:835-841.

81. Hooper DC, Scott GS, Zborek A, et al. Uric acid, a peroxynitrite scavenger, inhibits CNS inflammation, bolld CNS barrier permeability changes, and tissue damage in a mouse model of multiple sclerosis. *FASEB J* 2000;14:691-698.

82. Smith KJ, Kapoor R, Felts PA. Demyelination: the role of reactive oxygen and nitrogen species. *Brain Pathol* 1999;9:69-92.

83. Scott GS, Virag L, Szabo C, Hooper DC. Peroxynitrite-induced oligodendrocyte toxicity is not dependent on poly(ADP-ribose) polymerase activation. *Glia* 2003;41:102-116.

84. Touil T, Deloire-Grassin MS, Vital C, Petry KG, Brochet B. In vivo damage of CNS myelin and axons induced by peroxynitrite. *Neuroreport* 2001;12:3637-3644.

85. Santiago E, Perez-Mediavilla LA, Lopez-Moratalla N. The role of nitric oxide in the pathogenesis of multiple sclerosis. *J Physiol Biochem* 1998;54:229-237.

86. Yamashita Y, Fujimoto C, Nakajima E, Isagai T, Matsuishi T. Possible association between congenital cytomegalovirus infection and autistic disorder. *J Autism Dev Disord* 2003;33:455-459.

87. Ivarsson SA, Bjerre I, Vegfors P, Ahlfors K. Autism is one of several disabilities in two children with congenital cytomegalovirus infection. *Neuropediatrics* 1990;21:102-103.

88. Deykin EY, MacMahon B. Viral exposure and autism. Chess S. 1977 Follow-up report on autism in congenital rubella. *Am J Epidemiol* 1979;109:628-638.

89. Sweeten TL, Posey DJ, McDougle CJ. Brief report: autistic disorder in three children with cytomegalovirus infection. *J Autism Dev Disord* 2004;34:583-586.

90. Wilkerson DS, Volpe AG, Dean RS, Titus JB. Perinatal complications as predictors of infantile autism. *Int J Neurosci* 2002;112:1085-1098.

91. Barak Y, Kimhi R, Stein D, Gutman J, Weizman A. Autistic subjects with comorbid epilepsy: a possible association with viral infections. *Child Psychiatry Hum Dev* 1999;29:245-251.

92. Chess S. Follow-up report on autism in congenital rubella. *J Autism Child Schizophr* 1977;7:69-81.

93. Libbey JE, Sweeten TL, McMahon WM, Fujinami RS. Autistic disorder and viral infections. *J Neurovirol* 2005;11:1-10.

94. Shi L, Fatemi SH, Sidwell RW, Patterson PH. Maternal influenza infection causes marked behavioral and pharmacological changes in the offspring. *J Neurosci* 2003;23:297-302.

95. Pletnikov MV, Moran TH, Carbone KM. Borna disease virus infection of the neonatal rat: developmental brain injury model of autism spectrum disorders. *Front Biosci* 2002;7:d593-607.

96. Hornig M, Briese T, Lipkin WI. Bornavirus tropism and targeted pathogenesis: virus-host interactions in a neurodevelopmental model. *Adv Virus Res* 2001; 56:557-582.

97. Geier DA, Geier MR. A two-phased population epidemiological study of the safety of thimerosal-containing vaccines: a follow-up analysis. *Med Sci Monit* 2005;11:CR160-170.

98. Bernard S, Enayati A, Roger H, Binstock T, Redwood L. The role of mercury in the pathogenesis of autism. *Mol Psychiatry* 2002;7(Suppl)2:S42-S43.

99. Geier MR, Geier DA. Neurodevelopmental disorders after thimerosal–containing vaccines: a brief communication. *Exp Biol Med* 2003;228:660-664.

100. Blaxill MF, Redwood L, Bernard S. Thimerosal and autism? A plausible hypothesis that should not be dismissed. *Med Hypotheses* 2004;62:788-794.

101. Holmes AS, Blaxill MF, Haley BE. Reduced levels of mercury in first baby haircuts of autistic children. *Int J Toxicol* 2003;22:277-285.

102. Forstermann U, Goppelt-Strube M, Frolich JC, Busse R. Inhibition of acyl-coenzyme A: lysolecithin acyltransferase activated the production of endothelial-derived relaxing factor. *J Pharmacol Exp Therapeutics* 1986;238:252-259.

103. Forstermann U, Goppelt-Strube M, Frolich JC, Busse R. Thimerosal, an inhibitor of endothelial acyl-coenzyme A: lysolecithin acyltransferase, stimulates the production of a nonprostanoid endothelium-derived relaxing factor. *Adv Prostaglandin Thromboxane Leukot Res* 1987;17B:1108-1111.

104. Mulsch A, Bohme E, Busse R. Stimulation of soluble guanylate cyclase by endothelium-derived relaxing factor from cultured endothelial cells. *Eur J Pharmacol* 1987;135:247-250.

105. Beny JL. Thimerosal hyperpolarizes arterial smooth muscles in an endothelium-dependent manner. *Eur J Pharmacol* 1990;185:235-238.

106. Crack P, Cocks T. Thimerosal blocks stimulated but not release of endothelium-derived relaxing factor (EDRF) in dog isolated coronary artery. *Br J Pharmacol* 1992;107:566-572.

107. Chen YJ, Jiang H, Quilley J. The nitric oxide- and prostaglandin independent component of the renal vasodilator effect of thimerosal is mediated by epoxy-eicosatrienoic acids. *J Pharmacol Exp Ther* 2003;304:1292-1298.

108. Edelson SB, Cantor DS. Autism: xenobiotic influences. *Toxicol Ind Health* 1998;14:799-811.

109. McGinnis WR. Oxidative stress in autism. *Altern Ther Health Med* 2004; 10:22-36.

110. Blaylock RL. Interactions of cytokines, excitotoxins and reactive nitrogen and oxygen species in autism spectrum disorders. *J Am Neutraceutical Assoc* 2003; 6:21-35.

111. Angeli A, Minetto M, Dovio A, Paccotti P. The overtraining syndrome in athletes: a stress-related disorder. *J Endocrinol Invest* 2004;27:603-612.

112. Steinacker JM, Lormes W, Reissnecker S, Liu Y. New aspects of the hormone and cytokine response to training. *Eur J Appl Physiol* 2004;91:382-391.

113. Pearce PZ. A practical approach to the overtraining syndrome. *Curr Sports Med Rep* 2002;1:179-183.

114. MacKinnon LT. Special feature for the Olympics: effects of exercise on the immune system: overtraining effects on immunity and performance in athletes. *Immunol Cell Biol* 2000;78:502-509.

115. Pederson BK, Rohde T, Zacho M. Immunity in athletes. *J Sports Med Phys Fitness* 1996;36:236-245.

116. Lehmann M, Foster C, Dickhuth HH, Gastmann U. Autonomic imbalance hypothesis and overtraining syndrome. *Med Sports Exerc* 1998;30:1140-1145.

117. Smith LL. Cytokine hypothesis of overtraining: a physiological adaptation to excessive stress? *Med Sci Sports Exerc* 2000;32:317-331.

118. Robson P. Elucidating the unexplained underperformance syndrome in endurance athletes: the interleukin-6 hypothesis. *Sports Med* 2003;33:771-781.

119. Stefano GB, Prevot V, Cadet P, Dardik I. Vascular pulsations stimulating nitric oxide release during cyclic exercise may benefit health: a molecular approach (review). *Int J Mol Med* 2001;7:119-129.

120. MacDonald KL, Osterholm MT, LeDell KH, et al. A case-control study to assess possible triggers and cofactors in chronic fatigue syndrome. *Am J Med* 1996; 100:548-554.

121. Jackson MJ, Khassaf M, Vasilaki S, McArdle F, McArdle A. Vitamin E and theoxidative stress of exercise. *Ann NY Acad Sci* 2004;1031:158-168.

122. Ji LL, Gomez-Cabrera MC, Steihafel N, Vina J. Acute exercise activates nuclear factor (NF)-kappa B signaling pathway in rat skeletal muscle. *FASEB J* 2004;18:1499-1506.

123. Inhan N, Kamanli A, Ozmerdivenli R, Ilhan N. Variable effects of exercise intensity on reduced glutathione, thiobarbituric acid reactive substance levels, and glucose concentration. *Arch Med Res* 2004;35:294-300.

124. Aoi W, Naito Y, Takanami Y, et al. Oxidative stress and delayed-onset muscle damage after exercise. *Free Radic Biol Med* 2004;37:480-487.

125. Lauer N, Suvorava T, Ruther U, et al. Critical involvement of hydrogen peroxide in exercise-induced up-regulation of endothelial NO synthase. *Cardiovasc Res* 2005;65:254-262.

126. Karamouzis I, Christoulas K, Grekas D, et al. The response of muscle interstitial F2-isoprostane (8-ISO-PGF2alpha) during dynamic muscle contractions in humans. *Prostaglandins Leukot Essent Fatty Acids* 2004;71:87-90.

127. Bailey DM, Young IS, McEneny J, et al. Regulation of free radical outflow from an isolated muscle bed in exercising humans. *Am J Physiol Heart Circ Physiol* 2004;287:H1689-H1699.

128. Cavas L, Tarhan L. Effects of vitamin-mineral supplementation on cardiac marker and radical scavenging enzymes, and MDA levels in young swimmers. *Int J Sport Nutr Exerc Metab* 2004;14:133-146.

129. MacDonald KL, Osterholm MT, LeDell KH, et al. A case-control study to assess possible triggers and cofactors in chronic fatigue syndrome. *Am J Med* 1996; 100:548-554.

130. Hennekins CH, Lee IM, Cook NR, et al. Self-reported breast implants and connective tissue diseases in female health professionals. A retrospective cohort study. *JAMA* 1996;275:616-621.

131. Vasey FB. Clinical experience with systemic illness in women with silicone breast implants: comment on the editorial by Rose. *Arthritis Rheum* 1997;40:1545.

132. Brown SL, Pennello G, Berg WA, Soo MS, Middleton MS. Silicone gel breast implant rupture, extracapsular silicone, and health status in a population of women. *J Rheumatol* 2001;28:996-1003.

133. Brown SL, Duggirala HJ, Pennello G. An association of silicone-gel breast implant rupture and fibromyalgia. *Curr Rheumatol Rep* 2002;4:293-298.

134. Solomon G. A clinical and laboratory profile of symptomatic women with silicone breast implants. *Semin Arthritis Rheum* 1994;24(Suppl 1):29-37.

135. Cuellar ML, Gluck O, Molina JF, et al. Silicone breast implant-associated musculoskeletal manifestations. *Clin Rheumatol* 1995;14:667-672.

136. Vermeulen RC, Scholte HR. Rupture of silicone breast implants and symptoms of pain and fatigue. *J Rheumatol* 2003;30:2263-2267.

137. Blackburn WD Jr., Grotting JC, Everson MP. Lack of evidence of systematic inflammatory rheumatic disorders in symptomatic women with breast implants. *Plast Reconstr Surg* 1997;99:1054-1060.

138. Freundlich B, Altman C, Snadorfi N, Greenberg M, Tomaszewski J. A profile of symptomatic patients with silicone breast implants: a Sjogren's-like syndrome. *Semin Arthritis Rheum* 1994;24(Suppl 1):44-53.

139. Fenske TK. Human adjuvant disease revisited: a review of eleven post–augmentation mammoplasty patients. *Clin Exp Rheumatol* 1994;12:477-481.

140. Lipworth L, Tarone RE, McLaughlin JK. Breast implants and fibromyalgia: a review of the epidemiological evidence. *Ann Plast Surg* 2004;52:284-287.

141. Miller CS, Prihoda TJ. A controlled comparison of symptoms and chemical intolerances reported by Gulf War veterans, implant recipients and persons with multiple chemical sensitivity. *Toxicol Ind Health* 1999;15:386-397.

142. Shanklin DR, Smalley DL. Pathogenetic and diagnostic aspects of siliconosis. *Rev Environ Health* 2002;17:85-105.

143. Smalley DL, Shanklin DR, Hall MF, Stevens MV, Hanissian A. Immunologic stimulation of T lymphocytes by silica after use of silicone mammary implants. *FASEB J* 1995;9:424-427.

144. Castranova V. Signalling pathways controlling the production of inflammatory mediators in response to crystalline silica exposure: role of reactive oxygen/nitrogen species. *Free Radic Biol Med* 2004;37:916-925.

145. Misson P, van den Brule S, Barbarin V, Lison D, Huaux F. Markers of lymphocyte differentiation in experimental silicosis. *J Leukoc Biol* 2004;76:926-932.

146. Fubini B, Hubbard A. Reactive oxygen species (ROS) and reactive nitrogen species (RNS) generation by silica in inflammation and fibrosis. *Free Radic Biol Med* 2003;34:1507-1516.

147. Zeidler PC, Castranova V. Role of nitric oxide in pathological responses of the lung to exposure to environmental/occuopational *agents*. *Redox Rep* 2004; 9:7-18.

148. Chen F, Shi X. NF-kappa B, a pivotal transcription factor in silica-induced diseases. *Mol Cell Biochem* 2002;235:169-176.

149. Iribarren P, Correa SG, Sodero N, Riera CM. Activation of macrophages by silicones: phenotype and production of oxidant metabolites. *BMC Immunol* 2002;3:6.

150. Ojo-Amaize EA, Lawless OJ, Peter JB. Elevated concentrations of interleukin-1 beta and interleukin-1 receptor antagonist in plasma of women with silicone breast implants. *Clin Diagn Lab Immunol* 1996;3:257-259.

151. Mena EA, Kossovsky N, Chu C, Hu C. Inflammatory intermediates produced by tissues encasing silicone breast prostheses. *J Invest Surg* 1995;8:31-42.

152. Pollock JS, Webb W, Callaway D, et al. Nitric oxide synthase isoform expression in porcine model of granulation tissue formation. *Surgery* 2001;129: 341-350.

153. Gl. Paice E. Fortnightly review: reflex sympathetic dystrophy. *BMJ* 1995; 310:1645-1648.

154. Marsden CD, Obeso JA, Traub MM, et al. Muscle spasms with Sudeck's atrophy after injury. *Br Med J* 1984;288:173-176.

155. Veldman PHJM, Reynen HM, Arntz IE, Goris RJA. Signs and symptoms of reflex sympathetic dystrophy: a prospective study of 829 patients. *Lancet* 1993; 342:1012-1016.

156. Weber M, Neundorfer B, Birklein F. Sudeck's atrophy: pathophysiology and treatment of complex pain syndrome. *Dtsch Med Wochenshr* 2002;127:384-389.

157. Imanuel HM, Levy FL, Geldwert JJ. Sudeck's atrophy: a review of the literature. *J Foot Surg* 1981;20:243-246.

158. Cordioli E, Tondini C, Pizzi C, Premuda G. Sudeck's atrophy: a review of the literature. *Minerva Med* 1994;85:265-270.

159. Williams WR. Reflex sympathetic dystrophy. *Rheumatol Rehabil* 1977; 16:119-124.

160. Sarangi PP, Ward AJ, Smith EJ, Staddon GE, Atkins RM. Algodystrophy and osteoporosis after tibial fractures. *J Bone Joint Surg* 1993;75:450-452.

161. van der Laan L, Goris RJ. Sudeck's syndrome. Was Sudeck right? *Unfallchirurg* 1997;100:90-99.

162. Bruckbauer HR, Preac Mursic V, Herzer P, Hofmann H. Sudeck's atrophy in Lyme borreliosis. *Infection* 1997;25:372-376.

163. Sahin M, Bernay I, Canturk F, Demarcali AE. Reflex sympathetic dystrophy secondary to organophosphate intoxication induced neuropathy. *Ann Nucl Med* 1994;8:299-300.

164. Friedman LS, Brautbar N, Barach P, Wolfe AH, Richter ED. Creatine phosphate kinase elevations signaling muscle damage following exposures to anticholinesterases: 2 sentinel patients. *Arch Environ Health* 2003;58:167-170.

165. Lin TC, Wong CS, Chen FC, Lin SY, Ho ST. Long-term epidural ketamine and bupivacaine attenuate reflex sympathetic dystrophy neuralgia. *Can J Anaesth* 1998;45:175-177.

166. Schwartzman TJ, Popescu A. Reflex sympathetic dystrophy. *Curr Rheumatol Rep* 2002;4:165-169.

167. Von Eisenhart-Rothe R, Rittmeister M. Drug therapy in complex regional pain syndrome type I. *Orthopade* 2004;33:796-803.

168. Harden R, Norman MD. Pharmacotherapy of complex regional pain syndrome. *Pain Science Rational Polypharmacy* 2005;84(Suppl):S17-S28.

169. Tews DS, Apoptosis and muscle fibre loss in neuromuscular disorders. *Neuromuscul Disord* 2002;12:613-622.

170. Li YP, Atkins CM, Sweatt JD, Reid MB. Mitochondria mediate tumor necrosis factor-alpha/NF-kappa B signaling in skeletal muscle. *Antioxid Redox Signal* 1999;1:97-104.

171. Mentaverri R, Kamel S. Wattel A, Regulation of bone resorption andosteoclast survival by nitric oxide: possible involvement of NMDA receptor. *J Cell Biochem* 2003;88:1145-1156.

172. Hukkanen V, Broberg E, Salmi A, Eralinna JP. Cytokines in experimental herpes simplex virus infection. *Int Rev Immunol* 2002;21:355-371.

173. Imanishi J. Expression of cytokines in bacterial and viral infections and their biochemical targets. *J Biochem* 2000;127:525-530.

174. Skoldenberg B. Herpes simplex encephalitis. *Scand J Infect Dis Suppl* 1996;100:8-13.

175. Treede RD, Meyer RA, Raja SN, Campbell JN. Peripheral and central mechanisms of cutaneous hyperalgesia. *Prog Neurobiol* 1992;38:397-421.

176. Meller ST, Pechman PS, Gebhart GF, Maves TJ. Nitric oxide mediates the thermal hyperalgesia produced in a model of neuropathic pain in the rat. *Neuroscience* 1992;50:7-10.

177. Zimmermann M. Pathobiology of neuropathic pain. *Eur J Pharmacol* 2001; 429:23-37.

178. Wagner R, Myers RR. Endoneurial injection of TNF-α produces neuropathic pain behaviors. *Neuroreport* 1996;7:2897-2901.

179. Leung A, Wallace MS, Ridgeway B, Yaksh T. Concentration-effect relationship of intravenous alfentanil and ketamine on peripheral neurosensory thresholds, allodynia and hyperalgesia of neuropathic pain. *Pain* 2001;91:177-187.

180. Walker KM, Urban L, Medhurst SJ, et al. The VR1 antagonist capsazepine reverses mechanical hyperalgesia in models of inflammatory and neuropathic pain. *Pharmacol Exp Ther* 2003;304:56-62.

181. DeLeo JA, Colburn RW, Nichols M, Malhotra A. Interleukin-6-mediated hyperalgesia/allodynia and increased IL-6 expression is a rat mononeuropathy model. *J Interferon Cytokine Res* 1996;16:695-700.

182. Bonezzi C, Demartini L. Treatment options in postherpetic neuralgia. *Acta Neurol Scand Suppl* 1999;173:25-35.

183. Backonja M, Galnzman RL. Gabapentin dosing for neuropathic pain: evidence from randomized, placebo-controlled clinical trials. *Clin Ther* 2003;25:81-104.

184. Brill S, Sedgwick PM, Hamann W, Di Vadi PP. Efficacy of intravenous magnesium in neuropathic pain. *Br J Anaesth* 2002;89:711-714.

185. Douglas MW, Johnson RW, Cunningham AL. Tolerability of treatments for postherpetic neuralgia. *Drug Saf* 2004;27:1217-1233.

186. Klepstad P, Borchgrevink PC. Four years' treatment with ketamine and a trial of dextromethorphan in a patient with severe post-herpetic neuralgia. *Acta Anaesthesiol Scand* 1997;41:422-431.

187. Kotani N, Kudo R, Sakurai Y, et al. Cerebrospinal fluid interleukin 8 concentrations and the subsequent development of postherpteic neuralgia. *Am J Med* 2004;116:318-324.

188. Zak-Prelich M, McKenzie RC, Sysa-Jedrzejowska A, Norval M. Local immune responses and systemic cytokine responses in zoster: relationship to the development of postherpetic neuralgia. *Clin Exp Immunol* 2003;131:318-323.

189. Kotani N, Kushikata T, Hashimoto H, et al. Intrathecal methylprednisolone for intractable postherpetic neuralgia. *N Engl J Med* 2000;343:1514-1519.

190. Sterling M, Jull G, Vincenzino B, Kenardy J. Sensory hypersensitivity occurs soon after whiplash injury and its associated poor recovery. *Pain* 2003;104:509-517.

191. Haldorsen T, Waterloo K, Dahl A, et al. Symptoms and cognitive dysfunction in patients with the late whiplash syndrome. *Appl Neuropsychol* 2003;10:170-175.

192. Antepohl W, Kiviloog L, Andersson J, Gerdle B. Cognitive impairment in patients with chronic whiplash-associated disorder—a matched control study. *Neuro-Rehabilitation* 2003;18:307-315.

193. Bosma FK, Kessels RP. Cognitive impairments, psychological dysfunction and coping styles in patients with chronic whiplash syndrome. *Neuropsychiatry Neuropsychol Behav Neurol* 2002;15:56-65.

194. Sullivan MJ, Hall E, Barolacci R, Sullivan ME, Adams H. Perceived cognitive deficits, emotional distress and disability following whiplash injury. *Pain Res Manag* 2002;7:120-126.

195. Treleaven J, Jull G, Sterling M. Dizziness and unsteadiness following whiplash injury: characteristic features and relationship with cervical joint position error. *J Rehabil Med* 2003;35:36-43.

196. Wenzel HG, Haug TT, Mykletun A, Dahl AA. A population study of anxiety and depression among persons who report whiplash traumas. *J Psychosom Res* 2002;53:831-835.

197. Alexander MP. The evidence for brain injury in whiplash injuries. *Pain Res Manag* 2003;8:19-23.

198. Curatolo M, Petersen-Felix S, Arendt-Nielsen L, et al. Central hypersensitivity in chronic pain after whiplash injury. *Clin J Pain* 2001;17:306-315.

199. Banic B, Petersen-Felix S, Andersen OK, et al. Evidence for spinal cord hypersensitivity in chronic pain after whiplash injury and in fibromyalgia. *Pain* 2004; 107:7-15.

200. Klobas L, Tegelberg A, Axelsson S. Symptoms and signs of temporomandibular disorders in individuals with chronic whiplash-associated disorders. *Swed Dent J* 2004;28:29-36.

201. Ushida T, Tani T, Kanbara T, et al. Analgesic effects of ketamine ointment in patients with complex regional pain syndrome type I. *Reg Anesth Pain Med* 2002; 27:524-528.

202. Summers WK. Alzheimer's disease, oxidative injury and cytokines. *J Alzheimer's Dis* 2004;6:673-681.

203. Schmidt ML, Lee VM-Y, Saido T, et al. Amyloid plaques in Guam amyotrophic lateral sclerosis/parkinsonism-dementia complex contain species of Aβ similar to those found in the amyloid plaques in Alzheimer's disease and pathological aging. *Acta Neuropathol* 1998;95:117-122.

204. Brownson DM, Mabry TJ, Leslie SW. The cycad neurotoxicity amino acid, beta-N-methylamino-L alanine (BMAA), elevates intracellular calcium levels in dissociated rat brain cells. *J Ethnopharmacol* 2002;82:159-167.

205. Allen CN, Omelchenko I, Ross SM, Spencer P. The neurotoxin, beta-N-methylamino-L-alanine (BMAA) interacts with the strychnine-insensitive glycine modulatory site of the N-methyl-D-aspartate receptor. *Neuropharmacol* 1995;34: 651-658.

206. Khabazian I, Bains JS, Williams DE, et al. Isolation of various forms of stero?-D-glucoside from the seed of Cycas circinalis: neurotoxicity and implications of ALS-parkinsonism dementia complex. *J Neurochem* 2002;82:516-523.

207. Takahashi H, Snow BJ, Bhatt MH, et al. Evidence or a dopaminergic deficit in sporadic amyotrophic lateral sclerosis on positron emission scanning. *Lancet* 1993;342:1016-1018.

208. Hartman RE, Laurer H, Longhi L, et al. Apolipoprotein E4 influences amyloid deposition but not cell loss after traumatic brain injury in a mouse model of Alzheimer's disease. *J Neurosci* 2002;22:10083-10087.

209. Li YJ, Hauser MA, Scott WK, et al. Apolipoprotein E controls the risk and age of onset of Parkinson's disease. *Neurology* 2004;62:2005-2009.

210. Drory VE, Birnbaum M, Korczyn AD, Chapman J. Association of APOE ε4 allele with survival in amyotrophic lateral sclerosis. *J Neurol Sci* 2001;190:17-20.

211. Masliah E, Rockenstein E, Veinbergs I, et al. β-amyloid peptides enhance α-synuclein accumulation and neuronal deficits in a transgenic mouse model linking Alzheimer's disease and Parkinson's disease. *Proc Natl Acad Sci USA* 2001; 98:12245-12250.

212. Hageman G, van der Hoek J, van Hout M, et al. Parkinsonism, pyramidal signs, polyneuropathy and cognitive decline after long-term occupational exposure. *J Neurol* 1999;246:198-206.

213. Uitti RJ, Snow BJ, Shinotoh H, et al. Parkinsonism induced by solvent abuse. *Ann Neurol* 1994;35:616-619.

214. Ohlson CG, Hogstedt C. Parkinson's disease and occupational exposure to organic solvents, agricultural chemicals and mercury—a case-referent study. *Scand J Work Environ Health* 1981;7:252-256.

215. Kuriwaki R, Mitsui T, Fujiwara S, Nishida Y, Matsumoto T. Loss of postural reflexes in long-term occupational solvent exposure. *Eur Neurol* 2002;47:85-87.

216. Cintra A, Andbjer B, Finnman UB, et al. Subacute toluene exposure increases DA dysfunction in the 6-OH dopamine lesioned nigrostriatal dopaminergic system of the rat. *Neurosci Lett* 1996;217:61-65.

217. Kamel F, Hoppin JA. Association of pesticide exposure with neurologic dysfunction and disease. *Environ Health Perspect* 2004;112:950-958.

218. Langston JW, Ballard P, Tetrud JW, Irwin I. Chronic Parkinsonism in humans due to a product of mepiridine analog synthesis. *Science* 1983;219:979-980.

219. Lockwood AH. Pesticides and parkinsonism: is there an etiological link? *Curr Opin Neurol* 2000;13:687-690.

220. Uversky VN. Neurotoxicant-induced animal models of Parkinson's disease: understanding the role of rotenone, maneb and paraquat in neurodegeneration. *Cell Tissue Res* 2004;318:225-241.

221. Thiruchelavam M, Richfield EK, Goodman BM, Baggs RB, Cory-Slechta DA. Developmental exposure to the pesticides paraquat and maneb and the Parkinson's disease phenotype. *Neurotoxicology* 23:621-633.

222. Racette BA, McGee-Minnich L, Moerlein SM, et al. Welding-related parkinsonism: clinical features, treatment and pathophysiology. *Neurology* 2001; 56:8-13.

223. Hudness HK. Effects of environmental Mn exposures: a review of the evidence from non-occupational exposure studies. *Neurotoxicology* 1999;20:379-397.

224. Olanow CW. Manganese-induced parkinsonism and Parkinson's disease. *Ann NY Acad Sci* 2004;1012:209-223.

225. Lee JW. Manganese intoxication. *Arch Neurol* 2000;57:597-599.

226. Jakowec MW, Petzinger GM. 1-methyl-4-phenyl-1,2,3,6-tetrahydropyridine-lesioned model of Parkinson's disease, with emphasis in mice and nonhuman primates. *Comp Med* 2004;54:497-513.

227. Przedborski S, Vila M. The 1-methyl-4-phenyl-1,2,3,6-tetrahydropyridine mouse model: a tool to explore the pathogenesis of Parkinson's disease. *Ann NY Acad Sci* 2003;991:641-646.

228. Przedborski S, Jackson-Lewis V, Djaldetti R, et al. The parkinsonian toxin MPTP: action and mechanism. *Restor Neurol Neurosci* 2000;16:135-142.

229. Denicola A, Radi R. Peroxynitrite and drug-dependent toxicity. *Toxicology* 2005;208:273-288.

230. Tarabin V, Schwaninger M. The role of NF-κB in 6-hydroxydopamine- and TNFα-induced apoptosis of PC12 cells. *Naunyn Schiedebergs Arch Pharmacol* 2004;369:563-569.

231. Halasz AS, Palfi M, Tabi T, Magyar K, Szoko E. Altered nitric oxide production in mouse brain after administration of 1-methyl-4-phenyl-1,2,3,6-tetrahydropyridine or methamphetamine. *Neurochem Int* 2004;44:641-646.

232. Testa CM, Sherer TB, Greenamyre JT. Rotenone induces oxidative stress and dopaminergic neuron damage in organotypic substantia nigra cultures. *Brain Res Mol Brain Res* 2005;134:109-18.

233. Bhashkatova V, Alam M, Vanin A, Schmidt WJ. Chronic administration of rotenone increases levels of nitric oxide and lipid peroxidation products in rat brain. *Exp Neurol* 2004;186:235-241.

234. Vogt M, Bauer MK, Ferrari D, Schulze-Osthoff K. Oxidative stress and hypoxia/reoxygenation trigger CD95 (APO-1)/Fas) ligand expression in microglial cells. *FEBS Lett* 1998;429:67-72.

235. Zhou LZ, Johnson AP, Rando TA. NF-kappa B and AP-1 mediate transcriptional responses to oxidative stress in skeletal muscle cells. *Free Radic Biol Med* 2001;31:1405-1416.

236. Barlow BK, Lee DW, Cory-Slechta DA, Opanashuk LA. Modulation of antioxidant defense systems by the environmental pesticide maneb in dopaminergic cells. *Neurotoxicology* 2005;26:63-75.

237. Vaccari A, Saba P, Mocci I, Ruiu S. Dithiocarbamate pesticides affect glutamate transport in brain synaptic vesicles. *J Pharmacol Exp Ther* 1999;288:1-5.

238. Barhoumi R, Faske J, Liu X, Tjalkens RB. Manganese potentiates lipopolysaccharide-induced expression of NOS2 in C6 glioma cells through mitochondrial-dependent activation of nuclear factor kappa B. *Brain Res Mol Brain Res* 2004;122:167-179.

239. Jayakumar AR, Rama Rao KV, Kalaiselvi P, Norenberg MD. Combined effects of ammonia and manganese on astrocytes in culture. *Neurochem Res* 2004;29:2051-2056.

240. Filipov NM, Seegal RF, Lawrence DA. Manganese potentiates in vitro production of proinflammatory cytokines and nitric oxide by microglia through a nuclear factor kappa B-dependent mechanism. *Toxicol Sci* 2005;84:139-148.

241. Erikson KM, Aschner M. Manganese neurotoxicity and glutamate-GABA interaction. *Neurochem Int* 2003;43:475-480.

242. Hennekens CH, Buring JE. In: Mayrent SL ed. *Epidemiology in Medicine.* Boston: Little Brown and Co;1989.

243. Jellinger KA. Head injury and dementia. *Curr Opin Neurol* 2004;17:719-723.

244. Hinkebein JH, Martin TA, Callahan CD, Johnstone B. Traumatic brain injury and Alzheimer's: deficit profile similarities and the impact of normal aging. *Brain Inj* 2003;17:1035-1042.

245. Fleminger S, Oliver DL, Lovestone S, Rabe-Hesketh S, Giora A. Head injury as a risk factor for Alzheimer's disease: the evidence 10 years on: a partial replication. *J Neurol Neurosurg Psychiatry* 2003;74:857-862.

246. Baldi I, Lebailly P, Mohammed-Brahim B et al. Neurodegenerative diseases and exposure to pesticides in the elderly. *Am J Epidemiol* 2003;157:409-414.

247. Bidstrup P, Bonnel JA, Beckett AG. Paralysis following poisoning by a new organic phosphorus insecticide (Mipafox): report of two cases. *Br Med J* 1953; 1:1068-1072.

248. Fonseca RG, Resende LAL, Sillva MD, Camargo A. Chronic motor neuron disease possibly related to intoxication with organochlorine insecticides. *Acta Neurol Scand* 1993;88:56-58.

249. Burns CJ, Beard KK, Cartmill JB. Mortality in chemical workers potentially exposed to 2,4-dichlorophenoxyacetic acid (2,4-D) 1945-94: an update. *Occup Environ Med* 2001;58:24-30.

250. Bradberry SM, Proudfoot AT, Vale JA. Poisoning due to chlorophenoxy herbicides. *Toxicol Rev* 2004;23:65-73.

251. Brooks BR. Risk factors in the early diagnosis of ALS: North American epidemiological studies. ALS CARE GROUP. *Amyotroph Lateral Scler Other Motor Neuron Disord* 2000;1(Suppl 1):S19-S26.

252. Beckman JS, Estevez AG, Crow JP, Barbeito L. Superoxide dismutase and the death of motorneurons in ALS. *Trends Neurosci* 2001;24(11 Suppl):S15-S20.

253. Aslan M, Ozbun T. Oxidative stress in neurodegenerative diseases. In: Ozbun T, Chevion M. eds. *Frontiers in Neurodegenerative Disorders and Aging: Fundamental Aspects.* IOS Press;2004.

254. Dawson VL, Dawson TM. Nitric oxide neurotoxicity. *J Chem Neuroanat* 1996;10:179-190.

255. Torreilles F, Salman-Tabcheh S, Guerin M, Torreilles J. Neurodegerative disorders: the role of peroxynitrite. *Brain Res Brain Res Rev* 1999;30:153-163.

256. Heales SJ, Bolanos JP, Stewart VC, Brookes PS, Land JM, Clark JB. Nitric oxide, mitochondria and neurologic disease. *Biochim Biophys Acta* 1999;1410: 215-228.

257. Simonian NA, Coyle JT. Oxidative stress in neurodegenerative diseases. *Annu Rev Pharmacol Toxicol* 1996;36:83-106.

258. Di Matteo V, Esposito E. Biochemical and therapeutic effects of antioxidants in the treatment of Alzheimer's disease, Parkinson's disease, and amyotrophic lateral sclerosis. *Curr Drug Targets CNS Neurol Disord* 2003;2:95-107.

259. Takeuchi M, Mizuno T, Zhang G, et al. Neuritic beading induced activated microglia is an early feature of neuronal dysfunction toward neuronal death by inhibition of mitochondrial respiration and axonal transport. *J Biol Chem* 2005;280: 10444-10454.

260. Sonkusare SK, Kaul CL, Ramarao P. Dementia in Alzheimer's disease and other neurodegenerative disorders—memantine, a new hope. *Pharmacol Res* 2005; 51:1-17.

261. Hallett PJ, Standaert DG. Rationale for use of NMDA receptor antagonists in Parkinson's disease. *Pharmacol Ther* 2004;102:155-174.

262. Greenamyre JT, MacKenzie G, Peng TI, Stephans SE. Mitochondrial dysfunction in Parkinson's disease. *Biochem Soc Symp* 1999;66:85-97.

263. Hsu M, Srinivas B, Kumar J, Subramanian R, Anderson J. Glutathione depletion resulting in selective mitochondrial complex I inhibition in dopaminergic

cells is via an NO-mediated pathway not involving peroxynitrite: implications for Parkinson's disease. *J Neurochem* 2005;92:1091-1103.

264. Berg D, Youdin MB, Riederer P. Redox imbalance. *Cell Tissue Res* 2004; 318:201-213.

265. Tieu K, Ischiropoulos H, Przedborski S. Nitric oxide and reactive oxygen species in Parkinson's disease. *IUBMB* 2003;55:329-335.

266. Ebadi M, Sharma SK. Peroxynitrite and mitochondrial dysfunction in the pathogenesis of Parkinson's disease. *Antioxid Redox Signal* 2003;5:319-335.

267. Hirsch EC, Breidert T, Rousselet E, et al. The role of glial reaction and inflammation in Parkinson's disease. *Ann NY Acad Sci* 2003;991:214-228.

268. Mandel S, Grunblatt E, Riederer P, Gerlach M, Levites Y, Youdim MB. Neuroprotective strategies in Parkinson's disease: an update. *CNS Drugs* 2003; 17:729-762.

269. Griffin WS, Mrak RE. Interleukin-1 in the genesis and progression of and risk for development of neuronal degeneration in Alzheimer's disease. *J Leukoc Biol* 2002;72:233-238.

270. Bonfoco E, Krainc D, Ankarcrona M, Nicotera P, Lipton SA. Apoptosis and necrosis: two distinct events induced, respectively, by mild and intense insults with N-methyl-d-aspartate or nitric oxide/superoxide in cortical cell cultures. *Proc Natl Acad Sci USA* 1995;92:7162-7166.

271. Kreiger C, Lanius RA, Pelech SL, Shaw CA. Amyotrophic lateral sclerosis: the involvement of intracellular Ca^{2+} and protein kinase C. *Trends Pharmacol Sci* 1996;17:114-120.

272. Williamson KS, Gabbita SP, Mou S, et al. The nitration product 5-nitro-gamma-tocopherol is increased in the Alzheimer brain. *Nitric Oxide* 2002;6:221-227.

273. Migliori L, Fontana I, Colognato R, et al. Searching for the role of the most suitable biomarkers of oxidative stress in Alzheimer's disease and in other neurodegenerative diseases. *Neurobiol Aging* 2005;26:587-595.

274. Boll MC, Alcaraz-Zubeldia M, Montes S, Murillo-Bonilla L, Rios C. Raised nitrate concentration and low SOD activity in the CSF of sporadic ALS patients. *Neurochem Res* 2003;28:699-703.

275. Charbrier PE, Demerle-Pallardy C, Auguet M. Nitric oxide synthases: targets for therapeutic strategies in neurological diseases. *Cell Mol Life Sci* 1999;55: 1029-1035.

276. Antunes F, Nunes C, Larjinha J, Cadenas E. Redox interactions of nitric oxide with dopamine and its derivatives. *Toxicology* 2005;208:207-212.

277. Chung KK, Thomas B, Li X, et al. S-nitrosylation of parkin regulates ubiquitination and compromises parkin's protective function. *Science* 2004;304: 1328-1331.

278. Kao SC, Krichevsky AM, Kosick KS, Tsai LH. BACE1 suppression by RNA interference in primary cortical neurons. *J Biol Chem* 2004;279:1942-1949.

279. Tamagno E, Bardini P, Obbili A, et al. Oxidative stress increases expression and activity of BACE in NT2 neurons. *Neurobiol Dis* 2002;10:279-288.

280. Tamagno E, Guglielmotto M, Bardini P, et al. Dehydroepiandrosterone reduces expression and activity of BACE in NT2 neurons exposed to oxidative stress. *Neurobiol Dis* 2003;14:291-301.

281. Apelt J Bigl M, Wunderlich P, Schliebs R. Aging-related increase in oxidative stress correlates with developmental pattern of β-secretase activity and β-amyloid plaque formation in transgenic Tg2576 mice with Alzheimer-like pathology. *Int J Dev Neurosci* 2004;22:475-484.

282. Tong Y, Zhou W, Fung V, et al. Oxidative stress potentiates BACE1 gene expression and A(β) *J Neural Transm* 2005;112:455-469.

283. Parihar MS, Hemnani T. Alzheimer's disease pathogenesis and therapeutic interventions. *J Clin Neurosci* 2004;11:456-467.

284. Jang JH, Surh YJ. AP-1 mediates β-amyloid-induced iNOS expression in PC12 cells via the ERK2 and p38 MAPK signaling pathways. *Biochem Biophys Res Commun* 2005;331:1421-1428.

285. Floden AM, Li S, Combs CK. β-amyloid-stimulated microglia induce neuron death via synergistic stimulation of tumor necrosis factor alpha and NMDA receptors. *J Neurosci* 2005;25:2566-2575.

286. Kadowski H, Nishitoh H, Urano F, et al. Amyloid beta induces neuronal cell death through ROS-mediated ASK1 activation. *Cell Death Differ* 2005;12:19-24.

287. Keil U, Bonert A, Marques CA, et al. Elevated nitric oxide production mediates β-amyloid-induced mitochondrial failure. *Pol J Pharmacol* 2004;56:631-634.

288. von Bernhardi R, Eugenin J. Microglia reactivity to β-amyloid is modulated by astrocytes and proinflammatory factors. *Brain Res* 2004;1025:186-193.

289. Ma G, Chen S. Diazoxide and N-omega-nitro-L-arginine counteracted A beta 1-42-induced cytotoxicity. *Neuroreport* 2004;15:1813-1817.

290. Wang Q, Rowan MJ, Anwyl R. β-amyloid-mediated inhibition of NMDA receptor-dependent long-term potentiation induction involves activation of microglia and stimulation of inducible nitric oxide synthase and superoxide. *J Neurosci* 2004;24:6049-6056.

291. Tran MH, Yamada K, Nakajima A, et al. Tyrosine nitration of synaptic protein synaptophysin contributes to amyloid beta-peptide-induced cholinergic dysfunction. *Mol Psychiatry* 8:407-412.

292. Saez TE, Pehar M, Vargas M, Barbeito L, Maccioni RB. Astrocytic nitric oxide triggers tau hyperphosphorylation in hippocampal neurons. *In Vivo* 2004;18:275-280.

293. Wang DL, Ling ZQ, Cao FY, Zhu LQ, Wang JZ. Melatonin attenuates isoproterenol-induced protein kinase A overactivation and tau hyperphosphorylation in rat brain. *J Pineal Res* 2004;37:11-16.

294. Zhu LQ, Wang SH, Ling ZQ, Wang DL, Wang, JZ. Effect of inhibiting melatonin biosynthesis on spatial memory retention and tau phosphorylation in rat. *J Pineal Res* 2004;37:71-77.

295. Gomez-Ramos A, Diaz-Mido J, Smith MA, Perry G, Avila J. Effect of lipid peroxidation product acrolein on tau phosphorylation in neural cells. *J Neurosci Res* 2003;71:863-870.

296. Egana JT, Zambrano Cm Nunez MT, Gonzalez-Billaut C, Maccioni RB. Iron-induced oxidative stress modify tau phosphorylation patterns in hippocampal cell cultures. *Biometals* 2003;16:215-223.

297. Ho PI, Ortiz D, Rogers E, Shea TB. Multiple aspects of homocysteine neurotoxicity: glutamate excitotoxicity, kinase hyperactivation and DNA damage. *J Neurosci Res* 2002;70:694-702.

298. Mandelkow EM, Stamer K, Vogel R, Thies E, Mandelkow E. Clogging of axons by tau, inhibition of axonal traffic and starvation of synapses. *Neurobiol Aging* 2003;24:1079-1085.

299. Sanelli TR, Sopper MM, Strong MJ. Sequestration of nNOS in neurofilamentous aggregate bearing neurons in vitro leads to enhanced NMDA-mediated calcium influx. *Brain Res* 2004;1004:8-17.

300. Lin CL, Bristol LA, Dykes-Hoberg M, Crawford T, Clawson L, Rothstein JD. Aberrant RNA processing in neurodegerative disease: the cause for the absent EAAT2, a glutamate transporter in amyotrophic lateral sclerosis. *Neuron* 1998;20: 589-602.

301. Margakis NJ, Dykes-Hoberg M, Rothstein JD. Altered expression of the glutamate transported EAAT2b in neurologic disease. 2004 *Ann Neurol* 2004;55:469-477.

302. Hoogland G, va Oort RJ, Proper EA, et al. Alternative splicing of glutamate transporter EAAT2 RNA in neocortex and hippocampus of temporal lobe of epilepsy patients. *Epilepsy Res* 59:75-82.

Chapter 15

1. Logan AC, Wong C. Chronic fatigue syndrome: oxidative stress and dietary modifications. *Altern Med Rev* 2001;6:450-459.

2. Werbach M. Nutritional strategies for treating chronic fatigue syndrome. *Altern Med Rev* 2000;5:93-108.

3. Rigden S, Barrager E, Bland JS. Evaluation of the effect of a modified entero-hepatic resuscitation program in chronic fatigue syndrome patients. *J Adv Med* 1998;11:247-252.

4. Smith JD, Terpening CM, Schmidt SO, Gums JG. Relief of fibromyalgia following discontiuation of dietary excitotoxins. *Ann Pharmacother* 2001;35:702-706.

5. Blaylock RL. *Excitotoxins: The Taste That Kills* Santa Fe, NM: Health Press.

6. Miller CS, Mitzel HC. Chemical sensitivity attributed to pesticide exposure versus remodeling. *Arch Environ Health* 1995;50:119-129.

7. Teitelbaum J. *Effective treatment for CFS/FM - Part I & II*. Syllabus AAEM, 38th Annual Meeting, The Walking Wounded: Identifying the Causes and Exploring the Newest Treatment Options for Chronic Fatigue Syndrome, Fibromylagia and Environmental Sensitivities;2003:73-118.

8. Nicolson GL. *Nutritional supplement restores mitochondrial function and reduces moderately severe fatigue in aged subjects.* Syllabus AAEM, 38th Annual Meeting, The Walking Wounded: Identifying the Causes and Exploring the Newest

Treatment Options for Chronic Fatigue Syndrome, Fibromylagia and Environmental Sensitivities;2003:231-264.

9. Krop J. *Lyme disease: a missed diagnosis in chronic illness.* Syllabus AAEM, 38th Annual Meeting, The Walking Wounded: Identifying the Causes and Exploring the Newest Treatment Options for Chronic Fatigue Syndrome, Fibromylagia and Environmental Sensitivities;2003:265-280.

10. Rea WJ. *Chronic fatigue, fibromyalgia and environmental sensitivities:* oxygen extraction deficits and complex neurological immune dysfunction. An environmental medicine perspective. Syllabus AAEM, 38th Annual Meeting, The Walking Wounded: Identifying the Causes and Exploring the Newest Treatment Options for Chronic Fatigue Syndrome, Fibromylagia and Environmental Sensitivities;2003: 317-349.

11. Gerdes K. *Tips from the trenches: some useful tricks learned in practice.* Syllabus AAEM, 38th Annual Meeting, The Walking Wounded: Identifying the Causes and Exploring the Newest Treatment Options for Chronic Fatigue Syndrome, Fibromylagia and Environmental Sensitivities;2003:365-374.

12. Ionescu JG. *Oxidative therapies for severe infection, MCS and cancer.* Syllabus AAEM, 38th Annual Meeting, The Walking Wounded: Identifying the Causes and Exploring the Newest Treatment Options for Chronic Fatigue Syndrome, Fibromylagia and Environmental Sensitivities;2003:461-488.

13. LaCava NT. *A retrospective review of a therapeutic trial of IV alpha lipoic acid in chronically ill patients.* Syllabus AAEM, 38th Annual Meeting, The Walking Wounded: Identifying the Causes and Exploring the Newest Treatment Options for Chronic Fatigue Syndrome, Fibromylagia and Environmental Sensitivities; 2003:489-508.

14. Block MA. *First do no harm, next try magnesium.* Syllabus AAEM, 38th Annual Meeting, The Walking Wounded: Identifying the Causes and Exploring the Newest Treatment Options for Chronic Fatigue Syndrome, Fibromylagia and Environmental Sensitivities;2003:617-621.

15. Huang HY, Appel LJ. Supplementation of diets with α-tocopherol reduces serum concentrations of γ- and ϵ-tocopherol in humans. *J Nutr* 2003;133:3137-3140.

16. Olmedilla B, Granado F, Southon S, et al. A European multicentre, placebo-controlled supplementation study with α-tocopherol, carotene-rich palm oil, lutein or lycopene: analysis of serum responses. *Clin Sci* 2002;102:447-456.

17. Bates CJ, Chen SJ, Macdonald A, Holden R. Quantitation of vitamin E and carotenoid pigment in cataractous human lenses, and the effect of dietary supplement. *Int J Vitam Nutr Res* 1996;66:316-321.

18. Handelman GJ, Epstein WL, Peerson J, et al. Human adipose α-tocopherol and γ-tocopherol kinetics during and after 1 y of α-tocopherol supplementation. *Am J Clin Nutr* 1994;59:1025-1032.

19. Parker RS, Sontag TJ, Swanson JE, McCormick CC. Discovery, characterization, and significance of the cytochrome P450 omega-hydroxylase pathway of vitamin E catabolism. *Ann NY Acad Sci* 2004;1031:13-21.

20. Brigelius-Flohe R. Induction of drug metabolizing enzymes by vitamin E. *J Plant Physiol* 2005;162:797-802.

21. Christen S, Woodall AA, Shigenaga MK, et al. gamma-Tocopherol traps mutagenic electrophiles such as NO(x) and complements alpha-tocopherol: physiological implications. *Proc Natl Acad Sci USA* 1997;94:3217-3222.

22. Hoglen NC, Liegler DC. Products from reaction of peroxynitrite with gamma-tocopherol. *Methods Enzymol* 1999;301:483-490.

23. Wolf G. gamma-Tocopherol: an efficient protector of lipids against nitric oxide-initiated peroxidative damage. *Nutr Rev* 1997;55:376-378.

24. Sen CK, Khanna S, Roy S. Tocotrienol: the natural vitamin E to defend the nervous system? *Ann NY Acad Sci* 2004;1031:127-142.

25. Schaffer S, Muller WE, Eckert GP. Tocotrienols: constitutional effects in aging and disease. *J Nutr* 2005;135:151-154.

26. Kamat JP, Devasagayam TP. Tocotrienols from palm oil as potent inhibitors of lipid peroxidation and protein oxidation in rat brain mitochondria. *Neurosci Lett* 1995;195:179-182.

27. Snodderly DM. Evidence for protection against age-related macular degeneration by carotenoids and antioxidant vitamins. *Am J Clin Nutr* 1995;62(6 Suppl):1448S-1461S.

28. Richer S. Multicenter ophthalmic and nutritional age-related macular degeneration study—part2: antioxidant intervention and conclusions. *J Am Optometr Assoc* 1996;47:30-49.

29. Jampol LM, Ferris FL 3rd. Antioxidants and zinc to prevent progression of age-related macular degeneration. *JAMA* 2001;286:2466-1468.

30. Richer S, Stiles W, Statkute L, et al. Double-masked, placebo-controlled, randomized trial of lutein and antioxidant supplementation in the intervention of atrophic age-related macular degeneration: the Veterans LAST study. *Optometry* 2004;75:216-230.

31. Hogg R, Chakravarthy U. AMD and micronutrient antioxidants. *Curr Eye Res* 2004;29:387-401.

32. Head KA. Natural therapies for ocular disorders, part one: diseases of the retina. *Altern Med Rev* 1999;4:342-359.

33. Taylor HR, Tikellis G, Robman LD, et al. Vitamin E supplementation and macular degeneration: randomized controlled trial. *BMJ* 2002;325:11-16.

34. Packer L. α-Lipoic acid: a metabolic antioxidant which regulated NF-κB signal transduction and protects against oxidative injury. *Drug Metab Rev* 1998; 30:245-275.

35. Rahman I, Biswas SK, Jimenez LA, Torres M, Forman HJ. Glutathione, stress responses, and redox signaling in lung inflammation. *Antioxid Redox Signal* 2005;7:42-59.

36. Cos P, De Bruyne T, Heremans N, et al. Proanthocyanidins in health care: current and new trends. *Curr Med Chem* 11:1345-1359.

37. Rahman I, Marwick J, Kirkham P. Redox modulation of chromatin remodeling: impact on histone acetylation and deacetylation, NF-κB and pro-inflammatory gene expression. *Biochem Pharmacol* 2004;68:1255-1267.

38. Pande V, Ramos MJ. Nuclear factor kappa B: a potential target for anti-HIV chemotherapy. *Curr Med Chem* 2003;10:1603-1615.

39. Haddad JJ. Science review: redox and oxygen-sensitive transcription factors in the regulation of oxidant-mediated lung injury: role of nuclear factor-kappa B. *Crit Care* 2002;6:481-490.

40. Kretz-Remy C, Arrigo AP. Selenium: a key element that controls NF-κB activation and Iκ B half life. *Biofactors* 2001;14:117-125.

41. Yoshikawa T, Yoshida N. Vitamin E and leukocyte-endothelial cell interactions. *Antioxid Redox Signal* 2000;2:821-825.

42. Sen CK. Cellular thiols and redox-regulated signal transduction. *Curr Top Cell Regul* 2000;36:1-30.

43. Kodama M, Kodama T, Muramaki M. The value of the dehydroepiandrosterone-annexed vitamin C treatment in the clinical control of chronic fatigue syndrome I. A pilot study of the new vitamin C infusion treatment with volunteer CFS patients. *In Vivo* 1996;10:575-584.

44. Kodama M, Kodama T, Muramaki M. The value of the dehydroepiandrosterone-annexed vitamin C treatment in the clinical control of chronic fatigue syndrome II. Characterization of CFS patients with special reference to their reponse to a new vitamin C infusion treatment. *In Vivo* 1996;10:585-596.

45. Heuser G, Vojdani A. Enhancement of natural killer cell activity and T- and B-cell function by buffered vitamin C in patients exposed to toxic chemicals: the role of protein kinase C. *Immunopharmacol Immunotoxicol* 1997;19:291-312.

46. Conklin KA. Coenzyme Q10 for prevention of anthracycline-induced cardiotoxicity. *Integr Cancer Ther* 2005;4:110-130.

47. Chow CK. Dietary coenzyme Q10 and mitochondrial status. *Methods Enzymol* 2004;382:105-112.

48. Cooper JM, Schapira AH. Friedreich's ataxia: disease mechanisms, antioxidant and coenzyme Q10 therapy. *Biofactors* 2003;18:163-171.

49. Fosslien E. Review: mitochondrial medicine—cardiomyopathy caused by defective oxidative phosphorylation. *Ann Clin Lab Sci* 2003;33:371-395.

50. Zeviani M, Carelli V. Mitochodrial disorders. *Curr Opin Neurol* 2003;16:585-594.

51. Lisdero CL, Carreras MC, Meulmans A, et al. The mitochondrial interplay of ubiquinol and nitric oxide in endotoxemia. *Meth Enzymol* 2004;382:67-81.

52. Shopfer F, Riobo N, Carreras MC, et al. Oxidation of ubiquinol by peroxynitrite: implications for protection of mitochondria against nitrosative damage. *Biochem J* 2000;349:35-42.

53. Lass A, Sohal RS. The effect of coenzyme Q(10) and α–tocopherol content of mitochondria on the production of superoxide anions. *FASEB J* 2000;14:87-94.

54. Beal MF. Coenzyme Q10 administration and its potential for treatment of neurodegerative diseases. *Biofactors* 1999;9:261-266.

55. Dlugosz A, Sawicka E. The chemoprotective effect of coenzyme Q on lipids in the paint and laquer industry workers. *Int J Occup Med Environ Health* 11:153-163.

56. Chew GT, Watts GF. Coenzyme Q10 and diabetic endotheliopathy: oxidative stress and the 'recoupling hypothesis'. Also states that "long term safety and tolerability of CoQ supplementation has been consistently confirmed in several published animal and human trials." *Q J Med* 2004;97:537-548.

57. Bell DS. *The Doctor's Guide to Chronic Fatigue Syndrome.* Reading, MA: Addison Wesley Publishing Co.; 1995.

58. Lister RE. An open, pilot study to evaluate the potential benefits of coenzyme Q10 combined with Ginkgo biloba extract in fibromyalgia syndrome. *J Int Med Res* 2002;30:195-199.

59. Reinhard P, Schweinsberg F, Wernet D, Kotter I. Selenium status in fibromyalgia. *Toxicol Lett* 1998;96/97:177-180.

60. Klotz LO, Sies H. Defenses against peroxynitrite: selenocompounds and flavonoids. *Toxicol Lett* 2003;140-141:125-132.

61. Arteel GE, Mostert V, Oubrahim H, et al. Protection by selenoprotein P in human plasma against peroxynitrite-mediated oxidation and nitration. *Biol Chem* 1998;379:1201-1205.

62. Saito Y, Takahashi K. Characterization of selenoprotein P as a selenium supply protein. *Eur J Biochem* 2002;269:5746-5751.

63. Benton D. Selenium intake, mood and other aspects of psychological functioning. *Nutr Neurosci* 2002;5(6):363-374.

64. Panasenko OM, Sharov VS, Brivaba K, Sies H. Interaction of peroxynitrite with carotenoids in human low density lipoproteins. *Arch Biochem Biophys* 2000; 373:302-305.

65. Lavelli V, Hippeli S, Peri C, Elstner EF. Evaluation of radical scavenging activity of fresh and air-dried tomatoes by three model reactions. *J Agric Food Chem* 1999;47:3826-3831.

66. Kontush A, Weber W, Beisiegel U. Alpha- and beta-carotenes in low density lipoproteins are the preferred target for nitric oxide-induced oxidation. *Atherosclerosis* 2000;148:87-93.

67. Pannala AAS, Singh S, Rice-Evans C. Interaction of carotenoids and tocopherols with peroxynitrite. *Methods Enzymol* 1999;301:319-332.

68. Bohm F, Edge R, McGarvey DJ, Truscott TG. Beta-carotene with vitamins E and C offers synergistic cell protection against NOx. *FEBS Lett* 1998;436:387-389.

69. Scheidegger R, Pande AK, Bounds PL, Koppenol WH. The reaction of peroxynitrite with zeaxanthin. *Nitric Oxide* 1998;2:8-16.

70. Kikugawa K, Hiramoto K, Tomiyama S, Asano Y. β-Carotene effectively scavenges toxic nitrogen oxides: nitrogen dioxide and peroxynitrous acid. *FEBS Lett* 1997;404:175-178.

71. Edwards AM, Blackburn A, Christie S, Townsend A, David A. Food supplements in the treatment of fibromyalgia: a double-blind, crossover trial of anthocyanidins and placebo. *J Nutr Env Med* 2000;10:189-199.

72. Singal A, Kaur S, Tirkey N, Chopra K. Green tea extract catechins ameliorate chronic fatigue-induced oxidative stress in mice. *J Med Food* 2005;8:47-52.

73. Singh A, Naidu PS, Gupta S, Kulkarni SK. Effect of natural and synthetic antioxidants in a mouse model of chronic fatigue syndrome. *J Med Food* 2002;5:211-220.

74. Santos MR, Mira L. Protection by flavonoids against the peroxynitrite mediated oxidation of dihydrorhodamine. *Free Radic Res* 2004;38:1011-1018.

75. Yokozawa T, Rhyu DY, Cho EJ. (-)-Epicatechin 3-O-gallate ameliorates the damages related to peroxynitrite production by mechanisms distinct from those of other free radical inhibitors. *J Pharm Pharmacol* 2004;56:231-239.

76. Kim JY, Jung KJ, Choi JS, Chung HY. Hesperetin: a potent antioxidant against peroxynitrite. *Free Radic Res* 2004;38:761-769.

77. Olas B, Nowak P, Wachowicz B. Resveratrol protects against peroxynitrite-induced thiol oxidation in blood platelets. *Cell Mol Biol Lett* 2004;9:577-587.

78. Saint-Cricq De Gaulejac N, Provost C, Vivas N. Comparative study of polyphenol scavenging activities assessed by different methods. *J Agric Food Chem* 1999;47:425-431.

79. Behar-Cohen FF, Heydolph S, Faure V, et al. Peroxynitrite cytotoxicity on bovine retinal pigmented epithelial cells in culture. *Biochem Biophys Res Commun* 1996;226:842-849.

80. Mantle D, Eddeb F, Pickering AT. Comparison of relative antioxidant activities of British medicinal plant species in vitro. *J Ethnopharmacol* 2000;72:47-51.

81. Marcocci L, Maguire JJ, Droy-Lefaix MT, and Packer L. The nitric oxide-scavenging properties of Ginkgo biloba extract EGb 761. *Biochem Biophys Res Commun* 1994;201:748-755.

82. Pillai SP, Mitscher LA, Menon SR, Pillai CA, Shankel DM. Antimutagenic/antioxidant activity of green tea components and related compounds. *J Environ Pathol Toxicol Oncol* 1999;18:147-158.

83. Getha T, Garg A, Chopra K, Pal Kaur I. Delineation of antimutagenic activity of catechin, epicatechin and green tea extract. *Mutat Res* 2004;556:65-74.

84. Nakagawa T, Yokozawa T. Direct scavenging of nitric oxide and superoxide by green tea. *Food Chem Toxicol* 2002;40:1745-1750.

85. Yokozawa T, Rhyu DY, Cho EJ. (-)-Epicatechin 3-O-gallate ameliorates the damages related to peroxynitrite production by mechanisms distinct from those of other free radical inhibitors. *J Pharm Pharmacol* 2004;56:231-239.

86. Kruk I, Aboul-Enein HY, Michalska T, Lichszteld K, Kladna A. Scavenging of reactive oxygen species by the plant phenols genistein and oleuropein. *Luminescence* 2005;20:81-90.

87. VafeiAdou K, Weinberg PD. Antioxidant and free radical scavenging activity of isoflavone metabolites. *Xenobiotica* 2003;33:913-925.

88. Bahoran T, Gressier B, Trotin F, et al. Oxygen species scavenging activity of phenolic extracts from hawthorn fresh plant organs and pharmaceutical preparations. *Arzneimittelforschung* 1996;46:1081-1089.

89. Ichikawa H, Ichiyanagi T, Xu B, et al. Antioxidant activity of anthocyanin extract from purple black rice. *J Med Food* 2001;4:211-218.

90. Seki M, Kobayashi H. Inhibition of xanthine oxidase by flavonoids. *Biosci Biotech Biochem* 1999;63:1787-1790.

91. Feher J, Lang I, Nekam K, Gergely P, Muzes G. In vivo effect of free radical scavenger hepatoprotective agents on superoxide dismutase (SOD) activity in patients. *Tokai J Exp Clin Med* 1990;15:129-134.

92. Ghyczy M, Boros M. Electrophilic methyl groups present in the diet ameliorate pathologicl states induced by reductive and oxidative stress: a hypothesis. *Br J Nutr* 2001;85:409-414.

93. Sanchez-Perez AM, Montoliu C, Felipo V. Trialkylglycines: a new family of compounds with in vivo neuroprotection. *CNS Drug Reviews* 2003;9:263-274.

94. Llansola M, Erceg S, Hernandez-Viadel M, Felipo V. Prevention of ammonia and glutamate neurotoxicity by carnitine: molecular mechanisms. *Metab Brain Dis* 2002;17:389-397.

95. Bigini P, Larini S, Pasquali C, Muzio V, Menini T. Acetyl-L-carnitine shows neuroprotective and neurotrophic activity in primary culture of rat embryo motoneurons. *Neurosci Lett* 2002;329:334-338.

96. Llansola M, Felipo V. Carnitine prevents NMDA receptor mediated activation of MAP-kinase and phosphorylation of microtubule-associated protein 2 in cerebellar neurons in culture. *Brain Res* 2002;947:50-56.

97. Felipo V, Hermenegildo C, Montoliu C, Llansola M, Minana MD. Neurotoxicity of ammonia and glutamate: molecular mechanisms and prevention. *Neurotoxicol* 1998;19:675-681.

98. Ghyczy M, Torday C, Boros M. Simultaneous generation of methane carbon dioxide, and carbon monoxide from choline and ascorbic acid: a defensive mechanism against reductive stress? *FASEB J* 2003;17:1124-1126.

99. Fetrow CW, Avila JR. Efficacy of the dietary supplement S-adenosyl-L-methionine. *Annals Pharmacother* 2001;35:1414-1425.

100. Craig SA. Betaine in human nutrition. *Am J Clin Nutr* 2002;80:239-249.

101. Plioplys AV, Plioplys S. Amantadine and L-carnitine treatment of chronic fatigue syndrome. *Neuropsychobiology* 1997;35:16-23.

102. Vermeulen RC, Scholte HR. Exploratory open label, randomized study of acetyl- and proprionylcarnitine in chronic fatigue syndrome. *Psychosom Med* 2004;66:276-282.

103. Kuratsune H, Yamaguti K, Lindh G, et al. Brain regions involved in fatigue sensation: reduced acetylcarnitine uptake into the brain. *Neuroimage* 2002;17:1256-1265.

104. Kuratsune H, Yamaguti K, Lindh G, et al. Low serum levels of serum acylcarnitine in chronic fatigue syndrome and chronic hepatitis type C, but not other diseases. *Int J Mol Med* 1998;2:51-56.

105. Liu J, Head, E, Kuratsune H, Cotman CW, Ames BN. Comparison of the effects of L-carnitine and acetyl-L-carnitine on carnitine levels, ambulatory activity, and oxidative stress biomarkers in the brain of old rats. *Ann NY Acad Sci* 2004;1033:117-131.

106. Paradies G, Petrosillo G, Pistolese M, Ruggiero FM. Reactive oxygen species affect mitochondrial electron transport complex I activity through oxidative cardiolipin damage. *Gene* 2002;286:135-141.

107. Zanelli SA, Solenski NJ, Rosenthal RE, Fiskum G. Mechanisms of neuroprotection by acetyl-L-carnitine. *Ann NY Acad Sci* 2005;1053:153-161.

108. Binienda Z, Przybyla-Zawislak B, Virmani A, Schmued L. L-carnitine and neuroprotection in the animal model of mitochondrial dysfunction. *Neurosci Lett* 2004;367:264-267.

109. Inano A, Sai Y, Nikaido H, et al. Acetyl-L-carnitine permeability across the blood-brain barrier and involvement of carnitine transported OCTN2. *Biophar Drug Dispos* 2003;24:357-365.

110. Kuratsune H, Watanabe Y, Yanaguti K, et al. High uptake of [2-(11)] acetyl-L-carnitine into the brain: a PET study. *Biochem Biophys Res Commun* 1997;231: 488-493.

111. Ellithorpe RR, Settinery RA, Nicolson GL. Pilot study: reduction of fatigue by use of a supplement containing dietary glycophospholipids. *J Am Neutraceutical Assoc* 2003;6:23-28.

112. Agadjanyan M, Vasilevko V, Ghochikyan A, et al. Nutritional supplement (NT Factor) restores mitochondrial function and reduces moderately severe fatigue in aged subjects. *J Chronic Fatigue Syndr* 2003;11(4):1-12.

113. van der Kuy PH, Merkus FW, Lohman JJ, ter Berg JW, Hooymans PM. Hydroxocobalamin, a nitric oxide scavenger, in the prophylaxis of migraine: an open pilot study. *Cephalagia* 2002;22:513-519.

114. Delpre G, Stark P, Niv Y. Sublingual therapy for cobalamin deficiency as an alternative to oral and parenteral cobalamin supplementation. *Lancet* 1999;354: 740-741.

115. Sharabi A, Cohen E, Sulkes J, Garty M. Replacement therapy for vitamin B12 deficiency: comparison between the sublingual and the oral route. *Br J Clin Pharmacol* 2003;56:635-638.

116. Botez MI, Motez T, Leveille J, et al. Neuropsychological correlates of folic acid deficiency: facts and hypotheses. In: Botez MI, Reynolds EH, eds. *Folic Acid in Neurology, Pychiatry, and Internal Medicine.* New York: Raven Press;1979.

117. Kaslow JE, Rucker L, Onishi R. Liver extract-folic acid-cyanocobalamin vs placebo for chronic fatigue syndrome. *Arch Intern Med* 1989;149:2501-2503.

118. Stanger O, Weger M. Interactions of homocysteine, nitric oxide, folate and radicals in the progressively damaged endothelium. *Clin Chem Lab Med* 2003;41: 1444-1454.

119. Sawabe K, Wakasugi KO, Hasegawa H. Tetrahydrobiopterin uptake in supplemental administration: elevation of tissue tetrahydrobiopterin in mice following uptake of exogenously oxidized product 7,8-dihydrobiopterin and subsequent reduction of an anti-folate-sensitive process. *J Pharmacol Sci* 2004;96:124-133.

120. McCarty MF. Supplemental arginine and high-dose folate may promote bone health by supporting the activity of endothelial-type nitric oxide synthase in bone. *Med Hypoth* 2005;64:1030-1033.

121. Shi W, Meininger CJ, Haynes TE, Hatakeyama K, Wu G. Regulation of tetrahydrobiopterin synthesis and bioavailability in endothelial cells. *Cell Biochem Biophys* 2004;41:415-434.

122. Griffith TM, Chaytor AT, Bakker LM, Edwards DH. 5-methyltetrahydro-folate and tetrahydrobiopterin can modulate electronically mediated endothelium-dependent vascular relaxation. *Proc Natl Acad Sci USA* 2005;102:7008-7013.

123. Gorren AC, Schrammel A, Riethmuller C, et al. Nitric oxide-induced autoinhibition of neuronal nitric oxide synthase in the presence of the autoxidation-resistant pteridine 5-methyltetrahydrobiopterin. *Biochem J* 2000;347:475-484.

124. Stroes ES, van Faassen EE, Yo M, et al. Folic acid reverts dysfunction of endothelial nitric oxide synthase. *Circ Res* 2000;86:1129-1134.

125. Hyndman ME, Verma S, Rosenfeld RJ, Anderson TJ, Parsons HG. Interaction of 5-methyltetrahydrofolate and tetrahydrobiopterin on endothelial function. *Am J Physiol Heart Circ Physiol* 2002;282:H2167-H2172.

126. Ihlemann N, Rask-Madsen C, Perner A, et al. Tetrahydrobiopterin restore endothelian dysfunction induced by an oral glucose challenge in healthy subjects. *Am J Physiol Heart Circ Physiol* 2003;285:H875-882.

127. Shimizu S, Ishii M, Miyasaka Y, et al. Possible involvement of hydroxyl radical on the stimulation of tetrahydrobiopterin synthesis by hydrogen peroxide and peroxynitrite in vascular endothelial cells. *Int J Biochem Cell Biol* 2005;37:864-875.

128. Ebadi M, Gessert CF, Al-Sayegh A. Drug-pyridoxal phosphate interactions. *Q Rev Drug Metab Drug Interact* 1982;4:L289-331.

129. Kaneda K, Kikuchi M, Kashii S, et al. The effects of B vitamins on glutamate-induced neurotoxicity in retinal cultures. *Eur J Pharmacol* 1997;322:259-264.

130. Dawber, Diane. *Lifting the Bull: Overcoming Chronic Back Pain, Fibromyalgia and Environmental Illness.* Quarry Press;1999.

131. Wang HS, Kuo MF, Chou ML, et al. Pyridoxal phosphate is better than pyridoxine for controlling idiopathic intractable epilepsy. *Arch Dis Child* 2005;90:512-515.

132. Matsubara K, Mori M, Akagi R, Kato N. Anti-angiogenic effect of pyridoxal 5'-phosphate, pyridoxal and pyridoxamine on embryoid bodies derived from mouse embryonic stem cells. *In J Mol Med* 2004;14:819-823.

133. Hustad S, McKinley MC, McNulty H, et al. Riboflavin, flavin mononucleotide, and flavin adenine dinucleotide in human plasma and erythrocytes at baseline and after low-dose riboflavin supplementation. *Clin Chem* 2002;48:1571-1577.

134. Prentice AM, Bates CJ. A biochemical evaluation of the erythrocyte glutathione reductase (EC 1.6.4.2) test for riboflavin status 2. Dose-response relationships in chronic marginal deficiency. *Br J Nutr* 1981;45:53-65.

135. Clements JE, Anderson BB. Glutathione reductase activity and pyridoxine (pyridoxamine) oxidase activity in the red cell. *Biochem Biophys Acta* 1980;632:159-163.

136. Droge Wm Holm E. Role of cysteine and glutathione in HIV infection and other diseases associated with muscle wasting and immunological dysfunction. *FASEB J* 1997;11:1077-1089.

137. Bounous G, Molson J. Competition for glutathione precursors between the immune system and skeletal muscle: pathogenesis of chronic fatigue syndrome. *Med Hypoth* 1999;53:347-349.

138. Witschi A, Reddy S, Stofer B, Lauterburg BH. The systemic availability of oral glutathione. *Eur J Clin Pharmacol* 1992;43:667-669.

139. Kannan R, Mittur A, Bao Y, Tsuruo T, Kaplowitz N. GSH transport in immortalized mouse brain endothelial cells: evidence for apical localization of a sodium-dependent GSH transporter. *Neurochem* 1999;73:390-399.

140. Kannan R, Bao Y, Mittur A, Andley UP, Kaplowitz N. Glutathione transport in immortalized HLE cells and expression of transport in HLE cell poly(A)+ RNA injected Xenopus oocytes. *Invest Ophthalmol Vis Sci* 1998;39:1379-1386.

141. Kannan R, Mittur A, Bao Y, Tsuruo T, Kaplowitz N. GSH transport in immortalized mouse brain endothelial cells: evidence for apical localization of a sodium-dependent GSH transporter. *J Neurochem* 1999;73:390-399.

142. Zlokovic BV, Mackic JB, McComb JG, et al. Evidence for transcapillary transport of reduced glutathione in vascular perfused guinea-pig brain. *Biochem Biophys Res Commun* 1994;201:402-408.

143. Mathisen GA, Fonnum F, Paulsen RE. Contributing mechanims for cysteine excitotoxicity in cultured granule cells. *Neurochem Res* 1996;21:293-298.

144. Janaky R, Varga V, Hermann A, Saransaari P, Oja SS. Mechanisms of L-cysteine neurotoxicity. *Neurochem Res* 2000;25:1397-1405.

145. Piani D, Fontana A. Involvement of the cystine transport system xc- in the macrophage-induced glutamate-dependent cytotoxicity in neurons. *J Immunol* 1994; 152:3578-3585.

146. Warr O, Takahashi M, Attwell D. Modulation of extracellular glutamate concentration in rat brain slices by cystine-glutamate exchange. *J Physiol* 1999; 514:783-793.

147. http://www.cfsresearch.org/cfs/cheney/5.htm

148. http://www.cfsresearch.org/cfs/research/treatment/13.htm

149. http://www.cfsresearch.org/cfs/cheney/14.htm

150. http://www.cfsresearch.org/cfs/conferences/4.htm

151. Sen CK, Packer L. Thiol homeostasis and supplements in physical exercise. *Am J Clin Nutr* 2000;72(2 Suppl):653S-669S.

152. Smith AR, Shenvi SV, Widlanski M, Suh JH, Hagen TM. Lipoic acid as a potential therapy for chronic diseases associated with oxidative stress. *Curr Med Chem* 2004;11:1135-1146.

153. Wollin SD, Jones PJ. Alpha-lipoic acid and cardiovascular disease. *J Nutr* 2003;133:3327-3330.

154. Moini H, Packer L, Saris NE. Antioxidant and prooxidant activities of alpha-lipoic acid and dihydrolipoic acid. *Toxicol Appl Pharmacol* 2002;182:84-90.

155. Packer L, Kraemer K, Rimbach G. Molecular aspects of lipoic acid in the prevention of diabetes complications. *Nutrition* 2001;17:888-895.

156. Packer L, Tritschler HJ, Wessel K. Neuroprotection by the metabolic antioxidant alpha-lipoic acid. *Free Radic Biol Med* 1997;22:359-378.

157. Trujillo M, Folkes L, Bartesaghi S, et al. Peroxynitrite-derived carbonate and nitrogen dioxide radicals readily react with lipoic acid and dihydrolipoic acid. *Free Radic Biol Med* 2005;39:279-288.

158. Bast A, Haenen GR. Interplay between lipoic acid and glutathione in the protection of microsomal lipid peroxidation. *Biochim Biophys Acta* 1988;963:558-561.

159. Porras P, Pedrejas JR, Martinez-Galisteo E, et al. 2002 *Glutaredoxins cata-lyze the reduction of glutathione by dihydrolipoamide with high efficiency.*

160. Turner RE, Langkamp-Henken B, Littell RC, Lukowski MJ, Suarez MF. Comparing nutrient intake from food to the estimated average requirements shows middle- to upper-income pregnant women lack iron and possibly magnesium. *J Am Diet Assoc* 2003;103:461-466.

161. Vaquero MP. Magnesium and trace elements in the elderly: intake, status and recommendations. *J Nutr Health Aging* 2002;6:147-153.

162. Gullestad L, Nes M, Ronneberg R, et al. Magnesium status in healthy free-living elderly Norwegians. *J Am Coll Nutr* 1994;13:45-50.

163. Kubena KS, Durlach J. Historical review of the effects of marginal intake of magnesium in chronic experimental magnesium deficiency. *Magnes Res* 1990;3: 219-226.

164. Durlach J. Recommended dietary amounts of magnesium: Mg RDA. *Magnes Res* 1989;2:195-203.

165. Durlach J, Bac P, Durlach V, Rayssiguier Y, Bara M. Magnesium status and ageing: an update. *Magnes Res* 1998;11:25-42.

166. Abbott RD, Ando F, Masaki KH, et al. Dietary magnesium intake and future risk of coronary heart disease (the Honolulu Heart Program). *Am J Cardiol* 2003; 92:655-659.

167. Nair RR, Nair P. Alteration of myocardial mechanics in marginal magnesium deficiency. *Magnes Res* 2002;15:287-306.

168. Chakraborti S, Chakraborti T, Mandal M, et al. Protective role of magnesium in cardiovascular diseases: a review. *Mol Cell Biochem* 2002;238:163-179.

169. Landon RA, Young EA. Role of magnesium in lung function. *J Am Diet Assoc* 1993;93:674-677.

170. Seelig MS, Berger AR, Spielholz N. Latent tetany and anxiety, marginal magnesiumdeficit and normocalcemia. *Dis Nerv Syst* 1975;36:461-465.

171. Altura BM, Altura BT. Tension headaches and muscle tension: is there a role for magnesium? *Med Hypoth* 2001;57:705-713.

172. Sarchielli P, Coata G, Firenze V, et al. Serum and salivary magnesium levels in migraine and tension-type headache. Results in a group of adult patients. *Cephal-algia* 1992;12:21-27.

173. Held K, Antonijevic IA, Kunzel H, et al. Oral Mg(2+) supplementation reverses age-related neuroendocrine and sleep EEG changes. *Pharmacopsychiatry* 2002;35:135-143.

174. Penland JG. Quantitative analysis of EEG effects following experimental marginal magnesium and boron deprivation. *Magnew Res* 1995;8:341-358.

175. Cox IM, Campbell MJ, Dowson D. Red blood cell magnesium and chronic fatigue syndrome. *Lancet* 1991;337:757-760.

176. Manuel y Keenoy B, Moorkens G, Vertommen J, et al. Magnesium status and parameters of the oxidant-antioxidant balance in patients with chronic fatigue: effects of supplementation with magnesium. *J Am Coll Nutr* 2000;19:374-382.

177. Clague JE, Edwards RHT, Jackson MJ. Intravenous magnesium loading in chronic fatigue syndrome. *Lancet* 1992;340:124-125.

178. Seelig M. Review and hypothesis: might patients with chronic fatigue syndrome have latent tetany of magnesium deficiency. *J Chronic Fatigue Syndr* 1998; 4(2):77-118.

179. Kurup RK, Kurup PA. Hypothalamic digoxin, cerebral chemical dominance and myalgic encephalomyelitis. *Int J Neurosci* 2003;113:445-457.

180. Russell IJ, Michalek JE, Flechas JD, Abraham GE. Treatment of fibromyalgia syndrome with super malic: a randomized, double blind, placebo controlled crossover pilot study. *J Rheumatol* 1995;22:953-958.

181. Abraham GE, Flechas JD. Management of fibromyalgia: rationale for the use of magnesium and malic acid. *J Nutr Med* 1992;3:49-52.

182. Ho E, Ames BN. Low intracellular zinc induces oxidative DNA damage, disrupts p53, NF-κB and AP1 DNA-binding, and effects DNA repair in a rat glioma cell line. *Proc Natl Acad Sci USA* 2002;99:16770-16775.

183. Hennig N, Meerarani P, Toborek M, McClain CJ. Antioxidant-like properties of zinc in activated endothelial cells. *J Am Coll Nutr* 1999;18:152-158.

184. Hawk SN, Lanoue L, Keen CL, et al. Copper-deficient rat embryos are characterized by low superoxide dismutase activity and elevated superoxide ions. *Biol Reprod* 2003;68:896-903.

185. Uriu-Adams JY, Keen CL. Copper, oxidative stress, and human health. *Mol Aspects Med* 2005;26:268-298.

186. Pucheu S, Coudray C, Tresallet N, Favier A, de Leiris J. Effect of dietary antioxidant trace element supply on cardiac tolerance to ischemia-reperfusion in rat. *J Mol Cell Cardiol* 1995;27:2303-2314.

187. Evans P, Halliwell B. Micronutrients: oxidant/antioxidant status. *Br J Nutr* 2001;85(Suppl 2):S67-S74.

188. Johnson F, Giulivi C. Superoxide dismutases and their impact upon human health. *Mol Aspects Med* 2005;26:340-352.

189. Graven-Nielsen T, Aspegren Kendall SA, Henriksson KG, et al. Jetamine reduces muscle pain, temporal summation abd referred pain in fibromyalgia patients. *Pain* 2000;85:483-491.

190. Oye I, Rabben T, Fagerlund TH. Analgesic effect of ketamine in a patient with neuropathic pain. *Tidsskr Not Laegeforen* 1996;116:3130-3131.

191. Sorensen J, Bengtsson A, Backman E, et al. Pain analysis in patients with fibromyalgia. Effects of intravenous morphine, lidocaine and ketamine. *Scand J Rheumatol* 1995;24:360-365.

192. Bennett R. Fibromyalgia, chronic fatigue syndrome and myofascial pain. *Curr Opin Rheumatol* 1998;2:95-103.

193. Nicolodi M, Volpe AR, Sicuderi F. Fibromyalgia and headache: Failure of serotonergic analgesia and N-methyl-D-aspartate-mediated neuronal plasticity: their common clues. *Cephalalgia* 1998;18(Suppl 21):41-44.

194. Graven-Nielsen T, Aspergren Kendall S, Hensiksson KG, et al. Ketamine reduces muscle pain, temporal summation, and referred pain in fibromyalgia patients. *Pain* 200;85:483-491.

195. Stoll AL. Fibromyalgia symptoms relieved by flupirtine: an open label case series. *Psychosomatics* 2000;41:371-372.

196. Buskila D. Fibromyalgia, chronic fatigue syndrome and myofascial pain syndrome. *Curr Opin Rheumatol* 2001;13:117-127.

197. Henriksson KG, Sorensen J. The promise of N-methyl-D-aspartate receptor antagonists in fibromyalgia. *Rheum Dis Clin North Am* 2002;28:343-351.

198. Hocking G, Cousins MJ. Ketamine in chronic pain management: an evidence-based review. *Anesth Analg* 2003;97:1730-1739.

199. Staud SR, Vierck CJ, Robinson ME, Price DD. Effects of the N-methyl-d-aspartate receptors antagonist dextromethorphan on temporal summation of pain are similar in fibromyalgia patients and normal control subjects. *J Pain* 2005;6:323-332.

200. Goldstein JA. *Tuning the Brain: Principles and Practice of Neurosomatic Medicine*. Binghamton, NY: Haworth Medical Press;2004.

201. Dudley DL. MCS: trial by science. In: Matthews BL ed, *Defining Multiple Chemical Sensitivity*, Jefferson, NC: McFarland & Company;1998:9-26.

202. Chuang DM. Neuroprotective and neurotrophic actions of the mood stabilizer lithium: can it be used to treat neurodegenerative diseases? *Crit Rev Neurobiol* 2004;16:83-90.

203. Hashimoto R, Fujimaki K, Jeong MR, Christ L, Chuang DM. Lithium-induced inhibition of Src tyrosine kinase in rat cerebral cortical neurons: a role in neuroprotection against N-methyl-D-aspartate receptor-mediated excitoxicity. *FEBS Lett* 538:145-148.

204. McGeer EG, McGeer PL. Pharmacologic approaches to the treatment of amyotrophic lateral sclerosis. *BioDrugs* 2005;19:31-37.

205. Bensimon G, Doble A. The tolerability of riluzole in the treatment of patients with amyotrophic lateral sclerosis. *Expert Opin Drug Saf* 2004;3:525-534.

206. Snow RJ, Turnbull J, da Silva S, Jiang F, Tarnopolsky MA. Creatine supplementation and riluzole treatment provide similar beneficial effects in copper, zinc superoxide dismutase (G93A) transgenic mice. *Neuroscience* 2003;119:661-667.

207. Schiefer J, Landswehrmeyer GB, Luesse HG, et al. Riluzole prolongs survival time and alters nuclear inclusion formation in a transgenic mouse model of Huntington's disease. *Mov Disord* 2002;17:748-757.

208. Seppi K, Mueller K, Bodner T, et al. Riluzole in Huntington's disease (HD): an open label study with one year follow up. *J Neurol* 2001;248:866-869.

209. Fernandez-Espejo E. Pathogenesis of Parkinson's disease: prospects of neuroprotective and restorative therapies. *Mol Neurobiol* 2004;29:15-30.

210. Shwartz G, Fehlings MG. Secondary injury mechanisms of spinal cord trauma: a novel therapeutic approach for the management of secondary pathophysiology with the sodium channel blocker riluzole. *Prog Brain Res* 2002;137:177-190.

211. Jones MG, Cooper E, Amjad S, et al. Urinary and plasma organic acids and amino acids in chronic fatigue syndrome. *Clin Chim Acta* 2005;361:150-158.

212. Ziem GE. Profile of patients with chemical injury and sensitivity, Part II. *Int J Toxicol* 1999;18:401-409.

213. Larson AA, Giovengo SL, Russell IJ, Michalek JE. Changes in concentrations of amino acids in the cerebrospinal fluid that correlate with pain in patients with fibromyalgia: implications for nitric oxide pathways. *Pain* 2000;87:201-211.

214. Cozzi R, Ricordi R, Bartolini F, et al. Taurine and ellagic acid: two differently-acting natural antioxidants. *Environ Mol Mutagen* 1995;26:248-254.

215. Kim JW, Kim C. Inhibition of LPS-induced NO production by taurine chloramines in macrophages is mediated through Ras-ERK-NF-kappa B. *Biochem Pharmacol* 2005;70:1352-1360.

216. Serban V, Liu Y, Quinn MR. Production of nitric oxide by activated microglial cells is inhibited by taurine chloramines. *Adv Exp Med Biol* 2003;526: 357-364.

217. Elldrissi A, Trenkner E. Taurine as a modulator of excitatory and inhibitory neurotransmission. *Neurochem Res* 2004;29:189-197.

218. Lee NY, Kang YS. The brain-to-blood efflux transport of taurine and changes in the blood-brain barrier transport system by tumor necrosis factor-alpha. *Brain Res* 2004;1023:141-147.

219. Kuriyama K, Hashimoto T. Interrelationships between taurine and GABA. *Adv Exp Med Biol* 1998;442:329-337.

220. Olive MF. Interactions between taurine and ethanol in the central nervous system. *Amino Acids* 2002;23:345-357.

221. Song Z, Hatton GI. Taurine and the control of basal hormone release from rat neurohypophysis. *Exp Neurol* 2003;183:330-337.

222. Mori M, Gahwiler BH, Gerber U. Beta-alanine and taurine as endogenous agonists at glycine receptors in rat hippocampus in vitro. *J Physiol* 2002;539: 191-200.

223. Belluzzi O, Puopolo M, Benedusi M, Kratskin I. Selective neuroinhibitory effects of taurine in slices of the rat olfactory bulb. *Neurosci* 2004;124:929-944.

224. Hilgier W, Oja SS, Sansaari P, Albrecht J. Taurine prevents ammonia-induced accumulation of cyclic GMP in rat striatum by interaction with GABAA and glycine receptors. *Brain Res* 2005;1043:242-246.

225. Oja SS, Sansaari P. Modulation of taurine release by glutamate receptors and nitric oxide. *Prog Neurobiol* 2000;62:407-425.

226. Foos TM, Wu JY. The role of taurine in the central nervous system and the modulation of intracellular calcium homeostasis. *Neurochem Res* 2002;27:21-26.

228. Bayer K, Ahmadi S, Zeilhofer HU. Gabapentin may inhibit synaptic transmission in the mouse spinal cord dorsal horn through a preferential block of P/Q-type Ca^{2+} channels. *Neuropharmalogy* 2004;46:743-749.

229. Yoon MH, Choi JI, Jeong SW. Spinal gabapentin and antinociception: mechanisms of action. *J Korean Med Sci* 2003;18:255-261.

230. Ames BN, Cathcart R, Schwiers E, Hochstein P. Uric acid provides an antioxidant defense in humans against oxidant- and radical-caused aging and cancer: a hypothesis. *Proc Natl Acad Sci USA* 1981;78:6858-6862.

231. Ford E, Hughes MN, Wardman P. Kinetics of the reactions of nitrogen dioxide with glutathione, cysteine, and uric acid at physiological pH. *Free Radic Biol Med* 2002;32:1314-1323.

232. Kuzkaya N, Weissmann N, Harrison DG, Dikalov S. Interactions of peroxynitrite with uric acid in the presence of ascorbate and thiols: implications for uncoupling endothelial nitric oxide synthase. *Biochem Pharmacol* 2005;70:343-345.

233. Robinson KM, Morre JT, Beckman JS. Triuret: a novel product of peroxynitrite-mediated oxidation of urate. *Arch Biochem Biophys* 2004;423:213-217.

234. Teng RJ, Ye YZ, Parks DA, Beckman JS. Urate produced during hypoxia protects heart proteins from peroxynitrite-mediated protein nitration. *Free Radic Biol Med* 2002;33:1243-1249.

235. Whiteman M, Ketsawatsakul Halliwell B. A reassessment of the peroxynitrite scavenging activity of uric acid. *Ann NY Acad Sci* 2002;962:242-259.

236. Hooper DC, Scott GS, Zborek A, et al. Uric acid, a peroxynitrite scavenger, inhibits CNS inflammation, blood-CNS barrier permeability changes, and tissue damage in a mouse model of multiple sclerosis. *FASEB J* 2000;14:691-698.

237. Mattle HP, Lienert C, Greeve I. Uric acid and multiple sclerosis. *Ther Umsch* 2004;61:553-555.

238. Rentzos M, Nikolaou C, Anagnostouli M, et al. Serum uric acid and multiple sclerosis. *Clin Neurol Neurosurg* 2005;Sep 30 [Epub ahead of print].

239. Scott GS, Spitsin SV, Kean RB. Therapeutic intervention in experimental allergic encephalomyelitis by administration of uric acid precursors. *Proc Natl Acad Sci USA* 2002;99:16303-16308.

240. Spitsin S, Hooper DC, Leist T, et al. Inactivation of peroxynitrite in multiple sclerosis patients after oral administration of inosine may suggest possible approaches to therapy of the disease. *Mult Scler* 2001;7:313-319.

241. Scott GS, Cuzzocrea S, Genovese T, Koprowski H, Hooper DC. Uric acid protects against secondary damage after spinal cord injury. *Proc Natl Acad Sci USA* 2005;102:3483-3488.

242. Hoeldtke RD, Bryner KD, McNeil DR, et al. Nitrosative stress, uric acid, and peripheral nerve function in early type 1 diabetes. *Diabetes* 2002;51:2817-2825.

243. Schneider S, Klein HH. Inosine improves islet xenograft survival in immunocompetant diabetic mice. *Eur J Med Res* 2005;10:283-286.

244. Shen H, Chen GJ, Harvey BK, Bickford PC, Wang Y. Inosine reduces ischemic brain injury in rats. *Stroke* 2005;36:654-659.

245. Liu Z, Wang D, Xue Q, et al. Determination of fatty acid levels in erythrocyte membranes of patients with chronic fatigue syndrome. *Nutr Neurosci* 2003;6:389-392.

246. Horrobin DF. Post-viral fatigue syndrome, viral infections in atopic eczema, and essential fatty acids. *Med Hypoth* 1990;32:211-217.

247. Behan PO, Behan WM, Horrobin D. Effect of high doses of essential fatty acids on the postviral fatigue syndrome. *Acta Neurol Scand* 1990;82:209-216.

248. Pall ML. Elevated, sustained peroxynitrite levels as the cause of chronic fatigue syndrome. *Medical Hypoth* 2000;54:115-125.

249. Puri BK, Holmes J, Hamilton G. Eicosapentaenoic acid-rich essential fatty acid supplementation in chronic fatigue syndrome associated with symptom remission and structural brain changes. *Int J Clin Pract* 2004;58:297-299.

250. Puri BK. The use of eicosapentaenoic acid in the treatment of chronic fatigue syndrome. *Protaglandins Leukot Essent Fatty Acids* 2004;70:399-401.

251. Ozgocmen S, Catal SA, Ardicoglu O, Kamanli A. Effect of omega-3 fatty acids in management of fibromyalgia. *Int J Clin Pharmacol Ther* 2000;38:362-363.

252. Warren G, McKendrick M, Peet M. The role of essential fatty acids in chronic fatigue syndrome. A case-controlled study of red-cell membrane essential fatty acids (EFA) and a placebo-controlled study with high dose EFA. *Acta Neurol Scan* 1999;99:112-116.

253. Komatsu W, Ishihara K, Murata M, et al. Docosahexaenoic acid suppresses nitric oxide production and inducible nitric oxide synthase expression in interferon-γ plus lipopolysaccharide-stimulated murine macrophages by inhibiting oxidative stress. *Free Rad Biol Med* 2003;34:1006-1016.

254. Khair-El-Din T, Sicher SC, Vazquez MA, et al. Transcription of the murine iNOS gene is inhibited by docosahexaenoic acid, a major constituent of fetal and neonatal sera as well as fish oil. *J Exp Med* 1996;183:1241-1246.

255. Ohata T, Fukuda K, Takahashi M, et al. Suppression of nitric oxide production in lipopolysaccharide-stimulated macrophage cells by omega-3 polyunsaturated fatty acids. *Jpn J Cancer Res* 1997;88:234-237.

256. Takahashi M, Tsuboyama-Kasaoko N, Nakatani T, et al. Fish oil feeding alters live gene expression to defend against PPAR-activation and ROS production. *Am J Physiol Gastrointest Liver Physiol* 2002;282:G338-G348. And blocks NF-kappa B activation.

257. Zhao Y, Joshi-Barve S, Barve S, Chen LH. Eicosapentaenoic acid prevents LPS-induced TNF-α expression by preventing NF-κB expression. *J Am Coll Nutr* 2004;23:71-78.

258. Yoneda K, Yamamoto T, Ueta E, Osaki T. Suppression by azelastine hydrochloride of NF-kappa B activation involved in generation of cytokines and nitric oxide. *Jpn J Pharmacol* 1997;73:145-153.

259. Kempuraj D, Huang M, Kandere-Grzybowska K, et al. Azelastine inhibits secretion of IL-6, TNF-alpha and IL-8 as well as NF-kappa B activation and intracellular calcium ion levels in normal human mast cells. *Int Arch Allergy Immunol* 2003;132:231-239.

260. Bork PM, Schmitz ML, Kuhnt M, Escher C, Heinrich M. Sesquiterpene lactone containing Mexican Indian medicinal plants and pure sesquiterpene lactones as potent inhibitors of transcription factor NF-kappa B. *FEBS Lett* 1997;402:85-90.

261. Garcia-Pineres AJ, Lindenmayer MT, Merfort I. Role of cysteine residues of p65/NF-kappa B on the inhibition by the sesquiterpene lactone parthenolide and N-ethyl maleimide, and on its transactivating potential. *Life Sci* 2004;75:841-856.

262. Guzman ML, Rossi RM, Karnischky K. et al. The sesquiterpene lactone parthenolide induces apoptosis of human acute myelogenous leukemia and progenitor cells. *Blood* 2005;105:4163-4169.

263. Riggins RB, Zwart A, Nehra R, Clarke R. The nuclear factor kappa B inhibitor pathenolide restores ICI 182,780 (Faslodex;fulvestrant)-induced apoptosis in antiestrogen-resistant breast cancer cells. *Mol Cancer Ther* 2005;4:33-41.

264. Sandoval-Chacon M, Thompson JH, Zhang XJ, et al. Antiinflammatory action of cat's claw: the role of NF-kappa B. *Aliment Pharmacol Ther* 1998;12:1279-1289.

265. Akesson C, Lindgren H, Pero RW, et al. An extract of Uncaria tomentosa inhibiting cell division and NF-kappa B activity without inducing cell death. *Int Immunopharmacol* 2003;3:1889-1890.

266. Foster S, Tyler VE. *Tyler's Honest Herbal: A Sensible Guide to the Use of Herbals and Related Remedies.* Binghamton, NY: The Haworth Press;1998.

267. Biswas SK, McClure D, Jimenez LA, Megson IL, Rahman I. Curcumin induces glutathione biosynthesis and inhibits NF-kappa B activation and interleukin-8 release in alveolar epithelial cells: mechanisms of free radical scavenging activity. *Antioxid Redox Signal* 2005;7:32-41.

268. Kim JE, Kim AR, Chung HY, et al. In vitro peroxynitrite scavenging activity of diarylheptanoids from Curcuma longa. *Phytother Res* 2003;17:481-484.

269. Iwunze MO, McEwan D. Peroxynitrite interaction with curcumin solubilized in ethanolic solution. *Cell Mol Biol* 2004;50:749-752.

270. Vajragupta O, Boonchoong P, Berliner LJ. Manganese complexes of curcumin analogues: evaluation of hydroxyl radical scavenging ability, superoxide dismutase activity and stability towards hydrolysis. *Free Radic Res* 2004;38:303-314.

271. Barik A, Mishra B, Shen L, et al. Evaluation of a new copper(II)-curcumin complex as superoxide dismutase mimic and its free radical reactions. *Free Radic Biol Med* 2005;39:811-822.

272. Sumanont Y, Murakami Y, Tohda M, et al. Prevention of kainic acid-induced changes in nitric oxide level and neuronal cell damage in the rat hippocampus by manganese complexes of curcumin and diacetylcurcumin. *Life Sci* 2005;(Oct 30).

273. Merchant RE, Andre CA. A review of recent clinical trials of the nutritional supplement Chlorella pyrenoidosa in the treatment of fibromyalgia, hypertension and ulcerative colitis. *Altern Ther Health Med* 2001;7:79-91.

274. Merchant RE, Carmack CA, Wise CM. Nutritional supplementation with Chlorella pyrenoidosa for patients with fibromyalgia syndrome: a pilot study. *Phytother Res* 2000;14:167-173.

275. Shibata S, Natori Y, Nishihara T, et al. Antioxidant and anti-cataract effects of Chlorella on rats with streptozotocin-induced diabetes. *J Nutr Sci Vitaminol* 2003;49:334-339.

276. Guzman S, Gato A, Calleja JM. Antiinflammatory, analgesic and free radical scavenging activities of the marine microalgai, Chlorella Stigmatophora and Phaedactylum Triconutum. *Phytother Res* 2001;15:224-230.

277. Schubert H, Kroon BM, Matthijs HC. In vivo manipulation of the xanthophylls cycle and the role of zeaxanthin in the protection against photodamage in the green alga Chlorella pyrenoidosa. *J Biol Chem* 1994;269:7267-7272.

278. Pratt R, Johnson E. Vitamin C and choline content of Chlorella vulgaris and C. pyrenoidosa. *J Pharm Sci* 1967;56:536-537.

279. Wu LC, Ho JA, Shieh MC, Lu IW. Antioxidant and antiproliferative activities of Spirulina and Chlorella water extracts. *J Agric Food Chem* 2005;53:4207-4212.

280. Benedetti S, Benvenuti F, Pagliarani S, et al. Antioxidant properties of a novel phycocyanin extract from the blue-green alga Aphanizomenon flow-aquae. *Life Sci* 2004;75:2353-2362.

281. Halfen LN, Francis GW. The influence of culture temperature on the carotenoid composition of the blue-gree alga Anacystis nidulans. *Arch Mikrobiol* 1972;81:25-35

282. Bhat VB, Madyastha KM. Scavenging of peroxynitrite by phycocyanin and phycocyanobilin from Spirulina platensis: protection against oxidative damage to DNA. *Biochem Biophys Res Commun* 2001;285:262-266.

283. Hanninen O, Kaartinen K, Rauma A, et al. Antioxidants in vegan diet and rheumatic disorders. *Toxicology* 2000;155:45-53.

284. Yildiz S, Kiralp MZ, Akin A, et al. A new treatment modality for fibro-myalgia syndrome: hyperbaric oxygen. *J Int Med Res* 2004;32:263-267.

285. Van Hoof E, Coomans D, De Becker P, et al. Hyperbaric therapy in chronic fatigue syndrome. *J Chronic Fatigue Syndr* 2003;11:37-49.

286. Piantadosi CA, Tatro LG. Regional H_2O_2 concentration in rat brain after hyperoxic convulsions. *J Appl Physiol* 1990;69:1761-1766.

287. Rothfuss A, Dennog C, Speit G. Adaptive protection against the induction of oxidative DNA damage after hyperbaric oxygen treatment. *Carcinogenesis* 1998; 19:1913-1917.

288. Hink J, Jansen E. Are superoxide and/or hydrogen peroxide responsible for some of the beneficial effects of hyperbaric oxygen therapy? *Med Hypoth* 2001; 57:764-769.

289. Weinberg JM. The anti-inflammatory effects of tetracyclines. *Cutis* 2005; 75(4 Suppl):6-11.

290. Miyachi T, Yoshioka A, Imamura S, Niwa Y. Effect of antibiotics on the generation of reactive oxygen species. *J Invest Dematol* 1986;86:449-453.

291. Whiteman M, Kaur H, Halliwell B. Protection against peroxynitrite depend-ent tyrosine nitration and alpha-1antiproteinase inactivation by some anti-inflam-matory drugs and by the antibiotic tetracycline. *Ann Rheum Dis* 1996;55:383-387.

292. Kraus RL, Pasieczny R, Lariosa-Willingham K, et al. Antioxidant proper-ties of minocycline: neuroprotection in an oxidative stress assay and direct radical scavenging activity. *J Neurochem* 2005;94:819-827.

293. Zhu S, Stavrovskaya IG, Drozda M, et al. Minocycline inhibits cytochrome C release and delays progression of amyotrophic lateral sclerosis in mice. *Nature* 2002;417:74-78.

294. Kriz J, Nguyen MD, Julien JP. 2002 *Minocycline slows disease progression in a mouse model of amyotrophic lateral sclerosis.*

295. Lee SM, Yune TY, Kim SJ, et al. Minocycline inhibits apoptotic cell death via attenuation of TNF-a expression following iNOS/NO induction by lipopoly-saccharide in neuron/glia co-cultures. *J Neurochem* 2004;91:568-578.

296. Pi, R, Li W, Lee NTK, et al. Minocycline prevents glutamate-induced apoptosis of cerebellar granule neurons by differential regulation of p38 and Akt pathways. *J Neurochem* 2004;91:1219-1230.

297. Zhu S, Stavrovskaya IG, Drozda M, et al. Minocycline inhibits cytochrome C release and delays progression of amyotrophic lateral sclerosis in mice. *Nature* 2002;417:74-78.

298. Zhang W, Narayanan M, Friedlander RM. Additive neuroprotective effects of minocycline with creatine in a mouse model of ALS. *Ann Neurol* 2003;53:267-270.

299. Chem M, Ona VO, Li M, et al. Minocycline inhibits caspase-1 and caspase-3 expression and delays mortality in a transgenic mouse model of Huntington's disease. *Nat Med* 2000;6:797-801.

300. Pennington JAT. *Food Values of Portions Commonly Used.* 15th ed. Harper Perennial, 1989.

301. Andreassen OA, Jenkins BG, Dedeoglu A, et al. Increases in cortical glutamate concentrations in transgenic amyotrophic lateral sclerosis mice are attenuated by creatine supplementation. *J Neurochem* 2001;77:383-390.

302. Malcon C, Kaddurah-Daouk R, Beal MF. Neuroprotective effects of creatine administration against NMDA and malonate toxicity. *Brain Res* 2000;860:195-198.

303. Royes LF, Fighera MR, Furian AF, et al. Creatine protects against the convulsive behavior and lactate production elicited by the intrastriatal injection of methylmalonate. *Neuroscience* 2004;118:1079-1090.

304. Parnham M, Sies H. Ebselen: prospective therapy for cerebral ischaemia. *Expert Opin Investig Drugs* 2000;9:607-619.

305. Fujisawa S, Kadoma Y. Kinetic studies of radical-scavenging activity of ebselen, a seleno-organic compound. *Anticancer Res* 2005;25:3989-3994.

306. Nogueira CW, Quinhones EB, Jung EAC, Zeni G, Rocha JBT. Anti-inflammatory and antinociceptive activity of diphenylselenide. *Inflamm Res* 2003;52:56-63.

307. Herin GA, Du S, Aizenman E. The neuroprotective agent ebselen modifies NMDA receptor function via the redox modulatory site. *J Neurochem* 2001;78:1307-1314.

308. Kalayci M, Coskun O, Cagavi F, et al. Neuroprotective effects of ebselen on experimental spinal cord injury in rats. *Neurochem Res* 2005;30:403-410.

309. Fang J, Zhong L, Zhao R, Holmgren A. Ebselen: a thioredoxin reductase–dependent catalyst for alpha-tocopherol quinone reduction. *Toxicol Appl Pharmacol* 2005;207(2 Suppl):103-109.

310. Zhao R, Holmgren A. Ebselen is a dehydroascorbate reductase mimic, facilitating the recycling of ascorbate via mammalian thioredoxin systems. *Antioxid Redox Signal* 2004;6:99-104.

311. Asayama S, Nagaoka S, Kawakami H. Chemical modification of manganese porphyrins with biomolecules for new functional antioxidants. *J Biomater Sci Polym Ed* 2003;14:1169-1179.

312. Wu AS, Kiaei M, Aguirre N, et al. Iron porphyrin treatment extends survival in a transgenic animal model of amyotrophic lateral sclerosis. *J Neurochem* 2003;85:142-150.

313. Patel MN. Metalloporphyrins improve the survival of Sod2-deficient neurons. *Aging Cell* 2003;2:219-222.

314. Okado-Matsumoto A, Batinic-Haberle I, Fridovich I. Complementation of SOD–deficient Escherichia coli by manganes porphyrin mimics of superoxide dismutase. *Free Radic Biol Med* 2004;37:401-410.

315. Crow JP, Calingasan NY, Chen J, Hill JL, Beal MF. Manganese porphyrin given at symptom onset markedly extends survival of ALS mice. *Ann Neurol* 2005; 58:258-265.

316. Helme RD, Littlejohn GO, Weinstein C. Neurogenic flare responses in chronic rheumatic pain syndromes. *Clin Exp Neurol* 1987;23:91-94.

317. Morris V, Cruwys S, Kidd B. Increased capsaicin-induced secondary hyperalgesia as a marker of abnormal sensory activity in patients with fibromyalgia. *Neurosci Lett* 1998;250:205-7.

318. Staud R, Smitherman ML. Peripheral and central sensitization in fibromyalgia: pathogenetic role. *Curr Pain Headache Rep* 2002;6:259-266.

319. Pall ML, Anderson JH. The vanilloid receptor as a putative target of diverse chemicals in multiple chemical sensitivity. *Arch Environ Health* 2004;59:363-375.

320. McCarty DJ, Csuka M, McCarthy G, et al. Treatment of pain due to fibromyalgia with topical capsaicin: a pilot study. *Semin Arthritis Rheum* 1994; 23(Suppl 3):41-47.

321. Jung S-Y, Choi S, Ko Y-S, et al. Effects of ginsenosides on vanilloid receptor (VR1) channels expressed in Xenopus oocytes. *Mol Cells* 2001;12:342-346.

322. Hahn J, Nah SY, Nah J-J, Uhm D-Y, Chung S. Ginsenosides inhibit capsaicin–activated channel in rat sensory neurons. *Neurosci Lett* 2000;287:45-48.

323. Bennett RM, De Garmo P, Clark SR. A 1 year double blind placebo controlled study of guaifenesin in fibromyalgia. *Arth Rheum* 1996;39:S212.

324. Dicpinigaitis PV, Gayle YE. Effect of guaifenesin on cough reflex sensitivity. *Chest* 2003;124:2178-2181.

325. Reddy VP, Garrett MR, Perry G, Smith MA. Carnosine: a versatile antioxidant and antiglycating agent. *Sci Aging Knowledge Environ* 2005;2005:pe12.

326. Babishayev MA, Yermakova VN, Sakina NL, et al. N-alpha-acetylcarnosine is a prodrug of L-carnosine in ophthalmic application as an antioxidant. *Clin Chim Acta* 1997;254:1-21.

327. Fotana M, Pinnen F, Lucente G, Pecci L. Prevention of peroxynitrite-dependent damage by carnosine and related sulphanamido pseudodipeptides. *Cell Mol Life Sci* 2002;59:546-551.

328. Cacciatore I, Cocco A, Costa M, et al. Biochemical properties of new synthetic carnosine analogues containing the residue of 2,3-diaminopropionic acid: the effect of N-acetylation. *Amino Acids* 2005;28:77-83.

329. Chez MG, Buchanan CP, Aimonovitch MC, et al. Double-blind, placebo-controlled study of L-carnosine supplementation in children with autistic spectrum disorders. *J Child Neurol* 2002;17:833-837.

330. Pizzi M, Boroni F, Moraitis C, Memo M, Spano P. Neuroprotective effect of thyrotropin-releasing hormone against excitatory amino-acid-induced cell death in hippocampal slices. *Eur J Pharmacol* 1999;370:133-137.

331. Kinoshita K, Watanabe Y, Yamamura M, Matsuoka Y. TRH receptor agonists ameliorate 3-acetylpyridine-induced ataxia through NMDA receptors in rats. *Eur J Pharmacol* 1998;343:129-133.

332. Nakayama T, Hashimoto T, Nagai Y. Involvement of glutamate and gamma-aminobutyrate (GABA)-ergic systems in thyrotropin releasing hormone-induced cerebellar cGMP formation. *Eur J Pharmacol* 1996;316:157-164.

333. Koenig ML, Yourick DL, Meyerhoff JL. Thyrotropin-releasing hormone (TRH) attenuates glutamate-stimulated increases in calcium in primary neuronal cultures. *Brain Res* 1996;730:143-149.

334. http://virtualhometown.com/dfwcfids/medical/cheney.html#basic

335. Teitelbaum JE, Bird B, Greenfield RM, Weiss A, Muenz L, Gould L. Effective treatment of chronic fatigue syndrome and fibromyalgia: a randomized, double-blind, placebo-controlled, intent to treat study. *J Chronic Fatigue Syndr* 2002; 8(2):3-28.

336. Ellithorpe RR, Settinery RA, Nicolson GL. Pilot study: reduction of fatigue by use of a supplement containing dietary glycophospholipids. *J Am Neutraceutical Assoc* 2003;6:23-28.

337. Agadjanyan M, Vasilevko V, Ghochikyan A, et al. Nutritional supplement (NT Factor) restores mitochondrial function and reduces moderately severe fatigue in aged subjects. *J Chronic Fatigue Syndr* 2003;11(4):1-12.

339. http://www.cfidshealth.com/

340. http://home.earthlink.net/∼stompinangel/recovering.html#petrovic

341. Calderon C, Huang ZH, Gage DA, Sotomayor EM, Lopez DM. Isolation of a nitric oxide inhibitor from mammary tumor cells and its characterization as phosphatidyl serine. *J Exp Med* 1994;180:945-958.

342. DiNapoli MR, Calderon CL, Lopez DM. Phosphatidyl serine is involved in the reduced rate of transcription of the inducible nitric oxide synthase gene in macrophages from tumor-bearing mice. *J Immunol* 1997;158:1810-1817.

343. http://www.chemicalinjury.net/

344. Sackett DL. Evidence-based medicine: what it is and what it isn't. *BMJ* 1996;312:71-72.

Chapter 16

1. Kuhn, TS. *The Structure of Scientific Revolutions*, 3rd ed. Chicago: University of Chicago Press;1996.

Index

Page numbers followed by the letter "f" indicate a figure; those followed by the letter "t" indicate a table.

Explaining "Unexplained Illnesses"
© 2007 by The Haworth Press, Inc. All rights reserved.
doi:10.1300/5139_18

Order a copy of this book with this form or online at:
http://www.haworthpress.com/store/product.asp?sku=5139

EXPLAINING "UNEXPLAINED ILLNESSES"

Disease Paradigm for Chronic Fatigue Syndrome, Multiple Chemical Sensitivity, Fibromyalgia, Post-Traumatic Stress Disorder, Gulf War Syndrome, and Others

_____in hardbound at $89.95 (ISBN: 978-0-7890-2388-9)

_____in softbound at $39.95 (ISBN: 978-0-7890-2389-6)

439 pages plus index • Includes illustrations

Or order online and use special offer code HEC25 in the shopping cart.

COST OF BOOKS_____	☐ **BILL ME LATER:** (Bill-me option is good on US/Canada/Mexico orders only; not good to jobbers, wholesalers, or subscription agencies.)
	☐ Check here if billing address is different from shipping address and attach purchase order and billing address information.
POSTAGE & HANDLING_____ *(US: $4.00 for first book & $1.50 for each additional book)* *(Outside US: $5.00 for first book & $2.00 for each additional book)*	
	Signature_____
SUBTOTAL_____	☐ **PAYMENT ENCLOSED: $**_____
IN CANADA: ADD 6% GST_____	☐ **PLEASE CHARGE TO MY CREDIT CARD.**
STATE TAX_____ *(NJ, NY, OH, MN, CA, IL, IN, PA, & SD residents, add appropriate local sales tax)*	☐ Visa ☐ MasterCard ☐ AmEx ☐ Discover ☐ Diner's Club ☐ Eurocard ☐ JCB
	Account # _____
FINAL TOTAL_____ *(If paying in Canadian funds, convert using the current exchange rate, UNESCO coupons welcome)*	Exp. Date_____
	Signature_____

Prices in US dollars and subject to change without notice.

NAME_____

INSTITUTION_____

ADDRESS_____

CITY_____

STATE/ZIP_____

COUNTRY_____ COUNTY (NY residents only)_____

TEL_____ FAX_____

E-MAIL_____

May we use your e-mail address for confirmations and other types of information? ☐ Yes ☐ No
We appreciate receiving your e-mail address and fax number. Haworth would like to e-mail or fax special discount offers to you, as a preferred customer. **We will never share, rent, or exchange your e-mail address or fax number.** We regard such actions as an invasion of your privacy.

Order From Your Local Bookstore or Directly From

The Haworth Press, Inc.

10 Alice Street, Binghamton, New York 13904-1580 • USA
TELEPHONE: 1-800-HAWORTH (1-800-429-6784) / Outside US/Canada: (607) 722-5857
FAX: 1-800-895-0582 / Outside US/Canada: (607) 771-0012
E-mail to: orders@haworthpress.com

For orders outside US and Canada, you may wish to order through your local
sales representative, distributor, or bookseller.
For information, see http://haworthpress.com/distributors

(Discounts are available for individual orders in US and Canada only, not booksellers/distributors.)

PLEASE PHOTOCOPY THIS FORM FOR YOUR PERSONAL USE.
http://www.HaworthPress.com   BOF07

Dear Customer:

Please fill out & return this form to receive special deals & publishing opportunities for you! These include:
- availability of new books in your local bookstore or online
- one-time prepublication discounts
- free or heavily discounted related titles
- free samples of related Haworth Press periodicals
- publishing opportunities in our periodicals or Book Division

❑ OK! Please keep me on your regular mailing list and/or e-mailing list for new announcements!

Name _____

Address_____

_____

*E-mail address _____

*Your e-mail address will never be rented, shared, exchanged, sold, or divested. You may "opt-out" at any time.
May we use your e-mail address for confirmations and other types of information? ❑ Yes ❑ No

Special needs:
Describe below any special information you would like:
- Forthcoming professional/textbooks
- New popular books
- Publishing opportunities in academic periodicals
- Free samples of periodicals in my area(s)

Special needs/Special areas of interest:

_____

_____

_____

_____

Please contact me as soon as possible. I have a special requirement/project:

_____

_____

_____

_____

The Haworth Press Inc.

PLEASE COMPLETE THE FORM ABOVE AND MAIL TO:
Donna Barnes, Marketing Dept., The Haworth Press, Inc.
10 Alice Street, Binghamton, NY 13904–1580 USA
Tel: 1–800–429–6784 • Outside US/Canada Tel: (607) 722–5857
Fax: 1–800–895–0582 • Outside US/Canada Fax: (607) 771–0012
E-mail: orders@HaworthPress.com

GBIC07

Visit our Web site: www.HaworthPress.com